PHARMACOLOGY - RESEARCH, SAFETY TESTING AND REGULATION

INTRODUCTION TO DRUG DESIGNING AND DEVELOPMENT

Pharmacology - Research, Safety Testing and Regulation

Additional books in this series can be found on Nova's website under the Series tab.

Additional e-books in this series can be found on Nova's website under the e-book tab.

PHARMACOLOGY - RESEARCH, SAFETY TESTING AND REGULATION

INTRODUCTION TO DRUG DESIGNING AND DEVELOPMENT

RAJNISH KUMAR
ANJU SHARMA
AND
RAJESH KUMAR TIWARI
EDITORS

NOVA BIOMEDICAL

New York

For permission to use material from this book please contact us:
Telephone 631-231-7269; Fax 631-231-8175
Web Site: http://www.novapublishers.com

Library of Congress Cataloging-in-Publication Data

ISBN: 978-1-62948-556-0

Library of Congress Control Number: 2013952582

Published by Nova Science Publishers, Inc. † New York

Contents

Preface		**vii**
Acknowledgment		**ix**
Contributors		**xi**
Chapter 1	Drugs: Introduction and Definition *Rajnish Kumar*	**1**
Chapter 2	Pharmacokinetics *Rajnish Kumar*	**15**
Chapter 3	Pharmacodynamics *Rajnish Kumar*	**39**
Chapter 4	Plants As a Source of Lead Molecules *Mala Trivedi, Anju Sharma and Suresh Kumar Yadav*	**49**
Chapter 5	Animals As a Source of Lead Molecules *Gunjan Pandey and J. K. Srivastava*	**81**
Chapter 6	Drug Targets and Validation Techniques *Rajnish Kumar*	**99**
Chapter 7	Screening of Drugs *Swati Srivastava*	**111**
Chapter 8	Structure-Based Drug Designing *Anju Sharma and Rajnish Kumar*	**123**
Chapter 9	Concepts of Combinatorial Library *Anju Sharma*	**141**
Chapter 10	Quantitative Structure Activity Relationship *Anju Sharma*	**161**
Chapter 11	Pharmacophore Modeling *Rajnish Kumar*	**215**

Chapter 12	Drug Formulation and Dosage Forms *Prakash Deep and Amrit Kumar Singh*	**225**
Chapter 13	Drug Regulatory Affairs *Abhishek Kumar*	**235**
Chapter 14	Recent Advances in Healthcare and Development of Biomedical Sensors *Ashok Kumar Mishra*	**245**
Index		**259**

Preface

In recent years there has been an increased involvement of computers in drug design and development. New technologies have significantly reduced the total time taken by scientists, researchers and developers to derive a drug. However, basic theoretical knowledge about drugs and their designing is extremely important without which it is impossible to succeed in this field.

It gives us an immense pleasure to introduce this book to the readers who are starters in the field of drug design and development. This book starts with introduction and basic information about drugs. Pharmacokinetics and pharmacodynamics aspects are covered in initial chapters. Systemic descriptions of pharmacokinetic parameters such as absorption, distribution, metabolism, excretion etc. are explained in simple and easy language. Book demonstrates detailed concepts of lead molecules and their sources. In addition, drug target classification, identification and validation strategies, design and development of combinatorial libraries for new lead generation are also covered. Book contains various methodologies such as Structure based drug designing, Quantitative structure activity relationship, Pharmacophore modeling, docking studies etc. for screening and designing the drug candidates. This book will help in identification and designing of drugs that could be potentially useful in deriving the candidate drugs, which may have efficacy in animal models or cell culture, and thus the most effective compounds could be employed based on the above results for being moved through preclinical studies to clinical trials. Last couple of chapters describes dosage drug regulatory affairs and recent advancements in healthcare. Aim of this book is to provide comprehensive idea about overall drug design and development.

This book is result of three years of rigorous hard work and will be helpful to the students and researchers in the field of Biotechnology, Bioinformatics and Pharmaceutical sciences. Academically it can be a good handbook for Graduate and Postgraduate level students of science and technology.

Lucknow, UP, India
Editors

Acknowledgment

First and foremost, we thank God for his blessings. Because of him we were able to complete this book. In the urge of contributing to the society AMITY family has given the heritage of knowledge to world unconditionally.

We would like to take this opportunity to extend our sincere gratitude and deepest thanks to *Dr. Ashok Chauhan*, Founder President of AMITY University. We are also grateful to him to provide such an excellent platform to excel academically and professionally.

We are deeply grateful to *Mr. Aseem Chauhan*, Chancellor, AMITY University Haryana, AMITY University Rajasthan and Chairman AMITY University Uttar Pradesh, Lucknow Campus for providing us necessary facilities and support. He has been a perennial source of inspiration. We place on record our deep regards to him.

We would also like to extend our gratitude to *Maj. Gen. K.K Ohri*, AVSM (Retd.), Pro Vice Chancellor, Amity University, Uttar Pradesh Lucknow Campus for providing us valuable guidance and encouragement throughout the work. Maj Gen Ohri not only supported but also inspired us with his utmost level of devotion and dedication.

We owe a great many thanks to all our colleagues and support staffs. We thank all who helped and supported us directly or indirectly during writing this book. Their comments and suggestions kept us going from the very beginning of the work.

We place on record our sincere thanks to family members for their constant support and encouragement back home.

Finally, we would like to thank all authors who contributed with their chapter. Their endless effort and patience was truly motivating.

Contributors

Dr. Janmejai K. Srivastava, Professor
Amity Institute of Biotechnology
AMITY University, Uttar Pradesh
Lucknow campus, India
Email: jksrivastava@lko.amity.edu

Dr. Mala Trivedi, Asst. Professor
Amity Institute of Biotechnology
AMITY University, Uttar Pradesh
Lucknow campus, India
Email: mtrivedi@lko.amity.edu

Dr. Ashok K. Mishra, Professor
Amity School of Engineering and Technology, AMITY University Uttar Pradesh, Lucknow campus, India
Email: akmishra@lko.amity.edu

Mr. Rajnish Kumar, Lecturer
Amity Institute of Biotechnology
Amity Institute of Biotechnology
AMITY University, Uttar Pradesh
Lucknow campus, India
Email: rkumar2@lko.amity.edu

Ms. Anju Sharma, Lecturer
Amity Institute of Biotechnology
Amity Institute of Biotechnology
AMITY University, Uttar Pradesh
Lucknow campus, India
Email: asharma3@lko.amity.edu

Mr. Suresh Kumar Yadav, Lecturer,
Amity Institute of Biotechnology
Amity Institute of Biotechnology
AMITY University, Uttar Pradesh
Lucknow campus, India
Email: skyadav@lko.amity.edu

Gunjan Pandey
Nanoscience Centre, University of Jyvaskyla, P.O. Box 35, Finland
Email: genegunjan@gmail.com

Mr. Prakash Deep, Lecturer
Amity Institute of Pharmacy
AMITY University, Uttar Pradesh
Lucknow campus, India
Email: pdeep@lko.amity.edu

Mr. Amrit K. Singh, Lecturer
Amity Institute of Pharmacy
AMITY University, Uttar Pradesh
Lucknow campus, India
Email:aksingh5@lko.amity.edu

Ms. Swati Srivastava
Assistant Professor
Lovely Professional University-Phagwara, Punjab, India
Email: swati051@gmail.com

In: Introduction to Drug Designing and Development
Editors: R. Kumar, A. Sharma and R. Kumar Tiwari
ISBN: 978-1-62948-556-0

Chapter 1

Drugs: Introduction and Definition

Rajnish Kumar*
Amity Institute of Biotechnology, AMITY University-Uttar Pradesh,
Lucknow, Uttar Pradesh, India

Abstract

Drugs are an important and integral component of the health system. They are used for the prevention, mitigation or the cure of diseases. One has to be equipped with the basic information about drugs to understand the process of drug design. This chapter deals with basic information about drugs. This will help readers to understand the history, fundamental terminologies, nomenclature and classification of drugs.

Introduction

The word drug has originated from the French word "drogue" meaning dry herbs [1]. According to the World Health Organization (WHO), "Drug is a substance which is used or intended to be used to modify or explore the physiological system or pathological state for the benefit of recipients".

A substance used in the diagnosis, treatment or prevention of disease or as a component of medication recognized by the United States (U.S.) Food and drug administration (FDA).

According to another school of thought, a drug is a chemical compound which interacts with a biological molecule that leads to a physiological effect.

The drug can be a chemical or biological substance. It can be synthetic or non-synthetic.

The drug can be anything that affects the way organism works. It can be a substance which enhances function (Caffeine).

Phrase "drug like" is defined as a compound with sufficiently acceptable ADME and toxicity properties to survive through the completion of phase-I clinical trials.

* E-mail:12.rajnish@gmail.com, rkumar2@lko.amity.edu.

Most of the drugs are molecules which bind to protein receptor (ligands). They inhibit or enhance the function of a protein by blocking the active or allosteric site.

Drugs have an analogy with keys (figure 1). Similar to a key that opens a mechanical lock. Some components of biologically active molecule are essential while others are not. The role of non-essential element is to hold the essential elements in proper three-dimensional geometrical orientation.

History

- History of drugs appears to be started with Ayurveda. History of Ayurveda asserts that around 2nd millennium *BC*, Ayurveda's applied and fundamental principles were compiled and articulated. According to Indian history, Ayurveda traces its origin in the *Vedas*, particularly *Atharvaveda*. It is linked to Hindu religion. Atharvaveda is one of the four most ancient books of Indian culture. It contains 114 hymns (formulations) for the treatment of diseases. It is believed that these hymns are source of origin of Ayurveda. Ayurveda is believed by some to have divine origin. Indian medicine is one of the oldest organized systems of medicine. Its concepts are set out in the sacred writings called the Vedas. Dhanvantari was deified as the God of medicine. It is believed that Indian system of medicine was received by *Dhanvantari* from Hindu God *Brahma*. Sushrut saint wrote the Ayurveda by learning it from Lord Dhanwantari. Ayurveda contains eight (08) sections, that is why it is also known as Ashtang Ayurveda. The sections are as follows: Shalya tantra
- Shalakya tantra
- Kaya chikitsa
- Bhoot Vidya
- Kaumar bhutya tantra
- Agad tantra
- Rasayana Tantra
- Vajikaran tantra

Ayurveda contains information about the qualities of herbs and eatables, body science anatomy, surgery etc.

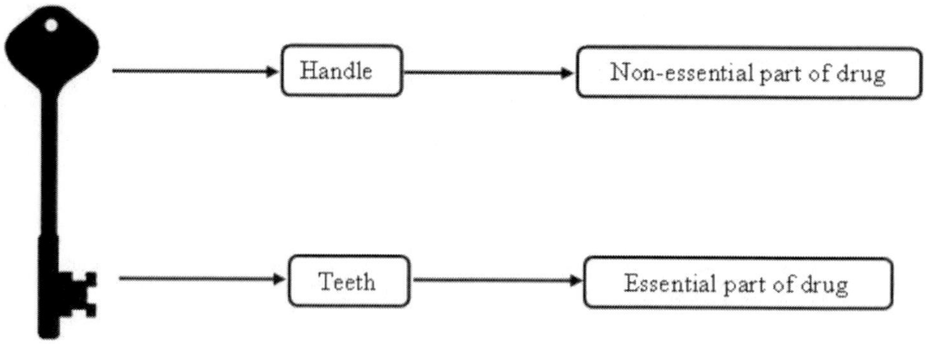

Figure 1. Key Model of drug parts.

According to Rishi Charak, Ayurveda is a subject that contains information about "age" on the basis of detrimental and beneficial foods, herbs and other factors that influence span of life. Sushruta defines Ayurveda as a means of increasing "life span and age."

Word 'Ayu' (Sanskrit) means age. Age is dependent on your karma (work). 100 years of age were considered as standard life span at that time. According to the 'Vedas' a man should have a lifespan of 100 years. *Ishopnishada* is a branch of 'Veda' that says; we must do karma yoga and strive to live for 100 years.

Ebers Papyrus (1500 BC) (figure 2) is an Egyptian medical papyrus oldest and most important medical papyrus of ancient Egypt. It is currently kept at the library of the University of Leipzig, in Germany. It contains Egyptian pharmacy and surgical practices. All diseases were considered as the wrath of God. Hippocrates (an ancient physician of Greek) is believed to be one of the most important contributors in the history of medicine.

Hippocrates is also known as the father of western medicine. This famous ambassador for medicine was believed to be born around 460 BC.

Hippocrates is credited with being the first person to believe that diseases were caused naturally. Hippocrates (figure 3) was credited by the disciples of Pythagoras of allying philosophy and medicine [2]. He separated the discipline of medicine from religion, believing and arguing that disease was not a punishment inflicted by the God, rather they are the product of environmental factors, diet, and living habits. Indeed there is not a single mention of a mystical illness in the Hippocratic Corpus. However, Hippocrates did work with many convictions that were based on what is now known to be incorrect anatomy and physiology, such as Humorism [3, 4, 5].

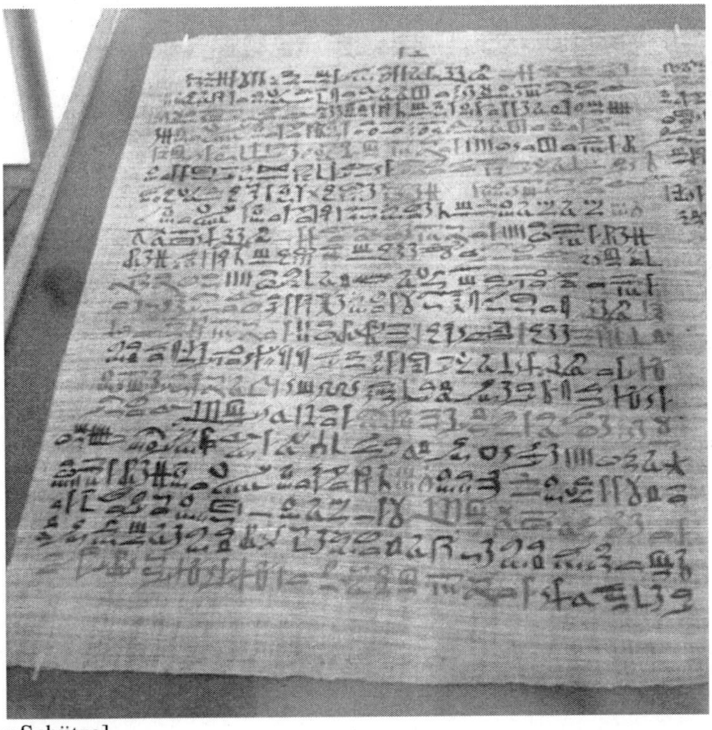

[curtsey: Einsamer Schütze].

Figure 2. Ebers Papyrus column 41 from ancient Egypt.

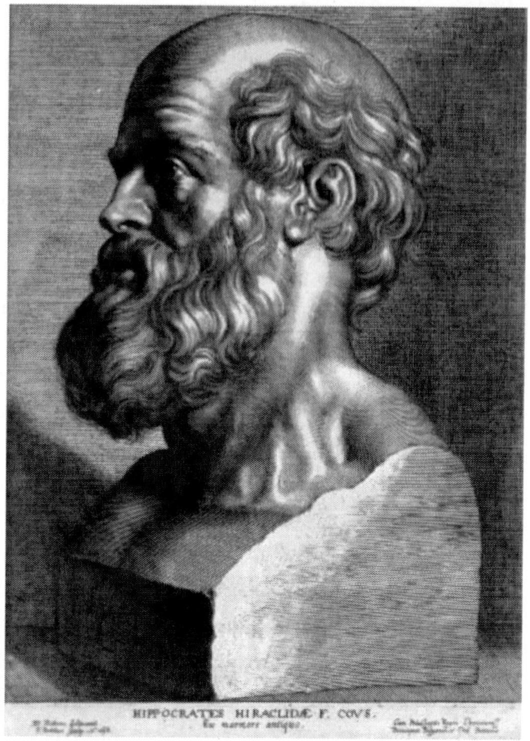

[Courtesy: National Library of Medicine-http://www.ihm.nlm.nih.gov/ihm/images/B/14/555.jpg].

Figure 3. Hippocrates, engraving by Peter Paul Rubens, 1638.

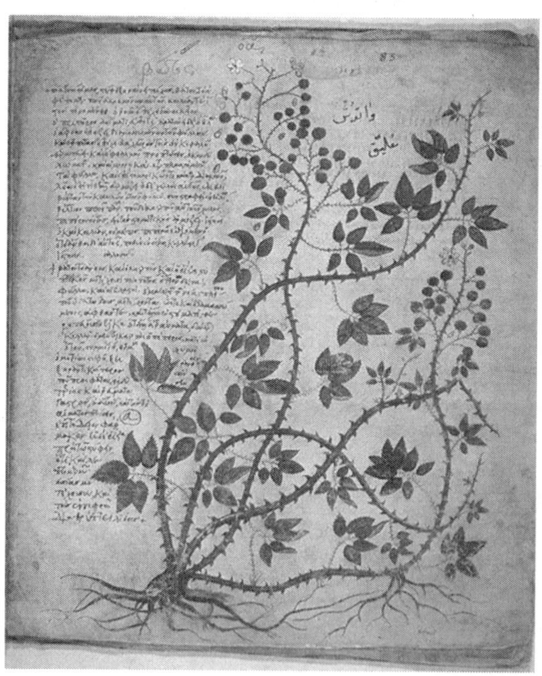

Figure 4. Page from the 6th century Vienna Dioscurides, an illuminated version of the 1st century De Materia Medica.

In the first century AD, Materia medica (figure 4) came into existence. Materia medica means medical substances. It contains information about therapeutic substances which are used for healing. De Materia Medica was the first extensive drug affinity system that included about a thousand natural product drugs (mostly plant-bases), 4,740 medicinal usages for drugs, and 360 medical properties (antiseptic, anti-inflammatory, stimulants, etc.) [6, 7]. An understanding of the mechanisms of action in drugs was not well-defined. This was due to the lack of methods to purify crude substances. Methods for testing hypotheses about the nature of drug actions were also missing.

In the second century AD, Galen, who was a proficient medical writer, pharmacist and physician, collected and compiled an extensive record of the medical knowledge of those days. He included the results of his own experimental observations. He has written about the structure of organs, the pulse and its relation with respiration, movement of blood in arteries etc. [8].

5th to 11th century is known as the Dark Age in European medicine. Magic and cosmology were followed extensively throughout the Europe. At the same time, Arabian and Chinese medicinal agents and herbal systems developed in a considerable manner. In the 11th century Avicenna, a Persian physician came to light and he is also referred as 'Father of clinical pharmacology'. He wrote 40 books on medicine. *Canon of Medicine* and *The Book of Healing are among his famous books*. These were used in various universities as medical textbooks. He also was the first to describe parasitic infection, to use urine for diagnostic purposes and discouraged physicians from the practice of surgery because it was too base and manual [9].

In the 16th century some of the major contributors to drug research emerged (Table1).

During the 18th century, smallpox vaccine was developed. Apart from it some other important events took place such as Digitalis (source of cardiac glycosides, Digoxin, Digitoxin) came to medicinal existence.

In the 19th century, important alkaloids such as Morphine, Quinine, Atropine and Codeine were isolated.

Table 1. Major contributors to drug research in the 16th century

Contributor	Details
Ermolao Barbaro	Italian physician and humanist (Much of his work was published after his death: In Dioscuridem Corelari, a work on Dioscorides)
Jean Ruel	Physician to King Francis I of France
Bruyerinus	Arabist, who translated the works of Avicena
Pietro Andrea Mattioli	Translation of De Materia Medica [10]
Andres Laguna	Physician, published his Annotations on Dioscorides of Anazarbus [11]
Valerius Cordus	German physician and botanist, identified and described several new plant species and varieties e.g. genus *Cordia* [12]
Martin Mathee	French physician, published a French translation of De Materia Medica [13]

In addition first generation anesthetics were made available. 20th century is known for application of synthetic and organic chemistry to drug discovery and development.

The most important breakthrough for treatment of diabetes mellitus occurred in the year 1922, "Insulin was isolated". During 1930-1940 oral antimicrobials (Sulfonamides) and antibiotics (Penicillin) were discovered. During 1940-1950 structure activity relationship studies were carried out on alpha and beta receptors. With the combination of antimicrobial agents, complete cure of tuberculosis started. In the year 1955 polio vaccines were developed and extensively used to eliminate paralysis and polio epidemics from earth.

In the 1960's treatment of Parkinson's disease was initiated using the levodopa. Swedish scientist Arvid Carlsson first demonstrated in the 1950's that administering levodopa to animals with Parkinsonian symptoms reduces their intensity and got a Noble prize for it in 2000 [14]. In 1970's antiviral medicinal agents came into existence for prevention and treatment of diseases caused by viruses. Cytotoxic substances and steroids were used to treat leukemia. The polymerase chain reaction (PCR) of the 1980's resulted in major advances in biotechnology that have had significant impact in drug discovery. In the 1990s, combinatorial chemistry, molecular modeling and bioinformatics contributed to the discovery of newer generation drugs based on genomics and proteomics [15]. Combinational therapy for AIDS, antineoplastic agents for treatment of cancer, antipsychotic drugs for treatment of schizophrenia etc. came into light in this period. Year 2000 onwards, lots of improved drugs came into the picture such as optically active drugs (chiral virson) Levobupivacain, Escitalopram, Genetically engineered agents (Insulin glargin), Latanoprost for treatment of glaucoma, Tyrosinekinase inhibitors, and Monoclonal antibodies (trastuzumab) in the treatment of cancer etc. [16].

Basic Terminologies Related to Drugs

Lead compound: A lead compound is representative of a compound series with sufficient potential (as measured by pharmacokinetics, potency, physicochemical properties, selectivity, novelty and absence of toxicity) to be marked as starting point of full drug development program.

Pharmacophore: (Pharmakon=drug + phore= to bear) A set of structural features in a molecule that is recognized by the receptor site and is responsible for that molecule's biological activity (by Gund 1977).

Pharmacokinetics: (Pharmakon=drug + Kinetics=Movement) It is what the body does to the drug. In other words study of the time course of substances and their relationship with an organism or system.

Pharmacodynamics: (Pharmakon=drug + Dynamics=Power) It is what the drug does to the body. In other words study of the biochemical and physiological effects of drugs, the mechanisms of drug action and the relationship between drug concentration and effect.

Prodrug: Drug which is taken in an inactive form. Prodrug is metabolized into a biologically active compound after administration in the body.

Receptor: These are macromolecules (DNA, mRNA, Proteins, Carbohydrates, Lipids, Cell membrane, Enzymes etc.) onto which drug binds. Receptors are generally activated by endogenous chemicals in the body.

QSAR: It is the acronym of Quantitative structure activity relationship. It works on the principle that biological activity of molecules is directly correlated with their structure. Physicochemical properties are used to derive a mathematical relationship, or quantitative structure-activity relationship, that can be used to predict the biological response of other chemical structures.

Drug action: When drug acts on the receptor, it brings out conformational changes in the receptor. This is known as drug action.

Drug effect: Final biological response of the drug is known as drug effect.

K_D: The equilibrium dissociation constant (K_D) represents the concentration of radio-ligand occupying half of the maximum receptor population. K_D is a measure of affinity.

B_{max}: The total number of receptors in a particular tissue.

Potency: Crudely defined as the dose range over which a response is produced.

ED_{50}: The dose of drug producing half the maximum response and is a measure of potency.

Efficacy: Crudely defined as the size or strength of a response produced by a particular agonist in a particular tissue.

E_{max}: Maximum response a particular agonist can produce in a particular tissue and is a crude measure of efficacy [17].

Agonist: Substance that has both affinity and intrinsic activity for the receptor and triggers the biological response.

Antagonist: Substance that has affinity but no intrinsic activity. In other words, antagonist binds with a receptor but it cannot alter the conformation of the receptor.

Inverse agonist: Substance that binds with the same receptor like agonist but leads to opposite pharmacological response with respect to agonist.

Neutral antagonist: A neutral antagonist has no activity in the absence of an agonist or inverse agonist but can block the activity of either [18].

Partial agonist: Drug that binds and activate the receptor but have only partial efficacy at the receptor in comparison to a full agonist.

Chemotherapy: It is a systemic treatment by using drugs that have selective toxicity for infective agents with minimal or no harm to the host cells.

Pharmacotherapeutics: It is the cumulative application of pharmacological information and knowledge of disease for its treatment, prevention or mitigation.

Pharmacy: It is a branch of science which deals with identification, collection, purification, isolation, synthesis, standardization, quality control, compounding and dispensing of medicinal agents.

Toxicity: Branch of science which deals with the study of poisons and adverse effect of chemical compounds and drugs. Toxicity is dose dependent.

Drug Nomenclature

In general a drug can be named using three categories:

(a) Brand name or Proprietary name
(b) Nonproprietary name
(c) Chemical name

The brand name is a trademark or property name given by a manufacturer. A drug can have multiple brand names as it depends upon the manufacturers. Brand name is kept in such a way so that it could be short, catchy, suggestive and easy to remember, e.g., Calpol, Pacimol, Metacin, Para, Crocin are some brand names for Paracetamol in India. Some brand names are inspired by the chemical name of drugs, e.g., chemical name of Paracetamol is Acetaminophen and has a brand name Acetalgin in Switzerland. Some brand names are suggestive, e.g., Tempra brand name of Paracetamol used in Mexico, the Philippines and Venezuela suggests that the drug deals with temperature of body.

Nonproprietary is a name accepted by competent scientific bodies, e.g., United States Adopted Name Council. Upon appearance in official publication list nonproprietary name becomes official name. The nonproprietary name is also known as approved name until it is included in pharmacopoeia. Uniformity in the nonproprietary name is maintained for newer drugs. However, many older drugs have a different nonproprietary name, e.g., Pethidine in India and UK has a different nonproprietary name in USA i.e., Meperidine.

Chemical name demonstrates the chemical nature of a medicinal agent, e.g., Acetamenophen for Paracetamol, Acetylsalicylic acid for Aspirin etc.

Adverse Effects of Drugs

Drugs can be beneficial or harmful depending on their effect. Drugs are chemical compounds, but that does not mean any chemical compound qualifies for being a drug. For a chemical compound to be qualified as a drug it must have the following characteristics:

(a) Safe
(b) Effective
(c) Stable (both chemically and metabolically)
(d) Deliverable (drug must be absorbed and makes its way to the site of action)
(e) Novel (patentable)

The adverse effect is any undesired response of the drug. It includes any unwanted or unintended noxious effect of drug after administration. As per Henri Manasse adverse drug effect can be defined as the iatrogenic hazard that is an inherent risk when drug therapy is indicated.

According to Karch, and Lasagna it can be defined as any response to a drug that is noxious and unintended, and occurs at doses used for prophylaxis, diagnosis, or therapy, excluding failure to accomplish the intended purpose [19]. Various types of adverse drug effects are shown in figure 5. According to the American Society of Health-System Pharmacists adverse drug reactions may lead to the following [20]:

(a) Discontinuation of the drug
(b) Change in the drug therapy
(c) Modification of dose
(d) Admission to the hospital
(e) Increased duration in a health care facility

(f) Requirement of supportive treatment
(g) Considerably complicates diagnosis
(h) Negatively affects diagnosis or output in temporary or permanent harm, disability, or death

Reactions due to drug withdrawal, drug abuse, poisoning, or drug complications are not included in the definition of the American Society of Health-System Pharmacists. Other terms that may be included as adverse drug reactions are drug intolerance, side effects, toxic reactions, idiosyncratic reactions, allergic reactions, or hypersensitivity reactions [21].

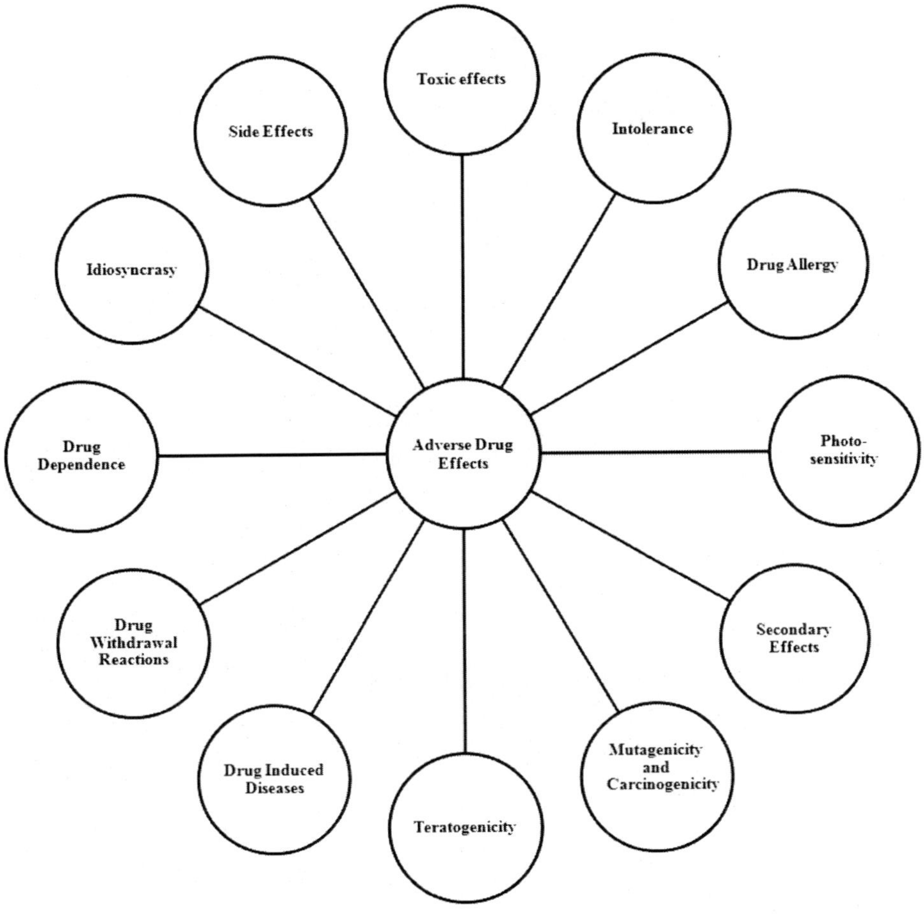

Figure 5. Different types of adverse drug reactions.

Side effects are unintended and unwanted reactions but are known pharmacological effects of the drug. Their frequency of occurrence is predictable. Drug intolerance is a mild reaction to a drug that results in no or little change in the management of the patient. Idiosyncratic response is an unexpected response that takes place with the usual dose of drug. Toxic reaction is a predictable response that results from higher than suggested drug concentration or drug dosages in the body. Unusual sensitivity to a drug is an immunologic reaction and it leads to allergic or hypersensitivity reaction. Various side effects are shown in figure 6.

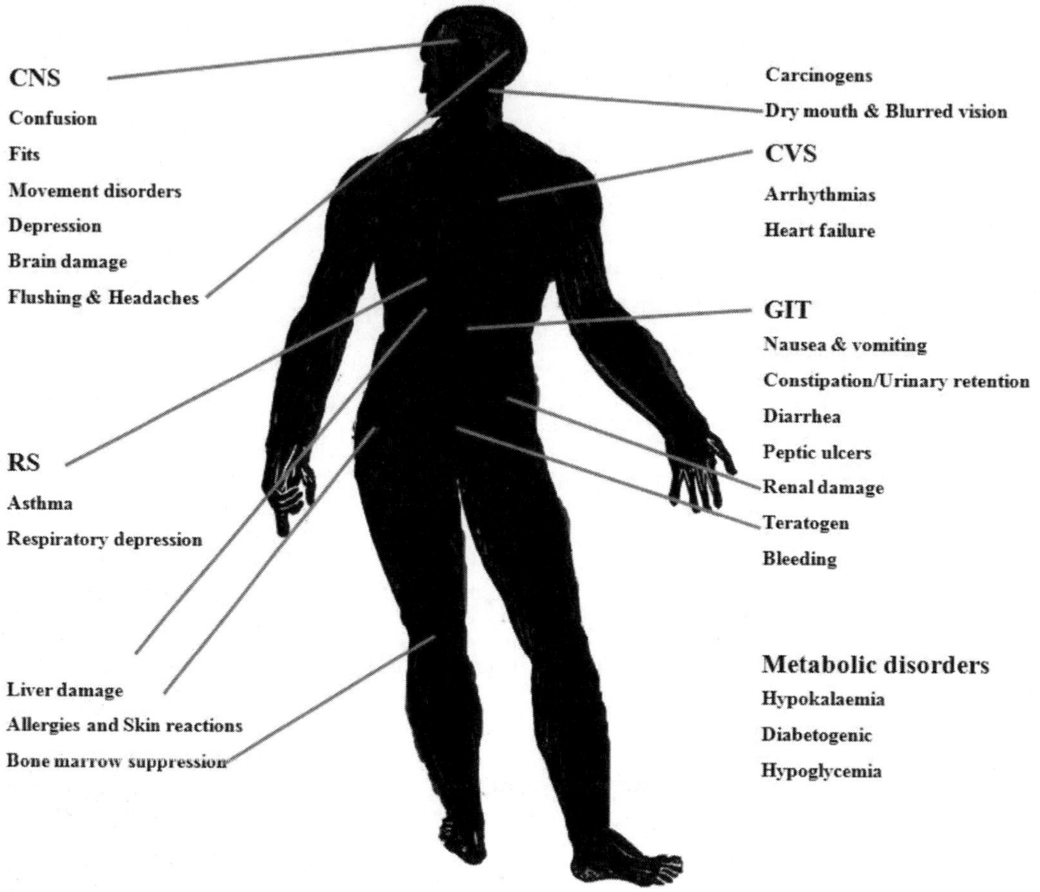

Figure 6. Various side effects of drugs.

Classification of Drugs

The drug can be classified on the basis of chemical nature or their pharmacological activities. Each drug can be classified into one or more drug classes. It is not possible for author to classify and quote all existing drugs in this text. However, a broad classification of drugs is given below which includes classes, therapeutic activity and examples of drugs (Table 2).

Table 2. Classification of Drugs based on their therapeutic activity

Classes of Drugs	Therapeutic Activity	Examples
Analgesic	Agents that relieve pain without causing loss of consciousness	Tylenol, Advil, Motrin
Anesthetic	Produces lack of feeling either local or general depending upon type and how administered	Lidocaine, Xylocaine, Novocain
Antacid	Neutralizes acid	Amphojel, Gelusil, Mylanta, Milk of Magnesia

Classes of Drugs	Therapeutic Activity	Examples
Anthelmintics	Used to treat worm infections	Albendazole, Mebendazole
Anti-impotence	Used to treat erectile dysfunction	Viagra, Levitra, Cialis
Anti-inflammatory	Prevents inflammation	Advil, Motrin, Naprosyn
Antianemic	Prevents or cures anemia	Ferrous Sulphate, Folic acid
Antianginal	Prevents or relieves angina attacks	Nitroglycerin, Isosorbide mononitrate
Antianxiety	Relieves anxiety and muscle tension	Librium, Valium
Antiarrhythmic	Controls cardiac arrhythmias	Lidocaine HCl, Xylocaine, Propranolol
Antibiotic	Destroys or inhibits growth of microorganisms	Kelfin, Rocephin, Pentids, Penicillins
Anticholinergic	Blocks parasympathetic nerve impulses; decreases oral and respiratory secretions	Atropine, Artane
Anticoagulant	Prevents or delays blood clotting	Heparin, Warfarin, Coumadin
Anticonvulsant	Prevents or relieves convulsions / seizures	Tegretol, Zarontin, Dilantin
Antidepressant	Prevents or relieves symptoms of depression	Tofranil, Marplan, Nardil
Antidiabetic	Used to manage diabetes	Biguanides, Insulin, Thiazolidinediones
Antidiarrheal	Prevents or relieves diarrhea; inhibits peristalsis and reduces fecal volume	Keopectate, Lomotil, Pepto-Bismol
Antidote	Counteracts poisons and their effects	Narcan
Antidysrhythmic	Controls and prevents cardiac dysrhythmias	Isoproterenol, Ephedrine
Antiemetic	Prevents or relieves nausea and vomiting	Dramamine, Marinol, Phenergan, Reglan, Tigan
Antiflatulent	Relieves gas and bloating in GI tract	Alpha-galactosidase
Antihistamine	Destroys or inhibits the action of histamine	Diflucan, Lamisil, Lotrimin, Monistat, Nizoral, Terazol
Antifungal	Kills or inhibits growth of fungi	Imidazole, Triazole, Thiazole
Antigout	Inhibits production of uric acid	Benzbromarone, Allopurinol
Antiallergic	Acts to prevent the action of histamine (allergies)	Pheniramine, Cetirizine
Antihyperlipidemic	Used to lower abnormally high blood levels of fatty substances (lipids).	Lipitor, Lopid, Mevacor, Nicobid, Zocor
Antihypertensive	Prevents or controls high blood pressure	Catapres, Aldomet, Lopressor
Antimanic	Used for treatment of manic episode of manic-depressive and bipolar disorder	Lithium
Antimigraine	Causes vasoconstriction in large intracranial arteries	Triptans
Antineoplastic	Prevents the replication of neoplastic cells; used to treat tumors	Myleran, Cytoxan
Antiparkinsonian	Used for palliative relief of major symptoms of Parkinson disease	L-Dopa, Requip, Symmetrel, Tasar
Antiprotozoal	Destroys protozoa	Eflornithine, Furazolidone, Melarsoprol, Metronidazole
Antipsychotic	Used to treat psychotic disorders	Phenothiazines, Butyrophenones
Antipyretic	Reduces fever	Tylenol, Aspirin
Antiretroviral	Used to manage HIV infections	Maraviroc and enfuvirtide

Table 2. (Continued)

Classes of Drugs	Therapeutic Activity	Examples
Antispasmodic	Controls hypermotility in IBS	Papaverine
Antituberculosis	Used in treatment of tuberculosis; inhibits growth of mycobacteria	INH, Myambutal, Mycobutin, Priftin, PZA, Rifadin, Streptomycin
Antitumor necrosis factor	Seems to slow if not halt altogether the destruction of joints by disrupting the activity of tumor necrosis factor (TNF)	Enbrel
Antitussive	Prevents or relieves cough	Codeine, Dextrometorphan
Antiulcer	Used in treatment of active duodenal ulcer and for pathological hypersecretory; controls stomach acid	Axid, Pepcid, Tagamet, Zantac
Antiviral	Combats a specific viral disease (e.g., herpes)	Denavir, Famivir, Relenza, Retrovir, Tamiflu, Zovirax
Bone resorption inhibitor	Treat and prevent osteoporosis	Alendronate
Bronchodilator	Dilates the bronchi	Proventil, Isuprel
Cardiac glycoside	Exerts a positive inotropic effect on the heart; increases strength and force of contractions and slows heart rate	Digitalis preps
Contraceptive	Device, method or agent that prevents conception	Ethinylnortestosterone
Corticosteroid	Supresses inflammation and modifies normal immune response	Betamethasone, Budesonide, Cortisone, Dexamethasone (Decadron)
COX-2 Inhibitor	Inhibits cyclooxygenase (COX-2) enzyme found in joints and other areas affected by inflammation	Aspirin, Ibuprofen
Decongestant	Reduces nasal congestion and/or swelling; produces vasoconstriction	Afrin, Sudafed
Disease-modifying antirheumatic drugs (DMARDs)	May influence the course of disease progression of rheumatoid arthritis	Arava, Cuprimine, Cytoxan, Rheumatrex, Ridaura
Diuretic	Increases the excretion of urine	Diuril, Lasix, Osmitrol
Electrolyte replacement	Treats or prevents electrolyte depletion	Endurolytes
Emetic	Used to induce vomiting	Apomorphine HCl, Ipecac syrup
Expectorant	Facilitates removal of secretion from broncho-pulmonary mucous membrane	Robitussin, Mucinex
Gastric acid-pump inhibitor	Suppresses gastric acid secretions; also used for gastroesophageal reflux disease (GERD)	Aciphex, Prevacid, Prilosec, Protonix
Hemostatic	Controls or stops bleeding	Amicar, Humafac, vitamin K
Classes of Drugs	Therapeutic Activity	Examples
Hormone replacement (HRT)	Treat vasomotor symptoms of menopause	Oestrogen, Progesterone
Hypnotic	Produces sleep or hypnosis; depresses CNS	Chloral hydrate, Placidyl, Seconal
Hypoglycemic	Lowers blood glucose level	Diabinese, Insulin

Classes of Drugs	Therapeutic Activity	Examples
Immunologic	Induces immunity and prevents infectious diseases; stimulates body to produce antibodies	DTP, MMR, Engerix-B, Varivax
Immunosuppressant	Treat and prevent rejection of transplanted organs	Methotrexate, Azathioprine
Laxative	Loosens and promotes normal bowel elimination; relieves constipation	Dulcolax, Metamucil
Leukotriene receptor antagonist blocker	Used for treatment and management of asthma	Singulair, Zyflo, Accolate
Lipid-lowering agent	Lowers cholesterol	Ezetimibe, Niacin, Mipomersen
Mucolytic	Breaks chemical bonds in mucus, lowering the viscosity	Mucomyst
Muscle relaxant	Produces relaxation of skeletal muscle	Norflex, Paraflex, Robaxin, Skelaxin, Valium
Neuroleptic	Modifies psychotic behavior	Risperdal, Zyprexa, Stelazine
Ophthalmic anti-infective	Treat eye infections	Levofloxacin, Azithromycin
Otic preparations	Treat ear conditions	Carbamide peroxide
Platelet inhibitor	Inhibits the ability of platelets to adhere to each other; similar to coagulant	Clopidogrel, Prasugrel (Effient), Ticagrelor (Brilinta), Ticlopidine (Ticlid)
Sedative	Produces calming effect without causing sleep; depresses CNS	Amytal, Buticaps, Phenobarbital
Selective serotonin reuptake inhibitors (SSRIs)	Selectively inhibits serotonin reuptake and results in potentiation of serotonergic neurotransmissions	Luvox, Paxilo, Prozac, Zoloft
Serotonin nonselective reuptake inhibitor (SNRI)	Inhibits the reuptake of both serotonin and norepinephrine	Effexor
Thrombolytic	Dissolves an existing thrombus (clot) when administered soon after its occurrence	Abbokinase, Activase, Eminase, Kabikinase, Streptase
Vasodilator	Produces relaxation of blood vessels; lowers BP	Isordil, Nitroglycerin
Vasopressor	Produces contraction of muscles of capillaries and arteries; elevates BP; used to treat allergic reactions	Aramine, Levophed

References

[1] Tripathi, K. D. (2003). *Essentials of medical pharmacology*, edition 5, pp 3. New Delhi: Jaypee brothers medical publishers Ltd.

[2] Adams, F. (1891). *The Genuine Works of Hippocrates*, pp 4. New York: William Wood and Company.

[3] Jones, W. H. S. (1868). *Hippocrates Collected Works*, pp 11. Cambridge Harvard University Press.

[4] Nuland, S. B. (1988). *Doctors: The Biography of Medicine*, pp 8-9. New York, Alfred A. Knopf.

[5] Garrison, F. H. (1966). *History of Medicine*, pp 93-94. Philadelphia: W.B. Saunders Company.
[6] Osbaldeston, T. A. (2000). *Dioscorides,* Johannesburg: IBIDIS Press.
[7] Collins, M. (2000). Medieval Herbals: The Illustrative Traditions, London: The British Library and University of Toronto Press.
[8] Parker, L. A. (1915). A Brief History of Materia Medica, *The American Journal of Nursing*, 5(9), 729-734.
[9] Le Wall, C. (1927). The Curious Lore of Drugs and Medicines: Four Thousand Years of Pharmacy. New York: Garden City Publishing Co. Inc.
[10] Genaust, H. (1976). Etymologisches Wörterbuch der botanischen Pflanzennamen. Basel: Birkhauser.
[11] De la Pena, A. (1963). Two great physicians of the sixteenth century. (Andres LAGUNA). *The Journal of the International College of Surgeons*, 2, 15-18.
[12] Durling, Richard J.-A catalogue of Sixteenth Century Printed Books in the National Library of medicine., Bethesda, MD, US Dept. of Health, NLM, 16thc.1967.
[13] Riddle, J. M. (1985). Dioscorides on pharmacy and medicine. Austin: University of Texas Press.
[14] Cotzias, G. C., Papavasiliou, P. S., Gellene, R. (1969). L-dopa in parkinson's syndrome. *The New England Journal of Medicine,* 281 (5): 272.
[15] http://www.uga-cdd.org/background.php [accessed on:08-05-2012].
[16] Bryant B. and Knights K. (2011). Introduction to pharmacology in Pharmacology for health professionals, edition 3. Elsevier publication Australia.
[17] Lambert, D. G. (2004). Drugs and receptors. *Continuing Education in Anaesthesia, Critical Care and Pain,* 4(6), 181-184.
[18] Kenakin, T. (2004). Principles: receptor theory in pharmacology. *Trends Pharmacol. Sci.,* 25 (4), 186–92.
[19] Karch, F. E. and Lasagna, L. (1975). Adverse drug reactions: a critical review. *JAMA*, 234, 1236–1241.
[20] American society of health-system pharmacists. (1998) .Suggested definitions and relationships among medication misadventures, medication errors, adverse drug events and adverse drug reactions. *Am. J. Health-Syst. Pharm.*, 55, 165–166.
[21] Edwards, I. R. (1997) Pharmacological basis of adverse drug. In Avery's Drug Treatment, edition 4; Speight, T., Holford, N., Eds.; ADIS International LTD: Auckland, New Zealand, pp 261–299.

In: Introduction to Drug Designing and Development
Editors: R. Kumar, A. Sharma and R. Kumar Tiwari
ISBN: 978-1-62948-556-0

Chapter 2

Pharmacokinetics

Rajnish Kumar*
Amity Institute of Biotechnology, AMITY University-Uttar Pradesh,
Lucknow, Uttar Pradesh, India

Abstract

Pharmacokinetics is the quantitative study of absorption, distribution, metabolism and excretion. These processes determine the fate of the substance inside the body. Hence, a detailed investigation of ADME properties is important during the drug discovery process. The biological, physiological, and physicochemical factors which influence the transfer of drugs in the body also influence the rate and extent of ADME properties of those drugs in the body. This chapter covers basic concepts of pharmacokinetics.

Introduction

Pharmacokinetic consists of two worlds; Pharmakon + Kinetic. Pharmakon is a Greek word, meaning drug and Kinetic meaning movement. In other words, pharmacokinetic studies deal with movement of drugs in the body. Pharmacokinetics offers a mathematical basis to study the effects of drugs and their time course inside the body.

Pharmacokinetic studies deal with 'what the body does to the drug'. These studies describe the movement of drug in the body in a quantitative manner. Pharmacokinetics cover a wide range of areas e.g., absorption, distribution, metabolism and excretion etc.

* E-mail: 12.rajnish@gmail.com, rkumar2@lko.amity.edu.

ADME Properties

A: Absorption
D: Distribution
M: Metabolism
E: Elimination

Drugs are handled by the body in four stages: Absorption, Distribution, Metabolism (Biotransformation), Elimination (Excretion). These properties are collectively known as ADME properties.

Absorption is the process by which drug reaches to systemic circulation. Distribution can be defined as dispersion of drugs in the body. Breakdown of active molecules into inactive forms is known as metabolism. It is an irreversible process. Elimination can be defined as the removal of substances from the body. Pharmacokinetic processes are illustrated in figure 2.1.

Large number of methods are available to represent the pharmacokinetics of a given drug. The most usual method is to simulate the body as it is made up of compartments and drug moves between these compartments. It assumes that the process of elimination of the drug occurs from these compartments. Rate constants are used to present the transfer of drug between these compartments.

Rates of Reaction

Rates of processes are important to explain the ADME properties. The rate of reaction (process) is defined as the velocity at which it takes place. This can be described as a zero-order or first-order.

Zero-Order Reaction

Assumptions:

1. Initial amount of drug is X.
2. The amount of the drug is decreasing at a constant rate. The rate of elimination of a drug X is the change of concentration of X over a time interval, t is:

   $-dX/dt = Ko$

   Where, Ko is the zero-order rate constant. A negative sign is because drug concentration is decreasing. Integration of the rate equation gives:

   $X=Kot$

A zero-order reaction plot for drug X against time 't' gives a straight line passing through the origin with a slope of Ko (figure 2).

The reaction takes place at a constant rate. It is independent of the concentration of drug X present in the body. An example is the elimination of Alcohol. Drugs that show this type of elimination are considered nonlinear pharmacokinetics and they tend to get accumulated in plasma levels.

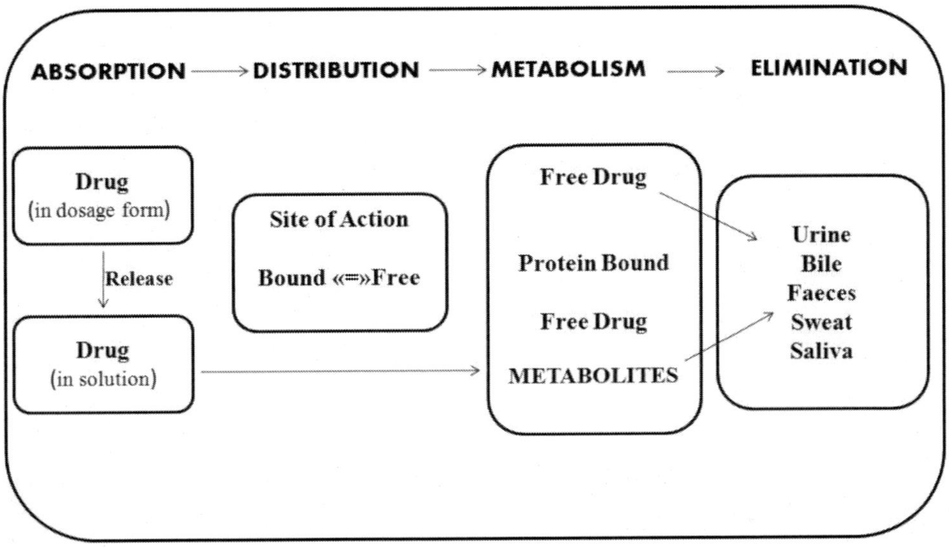

Figure 1. Illustration of Pharmacokinetic processes.

First-Order Reaction

When it is said that drug X gets eliminated by a first-order reaction, it means, the rate is proportional to the concentration of drug X at any particular time, i.e., rate ∝ [X].

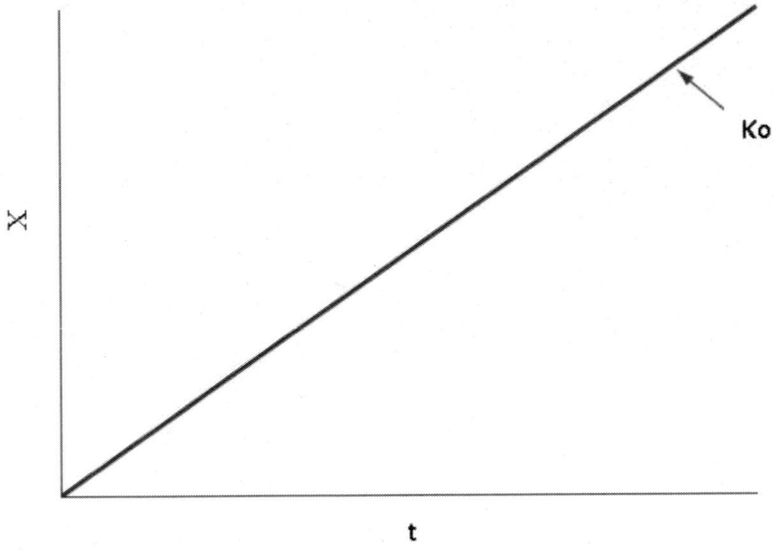

Figure 2. Plot of amount of drug eliminated against time for zero-order reaction.

The rate of reaction is therefore given by dx/dt = K1[X], where the proportionality constant, K1, is called the rate constant [1].

The first-order reaction rate depends on the concentration of one reactant. If the initial concentration of drug X is a mol dm–3 and if we find experimentally that x mol dm–3 of the drug has eliminated in time t, then the amount of drug remaining at a time t, i.e., [X], is

(a – x) mol dm–3 and the rate of elimination will become:

– d[X]/dt = –d(a – x)/dt = dx/dt,

where a is a constant and disappears after integration.

The rate equation is:

dx/dt = K1(a – x)

Integration of the rate equation gives:

K1= (2.303/t) log [a/ (a-x)]

Plot of time as ordinate against the logarithm of the amount remaining as abscissa is linear (figure 3). It is assumed that most drugs are eliminated by first-order reactions and the processes of ADME follow the same. Some exceptions are also present, for example phenytoin and high-dose salicylates. In essence, for drugs that show a first-order elimination process one can show that, as the amount of drug administered increases, the body is able to eliminate the drug accordingly and accumulation will not occur.

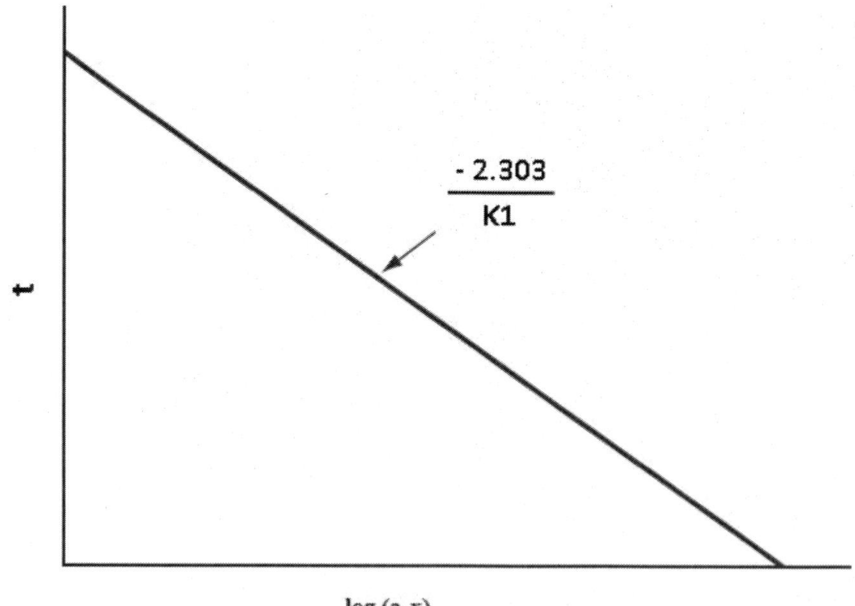

Figure 3. Plot of amount of drug eliminated against time for first-order reaction.

If you double the dose you will double the plasma concentration. However, if you continue to increase the amount of drug administered then all drugs will change from showing a first-order process to a zero-order process, for example in an overdose situation [2].

Models Associated with Pharmacokinetics

The overall kinetic process often can be described using different mathematical models e.g., compartment models, non-compartment models, and physiologically-based models. Fundamental knowledge of pharmacokinetic principles is vital. This is important for the clinician to understand basic patient-drug relationships. It is also important for the drug industries to assist the design of relevant studies for drug candidates and discovery. The inputs from designing proper pharmacokinetic studies can be useful in better therapy for the patient and long-term economic savings for the pharmaceutical industry can also be achieved [3].

Physiologically Based Pharmacokinetic Model

It is possible to analyze volumes and clearances for each organ in the body. Based upon these data set one can create models of pharmacokinetics by assembling the organ models into accurate models of the entire animal. In these models it is assumed that blood flows through the system as a zero-order process and drug transfers between the blood and tissues as a first-order process. The pharmacokinetics compartmental modeling helps in explaining the fate of a drug within the body, described as an entity separated into compartments. The drug leaves the site of administration (by the process of absorption) to enter in a central compartment, from which it is exchanged with peripheral compartments (by the process of distribution) and irreversibly eliminated (by the process of biotransformation and excretion Movement of drug from one compartment to another can be described by transfer rate constants: in linear kinetics, the rate of transfer is considered to be directly proportional to the drug amount available for transfer. In each compartment, characterized by its own volume, the drug concentrations are proportional to the amount. A compartment includes a number of organs/tissues and is kinetically homogenous. The drug is administered to the central compartment. The distribution of drug starts from this central compartment. Generally, all the compartments are connected to the central compartment. This compartment covers the initial dilution volume, which is usually composed of plasma and additional spaces. Drug diffuses extremely rapidly into this compartment. Elimination of drug occurs directly and exclusively from the central compartment.

Single Compartment Model

In single-compartment modeling, the drug is assumed to be distributed instantaneously into a single compartment in the body which is characterized by a distribution volume. It is considered as the drug achieves distribution throughout the body and the drug equilibrates instantaneously between tissues. Thus the drug concentration-time profile shows a single phase response. The drug entrance into this volume is dependent upon the dosage regimen. The output of the drug from this volume is described by an elimination constant rate (figure 4).

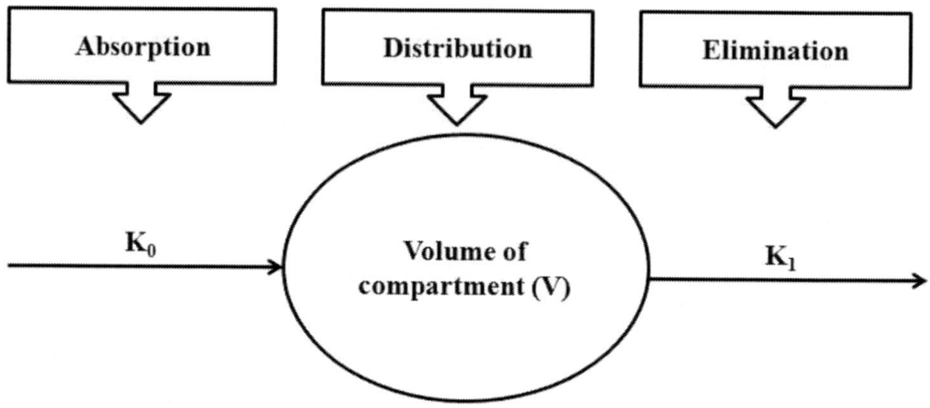

Figure 4. Diagram showing one compartment model, where K_0 and K_1 are rate constant for absorption and elimination respectively.

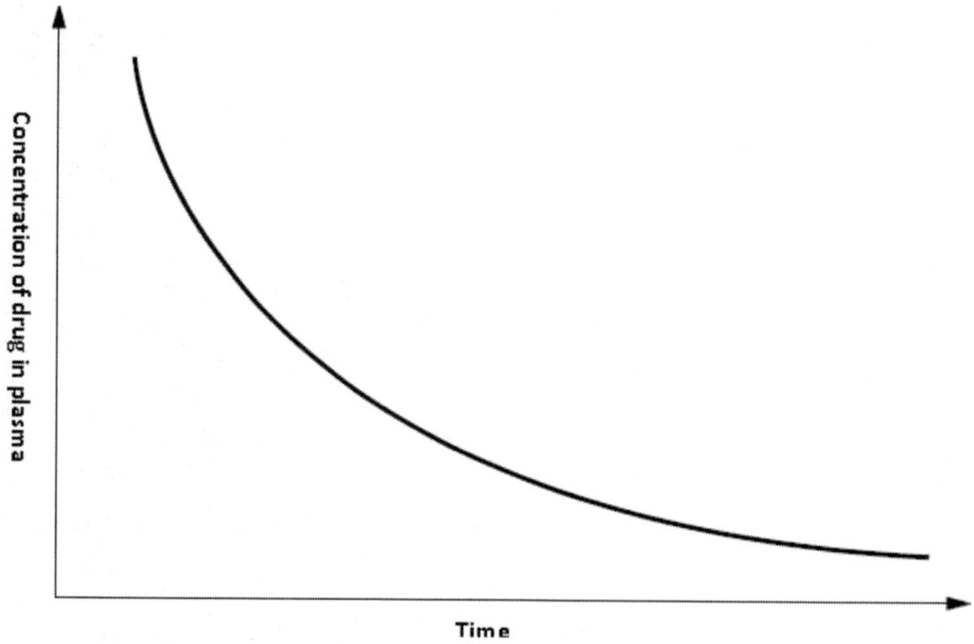

Figure 5. A plot for drug-concentration in plasma against time, for one-compartment model.

Assumptions:

Body homogeneous (one compartment)
Distribution instantaneous

Concentration proportional to dose (linear)
Rate of elimination proportional to how much is there (First order)

It is noteworthy that this does not imply that the drug concentration in plasma is equal to the drug concentration in the tissues. However, changes in the concentration of the drug in plasma numerically reflect changes in the tissues. It is further important to note that we know some of these assumptions are not true. It is of little consequence, as the data act as if these were true for many drugs. The visual image which is useful is one of a single box and a single arrow going out of the box depicting one compartment with linear kinetics (figure 5). The 'time-profile' of one-compartment model is showing a log of concentration of drug in plasma versus time (figure 6).

The dose is placed in the box and is eliminated by first order processes. In many cases, more complicated models (more boxes) are necessary to mathematically mimic the observed plasma versus time profile when one or more of these assumptions are not accurate. For example, the two-compartment (or multi-compartment) model results when the body is assumed to not be homogeneous and distribution is not instantaneous [4].

$$dA/dt = \text{Drug input} - (K_1 * A)$$

$$\text{Clearance (CL)} = K_1 * V$$

$$dC/dt = [\text{Drug input} - (CL * C)]/ V$$

where, K_1 = Rate of elimination
A = Amount of drug
V = Volume of distribution
C = Concentration in the volume

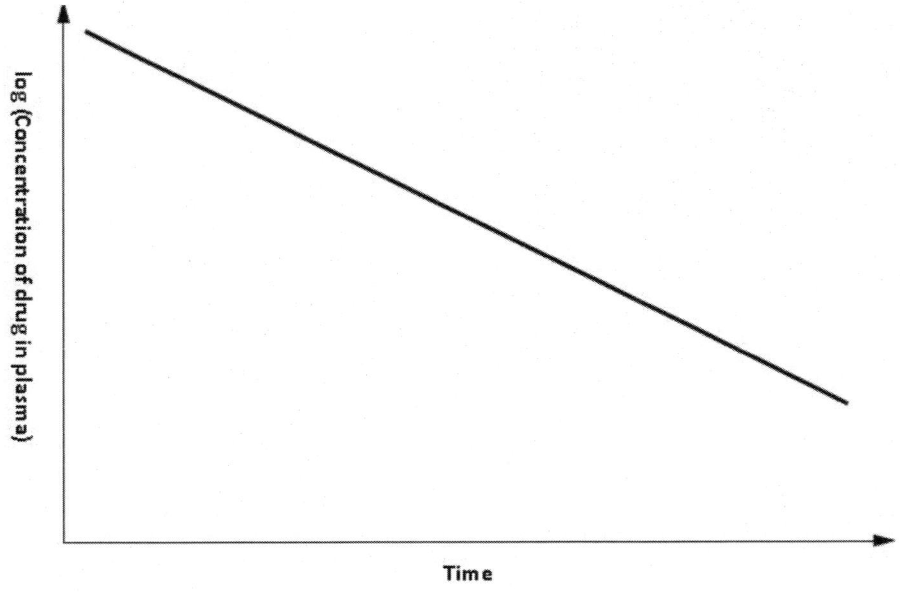

Figure 6. A plot showing logarithm of drug-concentration in plasma versus time.

Two-Compartment Model

According to the two-compartment model, the human body is considered to have a central compartment and a peripheral compartment. These compartments do not have any anatomical or physiological existence. The central compartment consists of high blood supply tissues such as heart, liver, kidney and peripheral compartment has comparatively less perfused tissues such as skin, muscle etc.

Two-compartment model comes into existence when the body is considered to not be homogeneous and distribution is not instantaneous. The dose is considered to be inducted in the central compartment; from here it moves to the peripheral compartment. Hence, at an initial phase concentration of drug rapidly decreases in central compartment and increases to a maximum in the peripheral compartment. After a time interval 't' drug concentration establishes equilibrium. All rates of transfer follow first order reaction.

Drug finally gets eliminated from the central compartment (figure 7). If we closely analyze the drug concentration in plasma versus time plot for a one- compartment model and the same for two-compartment model (figure 8), we can see the slight difference in the curve. As we know that in two-compartment model the drug concentration rapidly decreases initially in central compartment and drug moves through concentration gradient to peripheral compartment until the short term equilibrium establishes.

The removal of drugs take place from central compartment which establishes a concentration gradient in the opposite direction and this time drug travels from the peripheral compartment to central compartment. Due to this, the 'logarithm' of drug-concentration in plasma versus time plot (figure 9) shows a sudden break in the straight line.

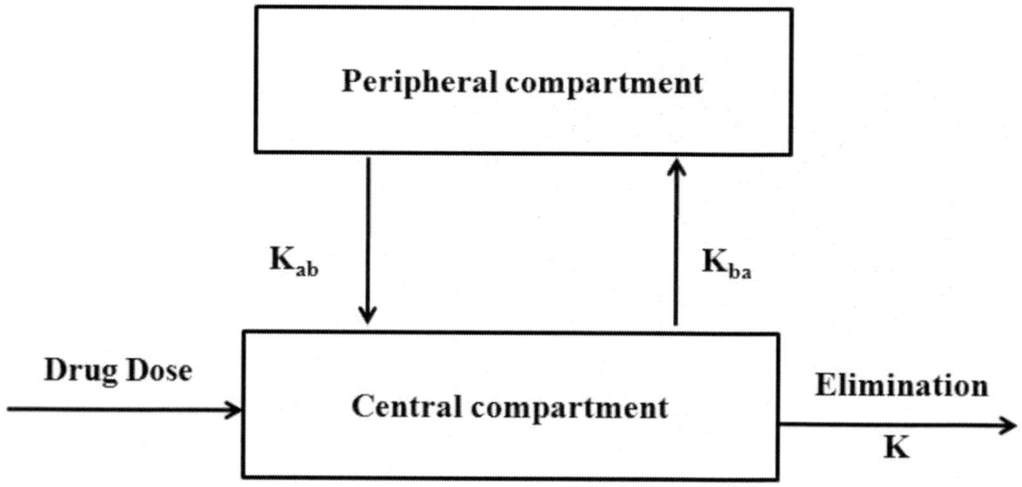

Figure 7. Two-compartment model: K_{ab}= Rate transfer from peripheral to central compartment, K_{ba}= Rate transfer from central to peripheral compartment, K= Rate of elimination from central compartment.

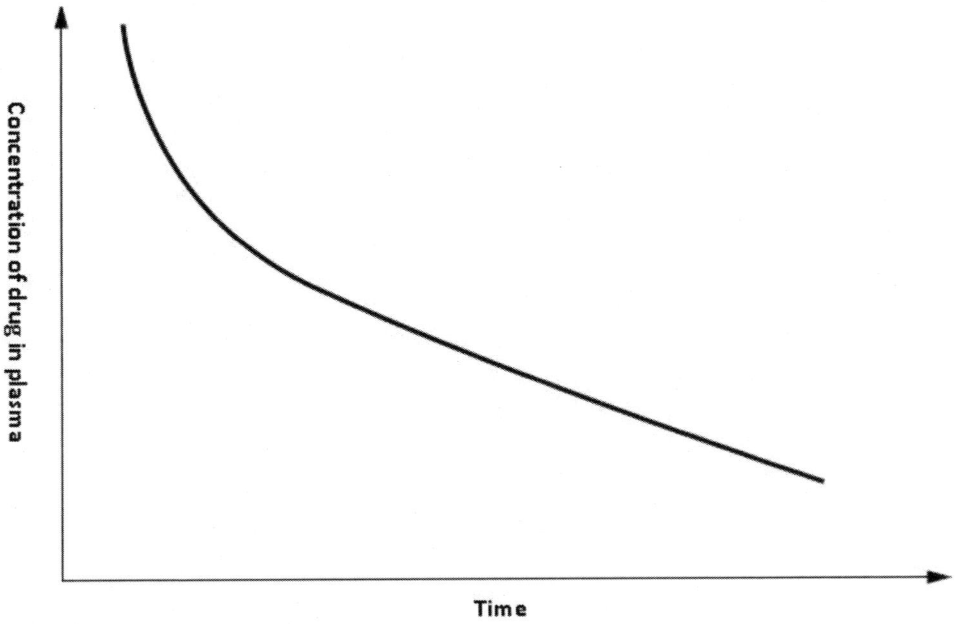

Figure 8. A plot for drug-concentration in plasma versus time for two-compartment model.

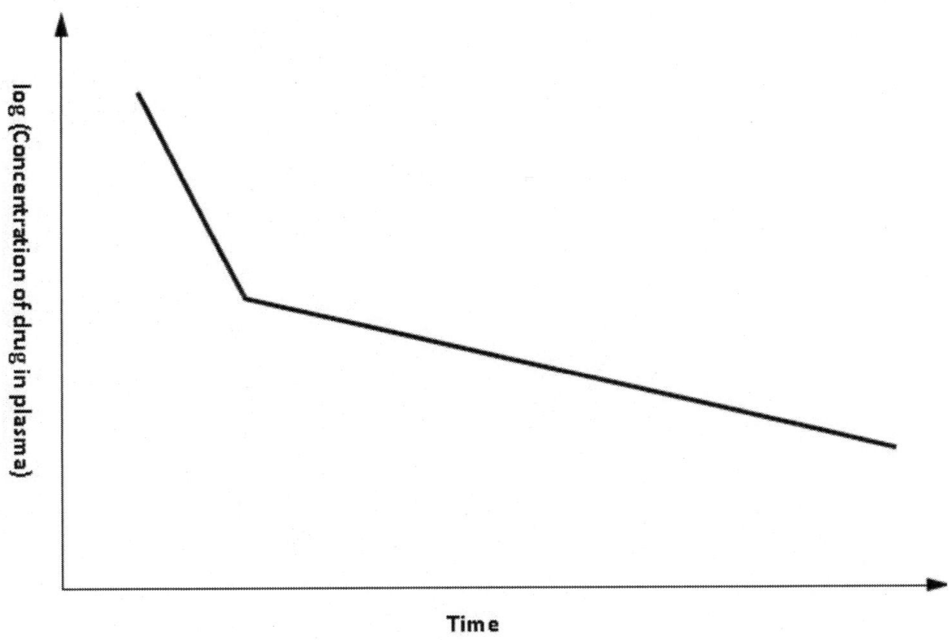

Figure 9. A plot for 'logarithm' of drug-concentration versus time for two-compartment model.

Absorption

In pharmacokinetics absorption can be defined as; a process by which drug molecule from the site of administration reaches to the blood stream.

Rate of absorption is equally important along with the amount of drug that reaches to circulation from administered dose. In case of intravenous (i.v.) route of administration, drug dose is directly injected into the systemic circulation. Hence, absorption is considered to be zero. In the rest of the cases drug has to pass different biological barriers to reach to the blood.

Factors Affecting Absorption

(a) *Biological factors* e.g., Biological membranes, local blood flow, stomach empty time, drug binding (with plasma and food).
(b) *Physiological factors* e.g., pH, route of administration, types of formulation etc.

Biological Membranes

The cell membrane consists of semi-permeable lipid bilayer. The lipids present in cell membranes are phospholipid and cholesterol molecules. Polar groups from the cholesterol molecules are oriented towards the outer two surfaces. The non-polar groups (hydrocarbon chains) are embedded inside the matrix along with intrinsic proteins. Polymeric sugars, amino-sugars or sialic acids are present on the surface of the membrane. The intrinsic proteins are present in the membranes in such a way so that they can float freely through the membrane [5]. Some of the proteins extend through the full thickness of membrane and surround the aqueous pores (figure 10).

Drugs are absorbed in the body by following processes:

(i) Passive diffusion
(ii) Active transport

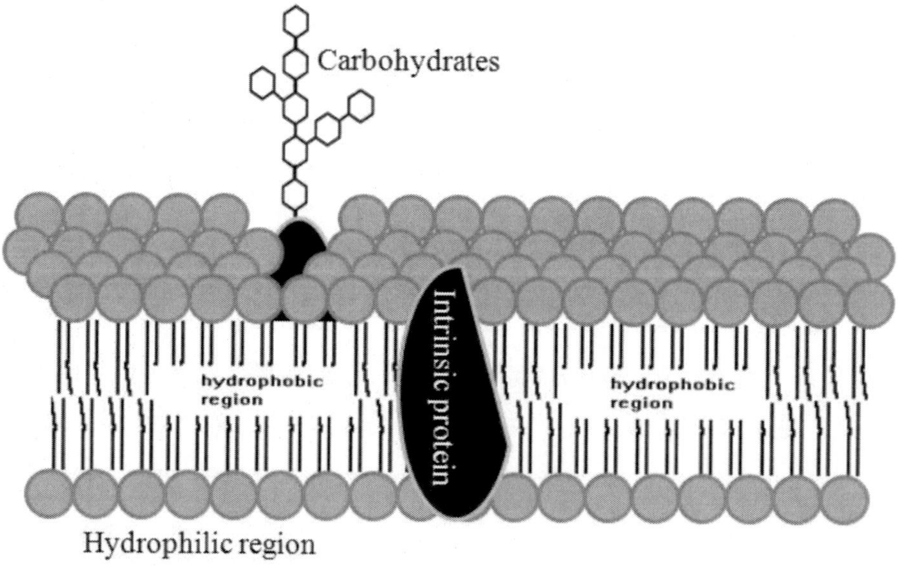

Figure 10. Illustration of components of cell membrane.

Passive Diffusion

In this type of diffusion drug diffuses in the direction of concentration gradient. In most of the tissues, passive aqueous diffusion occurs through channels provided molecules have less than 150-200 molecular weight. An exception is the endothelial capillary linings as they have comparatively large pores that allow molecules of 20-30,000 molecular weights to pass. However, the capillaries of most of the brain do not contain these large pores. Lipid soluble drug molecules get dissolved in the membrane and pass through the concentration gradient.

In facilitated diffusion drug passes from the region of high concentration to the region of low concentration but it specifically depends upon the protein carriers.

Active Transport

Active transport is the process by which the drug passes from the region of low concentration to the high concentration with the help of energy. Example: Methotrexate an anticancer agent transported through the process of active transport.

Local Blood Flow

Rate of absorption is highly dependent on blood flow. Continuous blood flow is necessary for maintaining the concentration gradient for passive diffusion of drugs. Drugs that are administered at the highly vascularized site get absorbed quickly. Orally administered hydrophilic drugs are absorbed into the portal vein.

This portal vain sends the drugs directly to the liver, where it may be partially deactivated. This is the first pass effect. First pass effect is discussed in detail in metabolism section of this chapter.

Stomach Empty Time

Food may interact chemically (process of chelation) or physically with drugs, by adsorbing the drug or acting as a barrier to assimilation. In general, gastrointestinal absorption of drug is favoured by an empty stomach, but the nature of drug-food interaction is complex and unpredictable; drug absorption may be delayed, reduced, enhanced or unaffected by the presence of food. Ampicillin, Aspirin, Atenolol, Captopril, Erythromycin, Ethanol, Hydrochlorothiazide, Penicillins, Tetracyclines etc. are examples of drugs with reduced absorption in presence of food. Acetaminophen, Cephalosporins, Diclofenac, Digoxin, Furosemide, Nitrofurantoin, Sulfadiazine, Sulfisoxazole etc. are drugs with delayed absorption in the presence of food.

There are a number of drugs who show an increase in absorption rate e.g., Chlorothiazide, Diazepam, Griseofulvin, Hydralazine, Labetalol, Metoprolol, Nitrofurantoin, Propranolol, Riboflavin etc. [6] Gastric emptying time differs among patients and contribute significantly to inter-subject variability in drug absorption.

Drug Binding

Number of drugs bind strongly to proteins in the blood or to food substances in the gut. Acidic drugs usually bind to the plasma protein named albumin. Basic drugs generally bind to alpha-one acid glycoprotein.

Binding to plasma proteins maintains the concentration gradient of free drug by increasing the rate of passive absorption. For many drugs, the gastrointestinal absorption rate, but not the extent of absorption, is reduced by the presence of food in the gut (as discussed in the last paragraph).

Some drugs are not affected by food, while the absorption of a third group of drugs is enhanced by food (bile secretion by the liver in response to food in GI tract increases drug absorption). Some drugs are irritating and should be administered with meals to reduce adverse effects.

Influence of pH

Acid can be defined as a substance that liberates hydrogen ions (H+) in solution. A substance that can bind H+ and remove them from solution is known as a base. pH is one of the primary influences on the solubility of most drugs that contain ionisable groups and hence influences the absorption.

Acidic drugs, such as the non-steroidal anti-inflammatory drugs (NSAID) e.g., Nimesulide, Ibuprofen, Diclofenac etc. are less soluble in acidic solutions in comparison to alkaline solutions.

This is because of the predominant undissociated species cannot interact with water molecules to the same extent as the ionized form which is readily hydrated. The equation for the pH of the solution of an acidic drug is as follows:

$$pH - pK_a = \log [(S-S_o)/S_o]$$

where, S= Solubility of acidic drug; S_o= Solubility of unassociated drug.

Basic drugs are more soluble in acidic solutions. Here drugs predominantly exist in the ionized form. The equation relating the solubility S, of a basic drug in the pH of the solution is:

$$pH - pK_a = \log [S_o/(S-S_o)]$$

where, S= Solubility of basic drug; S_o= Solubility of unassociated drug.

Many drugs are weak organic acids e.g., Aspirin, or weak organic bases e.g., procaine or their salts e.g., Ephedrine hydrochloride. Strong acid or strong base is completely ionized, whereas, a weak acid or weak base is only slightly ionized in solution. The pH is deciding factor for the degree of ionization of any weak acid or strong alkali. Some notable exceptions to the above statement are non-electrolytes e.g., steroids, and the quaternary ammonium compounds, which are completely ionized at all pH values and due to this fact they act as strong electrolytes. The extent of ionization of a drug has a significant effect on its absorption, distribution and elimination.

Table 2.1. List of weak acid drugs and weak base drugs

Weak acid drugs	Weak base drugs
Aspirin	Erythromycin
Penicillin	Quinine
Tetracycline	Atropine
Sulfathiazole	Tolbutamide
phenytoin	Quinidine
Barbiturates	Codeine
Phenylbutazone	Pilocarpine

The pH Partition Theory

The pH - partition theory was proposed by Brodie et al. It explains that extent of drug transfer or drug absorption is influenced by gastrointestinal pH and drug pKa. According to Brodie when a drug is in ionized form, it will not pass through the lipid membrane. When a drug is not ionized it can pass through therefore lipid bilayer membrane and hence greater lipid solubility exists [7].

Varied concentration of the drug was injected into the intestine of rats intravenously by Brodie. It was done until there was no net transfer of drug across the lining of the digestive tract. He then determined the ratio, D as:

$$D \frac{\text{Total concentration of drug in blood}}{\text{Total concentration in gastrointestinal tract}}$$

Influence of Route of Administration on Absorption

Apart from the extent and rate of dissolution and the rate of gastric emptying, site of absorption plays a vital role in determining the absorption rate of drugs. Various routes of administration and their effect on drug absorption are discussed below:

The Oral Route and Oral Absorption

Oral route is most widely used route of administration in drug delivery system. A variety of dosage forms such as tablet, capsule, emulsion; suspension and syrup are given by oral route of administration. In these dosage forms syrups are absorbed at a faster rate as compared to rest of the oral dosage forms. In case of tablets or capsules, they first need to get disintegrate followed by dissolution of the dose.

Due to these two processes drug takes comparatively larger durations to get absorbed to reach the systemic circulation. In case of syrups drugs are already dissolved and exist in the form of solution. Hence, drugs in the form of solution get absorbed at comparatively faster rate. An absorption rate of emulsion and suspension lie in-between the tablet and syrup.

Buccal and Sublingual Absorption

The absorption of drug through buccal and sublingual route takes place by oral mucosa and provides a route for systemic administration. As this route does not follow gastrointestinal tract, drugs bypass the liver and so avoid first pass metabolism through the liver. Drugs through these routes have direct access to the systemic circulation. A classical example is glyceryl trinitrate which have been administered in this way. This drug gets absorbed at a very fast rate and gives pharmacological action within one to two minutes after sublingual administration. Mucosal adhesive systems are utilized for administration of buprenorphine through the gums. In this route of administration most of the drugs get absorbed by the process of simple diffusion. For homologous series of drugs, there is a linear relationship between absorption percentage through the buccal cavity epithelium and partition coefficient.

Intramuscular and Subcutaneous Injection

These routes of administration are used for selective drugs as some of the drugs are not released and larger portion of the drug remain unabsorbed. Subcutaneous route of administration is rich in vascularisation due to the presence of a large number of capillaries. Due to rich the capillary supply drug diffuses through the capillary walls and reaches to the systemic circulation.

Inhalational Route of Administration

In this route of administration, absorption takes place through the respiratory system. High capillary supply and large surface area of alveoli provide rapid absorption of drugs. In some of the medicinal treatments, this route of administration minimizes the side effects e.g., epinephrine suspensions. Drugs with lipophilic nature absorbed significantly through this route. Pressurized aerosols and Nebulizers are used for drug delivery through this route of administration.

Nasal Route

This route of administration is used for the drugs that are destroyed in the gastrointestinal tract. Nasal route is used as an alternative to the injections. It bypasses the first-pass metabolism by the liver and rapid absorption of drugs take place.

Rectal Route

Dosage forms used by this route are known as suppositories. Suppositories are placed in the rectal cavity. Veins of the inferior part of the sub-mucous plexus become the rectal veins.

The Venous network provide the site of absorption of the drugs. Superior haemorrhoidal veins are connected with portal vein but drugs get absorbed in inferior veins that enter into inferior vena-cava. Due to this fact drugs taken by the rectal route bypasses the liver and hence first pass metabolism.

Vaginal Route

Conventional vaginal delivery systems include vaginal tablets, foams, gels, suspensions and pessaries. It is not preferred route for systemic absorption of drugs. Steroids, prostaglandins, iodine, few antibiotics and antifungals are appreciably absorbed through this route of administration. As absorptive surface changes constantly so absorption is also variable through this route. This route of administration is sometimes used to deliver contraceptive steroids using vaginal rings.

Bioavailability

Bioavailability may be defined as the rate or extent by which drug reaches to the systemic circulation unchanged. Bioavailability is defined as the percentage of drug dose that proceeds in an unchanged form, from a site of drug administration to site of its action, to carry out its pharmacological and therapeutic effect. It indicates about two aspects, first is rate by which drug get absorbed and the second is the total quantity of drug that reaches to the systemic circulation.

Once a drug is administered into the body, it has to undergo very complicated and long path before producing the desired therapeutic effect. A drug which is aimed to be given orally should have an ideal balance between the pharmacokinetics, safety and appropriate drug delivery. Oral bioavailability is denoted by the letter F [8].

Oral dosage forms are prescribed most widely and they have found a hugely effective way of giving drugs to patients. One of the important considerations of the drug development process is to develop molecules having high oral bioavailability. Factors that influence oral bioavailability are enormous, for example first pass metabolic activity in liver, permeation by intestinal membrane, gastrointestinal absorption etc. During metabolism drug is exposed to a variety of enzymes resulting in chemical alteration in drug thereby either increasing or decreasing its therapeutic effect.

Drug permeation through the intestinal membrane rely upon several things like total lipophilicity of drug molecules, flexibility, hydrogen bonds formed, size and shape of drug molecules. Various factors influence rates of absorption are circulatory states, solubility, body pH, concentration, interactions with transporters and metabolizing enzymes. Bioavailability of drugs is also dependent on a number of other physiological factors including the composition of gastrointestinal fluid, transport dynamics, transit and motility, each of which varies with age, race, gender, food and disease [9].

Lipinski Rule of Five

In 1997 Christopher A. Lipsinki [10] published a paper mentioning a number of features commonly present in oral drugs. The features he identified, commonly referred as Lipsinki's Rule of Five and are considered as rule of vital importance to find, whether a molecule is orally bioavailable or orally non-bioavailable. Lipsinki's "Rule-of-Five" pioneered the in-silico prediction of oral bioavailability. A molecule is said to have poor absorption or permeability if any two out of the following parameters are not fulfilled:

Molecular weight under 500
Hydrogen bond donors not more than 5
Hydrogen bond acceptors not greater than 10
logP value less than 5

After the influential work of Lipsinki's et al., there exists abundant of research to predict oral bioavailability of drugs. Several research groups exploited the above mentioned properties and tried to uncover other factors influencing oral bioavailability, indicating it to be an incredibly rich area of interest.

Distribution

Distribution is the process by which drugs become disseminated to all parts of the body after absorption. It is process of distribution of a drug from the systemic circulation to organs and tissue.

Conditions that affect distribution include:

Normally, the drug concentration is much lesser than protein-binding capacity; as a result the free fraction is generally constant.

Only unbound drugs pass through the cell membranes. Many drugs bind to the plasma proteins like albumin, and there is a dynamic equilibrium between bound and free drug molecules.

Drug + Protein = Drug-Protein Complex
Bound Drug «=» Free Drug
Free Drug= Active
Bound Drug= Inactive

Free content of drug increases due to competition between the drug plasma protein binding site by the process of drug displacement. The placenta may serve as a barrier to distribution of drugs. Drugs with small molecular weight cross the placental barrier to reach to fetal blood levels. However, the concentration of the drug in blood of the fetus is generally lower than maternal. Blood brain barrier (BBB) is permeable only to lipid-soluble drugs or those of very low molecular weight. Example: steroidal drugs. It is a well know fact that transport of drug molecules from the blood to different tissues of organisms occur either by transcellular transport (through the endothelial cells) or by paracellular transport (through gaps between the endothelial cells). The selective BBB permeability of few drug molecules leads to Edwin Goldmann's hypothesis. According to the hypothesis, "The cerebral capillaries provide the anatomical basis for a physiological barrier between the brain and the rest of the body". This hypothesis has been further confirmed with the advent of electron microscopy i.e., the outermost layers of the endothelial cells in the brain capillaries are fused together. The tight junctions of brain endothelial cells form a selective BBB to facilitate homeostatic regulation which ensures that fluctuations in the concentration of nutrients, hormones or ions cannot directly affect the synaptic functions of the nerve cells. Thus, while the BBB is beneficial in maintaining regular cerebral functions, it represents an obstacle to drug therapies designed to tackle several disorders of central nervous system (CNS). It has been seen that few lipophilic antibiotics such as chloramphenicol can cross the BBB whereas, passage of hydrophilic antibiotics like penicillin is hindered. It is also interesting to know that more than 98% of all small drug molecules and around 100% of large drug molecules do not cross the BBB (Garg et al., 2008; Pardridge, 2001; Pardridge, 2003). Therefore, in the discovery of the CNS acting drug, the degree to which a molecule penetrates through BBB is most crucial aspect of its absorption distribution metabolism and excretion (ADME) consideration.

An ideal therapeutic agent on molecular targets (present in the CNS) should cross the BBB. Whereas, for a peripherally acting agent it should not cross the BBB to avoid CNS related side effects. In both circumstances, the prediction of the BBB permeability index has been proved to be an efficient tool for drug discovery and development. BBB permeability is expressed as log (C_{brain}/C_{blood}) i.e., ratio of the steady-state concentrations of the drug molecule in the brain and in the blood. Recently it has also been quantified as logPS i.e., permeability and surface area product.

Apparent Volume of Distribution (Vd)

It is theoretically calculated value and not the real volume by nature. It is useful while calculating the loading dose of a drug. Apparent volume of distribution is expressed as liters per kilogram.

It is a kinetic parameter of a drug that relates dose with plasma level at t=0.

Vd is that volume of plasma in which the total amount of drug in the body would be required to be dissolved to reflect the drug concentration attained in plasma.

V_d = Total amount of drug (X)/ Plasma concentration of drug (C_P)

If the drug present throughout the body as the same concentration in plasma, then the volume of distribution reflects the total amount of drug in the body.

Vd is low when a high amount of a drug is bound with plasma proteins. When a large percentage of a drug is free and passes in tissues then Vd is considered to be high. This increases the possibility of displacement of drug by other agents e.g., Digoxin can be displaced by quinidine from tissue binding sites. Apart from crossing the BBB, lipid-soluble (steroidal) drugs redistribute into fat tissues before elimination As the plasma concentration falls, the drug readily diffuses back into the circulation to be quickly redistributed to other tissues with high blood-flow rates, such as the muscles; then, over time, the drug also becomes deposited in lipid-rich tissues with poor blood supplies, such as the fat depots. In case of drugs acting on the CNS, the duration of action of an initial dose may depend more on the rate of redistribution than on the half-life of a drug. On the administration of the second dose, the rate of redistribution is less as the available blood/fat is less. Due to this fact the second dose has a longer duration of action. Most drugs are not distributed equally throughout the body but tend to accumulate in certain specific tissues or fluids. The general principles that govern the movement and distribution of drugs across cellular membranes are applicable. Basic drugs tend to accumulate in tissues and fluids with pH values lower than the pKa of the drug; conversely, acidic drugs concentrate in regions of higher pH, provided that the free drug is sufficient lipid soluble to be able to penetrate the membranes that separate the compartments.

Compounds that permeate freely through cell membranes become distributed, in the body water, both intracellular and extracellular. Compounds are distributed into the extracellular fluid space if they pass through capillary endothelial cells, but not able to go through other cell membranes. Sometimes the drug molecule may be very large or very highly bound to plasma proteins that it remains in the intravascular space after intravenous administration. Binding to large molecules like protein components of cells or fluids, dissolution in adipose tissue, formation of non-diffusible complexes in tissues such as bone, incorporation into specific storage granules, or binding to 'selective sites' in tissues all delay movement of drugs in the body and account for differences in the cellular and organ distribution of particular drugs. Medicinal compounds may also be a carried by carrier-mediated systems through to certain cellular membranes. This leads to higher concentration gradient on one side than the other. Some examples of these nonspecific transport mechanisms can be seen in renal tubular hepatocytes, epithelial cells, and the choroid plexus.

Only the unbound or free part of a drug can pass through capillaries to reach into tissues. Proteins that bind to drugs in the circulatory system are plasma albumin, globulins and, α-1 acid glycoprotein (for bases) and they play a significant role. Degree of drug binding to plasma proteins depends upon a number of factors, e.g., plasma pH, concentration of plasma proteins, concentration of the drug, the presence of another agent with a greater affinity for the limited number of binding sites, and the presence of acute-phase proteins during active inflammatory conditions. The degree of plasma-protein binding has great clinical significance in some and the affinity of a drug for the nonspecific protein-binding sites are of great clinical significance in some cases and has lesser significance in other. For example, Dicumarol (potentially toxic compound) may be 98% bound. Due to any reason it becomes 96% bound then the concentration of the unbound active drug that becomes available in the plasma is doubled, and may lead to very harmful results. Drug overdose may lead to exceed of the binding capacity of the plasma protein and result in an excess of free drug, which can pass into various target tissues by the process of diffusion and produce exaggerated effects. Another important factor is the readiness of drug with which drugs dissociate from plasma proteins.

Tightly bound drugs have tendency for having much longer elimination half-lives because they are released gradually from the plasma protein. The long-acting antimicrobial agents like sulfonamides are good examples of this phenomenon. During distribution and elimination from the body, a drug may or may not penetrate certain blood-brain, placental, and mammary barriers. Drugs penetrate into the cortex more rapidly than in white matter, probably because of the greater delivery rate of drug via the bloodstream to the tissue.

The pharmacological factors and their influence on CNS for drug permeability are following:

1) Water soluble ionized drugs will not cross the CNS
2) Low ionization, low plasma-protein binding, and a fairly high lipid-water partition coefficient leads to permeability
3) Direct drug delivery into the CSF using injections often produces unexpected effects
4) Meningoencephalitis can substantially alter the permeability of the blood-brain barrier

During pregnancy, placental barrier should be considered while therapeutic treatment. The potential teratogenicity of any drug (agents that can interfere with normal embryonic development) needs to be investigated before its administration. If the drug is to be used during the late gestation period, its effects on the fetus and on the process of parturition should be taken into consideration. Placenta allows nutrients, such as minerals, glucose, amino acids, and some vitamins to pass across the placenta. The passage of drugs across the placenta is largely by lipid diffusion. The distribution of drugs within the fetus follows essentially the same pattern as in the adult, with some differences with respect to the volumes of drug distribution, plasma-protein binding, blood circulation, and greater permeability of interceding membranous barriers.

Like other biologic membranes epithelium of a mammary gland acts as a lipid barrier and many drugs readily diffuse from the plasma into milk [11].

Metabolism

The process of chemical modification of drugs by enzymes present in the body is known as metabolism or biotransformation. Metabolism of drugs in the body is primarily done by the liver. For some of the drugs lungs, kidneys and intestinal mucosa are also involved in metabolism process within the body. Drug metabolism has great biological significance. It converts the active form of drug into an inactive form so that it can be easily eliminated from the body. In most of the cases drugs are converted to water soluble forms (metabolites). It helps the drug elimination by the process of excretion. In some cases body metabolism changes inactive form of drug into an active one, e.g., prodrugs such as Acetylsalicylic acid, Solindac, Losartan etc. These prodrugs get metabolized in the liver.

First Pass Metabolism

Most of the compounds absorbed from the stomach and intestines enter the systemic circulation.

But prior to reaching to systemic circulation, drug reaches to the liver via the hepatic portal vain. Compounds absorbed via this route must therefore pass through the liver. A hepatic metabolism generally follows first order kinetics. A large proportion of any orally administered drug that is highly and efficiently metabolized in the liver will be cleared during the initial first pass. Hence, there is strong possibility that a drug could be efficiently absorbed from the gastrointestinal tract and yet poorly available to the general circulation as a result of first-pass metabolism in the liver.

Metabolism in the body can be classified into two types:

(1) Phase I reactions or Non-synthetic reactions
(2) Phase II reactions or Synthetic reactions

Phase I Reactions or Non-Synthetic Reactions

This class of reactions includes oxidation, reduction, hydrolysis, cyclization, decyclization etc.

Oxidation: It is reaction that involves the addition of oxygen or loss of hydrogen or loss of electrons.

It is the most important reaction in metabolism process in the body. Cytochrom P-450 in the liver plays vital role in the oxidation of drugs. There are more than 100 cytochrome P-450 enzymes are identified till date e.g., CYP1A1/2, CYP2C8/9, CYP2C19, CYP2D6, CYP2E1, CYP3A4/5 etc. The amount of cytochrome P-450 differs from species to species and in some cases individual to individual in the same species. This is one of the major reasons for differences in drug metabolism between two species or individuals of the same species. Drugs that metabolized by the process of oxidation are Nifedipine, Tolbutamide etc.

Reduction: It is reaction which involves the addition of hydrogen or loss of oxygen or gain of electrons.

Drugs reduced in the body are Chloramphenicol, Halothane etc.

Hydrolysis: It takes place by the addition of water molecule and leads to cleavage of drug molecules. Liver, intestine, plasma and other tissues are sites for hydrolysis. Most of the esters get hydrolyzed in the body to give acids and alcohols. Drugs that get hydrolyzed in body are Lidocain, Procain, Choline esters etc.

Cyclization: Straight chain compounds form ring structures by the process of cyclization, e.g., Proguanil.

Decyclization: This reaction leads to opening of ring structures. Cyclic drugs like Barbiturates, Phenytoin etc. follow this minor pathway for metabolism.

Phase II Reactions or Synthetic Reactions

Phase II reactions are energy driven conjugation reactions. Conjugation takes place between phase I reaction metabolites of the drugs with endogenous substrates such as glucuronic acid, glycine, sulfate etc. These endogenous substrates are derived from amino acids and carbohydrates in the body. These conjugation reactions lead to the formation of water soluble, highly polar organic acids which can be excreted easily out of the body.

Some conjugation reactions are briefly explained below:

Glucuronide conjugation: Glucuronide is derived from glucose. Hydroxyl or carboxylic acid group containing compounds conjugates with glucuronic acid to give water soluble compounds. This is a most important synthetic reaction in the body. Drugs that follow glucuronide conjugations are Aspirin, Morphine, Metronidazole etc.

Acetylation: It takes place with the help of acetyl coenzyme-A. Compounds with amino or hydrazine groups get conjugated with acetyl coenzyme-A. Drugs that are metabolized by this process are Hydralazine, Isoniazid, Sulfonamides etc.

Glycine conjugation: Drugs with carboxylic acid are conjugated with amino acid glycine e.g., Salicylate drugs. It is not a major pathway for drug metabolism.

Glutathione conjugation: It is a minor pathway for drug metabolism. Drugs like paracetamol for highly reactive epoxides or quinines that are inactivated by the process of glutathione conjugation.

Apart from the above reactions, methylation, sulfate conjugation, ribonucleoside/ ribonucleotide synthesis etc. also take part in phase II or synthetic metabolism of drugs in the body.

Metabolism process can be summarized in figure 11.

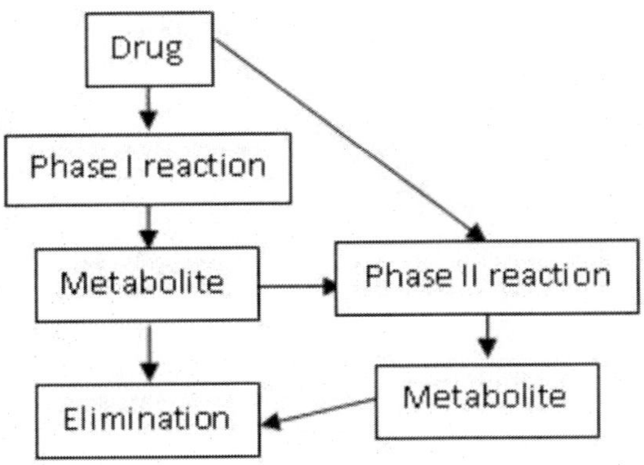

Figure 11. Sequential presentation of drug metabolism in the body.

Elimination

Removal of drugs from the body is known as drug elimination. Drugs get eliminated from the body via kidney, bile, sweat, saliva, exhaled air, or milk. Major elimination of drugs is done by the kidney. As discussed in the initial part of this chapter elimination is a first order process. Drugs can be eliminated in one of the following forms:

Urinary excrete: It is the most important way of elimination of most of the drugs. The excretion of drugs by the kidney utilizes three processes. All of these processes occur in the nephron which is a microscopic functional unit of the kidney. These processes are:

1) Glomerular filtration
2) Tubular secretion and
3) Tubule reabsorption.

Glomeruli allow the passing of majority of drug molecules, but limit the movement of drugs that are bound to the protein. Larger drugs or the drugs bound to plasma proteins are not able to filter and hence poorly excreted by glomerular filtration. Changes in glomerular filtration rate affect the rate of elimination of drugs which are generally eliminated by the process of filtration.

Tubule secretion involves two carrier systems:

(a) Basic carriers: For transport basic drugs e.g., Dopamine, Histamine etc.
(b) Acidic carriers: For acidic drugs e.g., Indomethacin, Frusemide, Penicillin etc.

Biliary Excrete: Very less is known about hepatic elimination of drugs. Many drugs and their metabolites reach to the small intestine through bile and may undergo enterohepatic cycling. Most of the drugs present in feces are derived from bile.

Respiratory exhaled air: In case of inhaled anesthetics excretion happens mainly in exhaled air. Volatile drugs and gases are inhaled and excreted via the lungs. Excretion from the lungs is dependent upon the rate of respiration and deep breathing or exercise. It causes in increase in cardiac output and subsequent increase in pulmonary blood flow and promoting excretion. Volatile substances, such as ethyl alcohol (highly soluble in blood) are excreted in limited amounts by the lungs. In case of ethyl alcohol pulmonary excretion is the basis of alcohol breath test.

Saliva and sweat: Some drugs are excreted in saliva and sweat but amount of drug excreted via them is of less importance because this process is very slow and presents only minor proportion of drug in total excretion. Sometimes, excretion of drugs in sweat is responsible for adverse drug effects which lead to dermatitis and skin reactions.

Milk: Drugs or their metabolites pass through the epithelial cells of mammary glands and are excreted in breast milk. The excretion of drugs in breast milk is significant only because the drug may affect the breastfeeding infant.

Clearance (CL)

Drug clearance (CL) is defined as the volume of plasma in the vascular compartment cleared of drug per unit time by the processes of excretion. If the drug is eliminated by first-order kinetics, clearance of a drug is constant. The drug can be cleared by renal excretion or by metabolism or both. With respect to the kidney and liver, the clearances are additive by nature:

$$CL\ (total) = CL\ (renal) + CL\ (non\text{-}renal)$$

Clearance is the product of the first-order elimination rate constant (k) and the apparent volume of distribution (V_d):

$$CL\ (total) = k * V_d$$

Clearance is related to half-life by:

$$t_{1/2} = (0.693 * V_d)/CL$$

Plasma Half Time

Half life a drug is defined as total duration of drug action. This is the time period at which amount or concentration of drug in the body is reduced by one-half. The half life of a drug is calculated in relation to the amount of the drug in plasma. The speed of drug is the elimination from the plasma determines plasma half life. A drug molecule that leaves plasma may follow one of the following:

(1) It can be eliminated from the body
(2) It can be translocated to another body fluid compartment such as the intracellular fluid
(3) It can be destroyed in the blood.

As discussed in previous pages that the removal of a drug from the plasma is known as clearance and the distribution of the drug in the various body tissues is known as the volume of distribution. Both of these pharmacokinetic factors are extremely important in determining the half life of a drug. The half life of a drug is presented by symbol: $t_{1/2}$

Half life can be determined by using the following steps:

(1) Give a single dose intravenously to the animal under investigation.
(2) Measure the plasma concentration of the drug at regular intervals. The concentration of the drug will reach a peak value in the plasma and will then fall as the drug is broken down and cleared from the blood.
(3) Calculate the time taken for the plasma concentration to become half in the plasma. It is the half life of that drug.

Drugs that are cleared from the blood with considerably high speed have a short span of half life time. These drugs should be given at regular intervals to have enough concentration in blood. It helps drug to exert their therapeutic activity effectively. Nonsteroidal anti-inflammatory drug such as ibuprofen is an example of short half life drug. Repeated dose administration builds required plasma concentration of drug and lead to the steady state. Steady state is a balance between therapeutically effective concentration level of blood and clearance of the drug. The time taken by a drug to reach steady state is generally about five folds greater than half life. Drugs like with a long half life (e.g., Digoxin, Warfarin etc.) have longer duration to achieve a steady state in comparison to drugs with a shorter half life.

Sometimes a loading dose (higher dose) may be administered to achieve steady state more quickly and after first loading dose, smaller maintenance doses are given to make sure that the drug level in the blood stays within the steady state.

References

[1] Attwood, D., Florence, A. T. (2008). *Physical Pharmacy*, pp 31-32. London: Pharmaceutical Press.

[2] Dhillon, S., Gill, K. (2006). Basic pharmacokinetics. In: Dhillon S., Kostrzewski A. J., eds. Clinical Pharmacokinetics pp 1-44. London: Pharmaceutical Press.

[3] Benet, L. Z., Mancinelli, L. (2006). Clinical Pharmacokinetics and Pharmacodynamics. In: Swarbrick. J. *Encyclopedia of Pharmaceutical Technology*. 3rd edition. pp 572-590. London: Informa Healthcare USA, Inc.

[4] Makoid, M. C., Vuchetich, P. J., Banakar, U. V. (1999). *Basic Pharmacokinetics.* Creighten University: The Virtual University Press.

[5] Tripathi, K. D. (2003). Essentials of medical pharmacology, edition 5, pp 3. New Delhi: Jaypee brothers medical publishers Ltd.

[6] Welling, P. G. (1986). Pharmacokinetics, Processes and Mathematics, American Chemical Society, Washington D.C.

[7] Shore, P. A., Brodie, B. B., Hogben, C. A. M. (1957). The Gastric Secretion of Drugs: A pH Partition Hypothesis, *J. Pcol., Exp., Therap*., 119, 361-369.

[8] Kumar, R., Sharma, A., Varadwaj, P. K. (2011). *Machine Learning and Biological data: A Research Overview,* pp7-10. Saarbrucken, Germany: Lambert Academic Publishing GmbH and Co. KG.

[9] Masoud, J., Dabid, T. et al. (2009). Population based mechanistic prediction of oral drug absorption. *The AAPS Journal*, 1, E27-40.

[10] Lipsinki, C. A., Lomabardo, F., Dominy, B. W., Feeney, P. J. (1997). Experimental and computational approaches to estimate solubility and permeability in drug discovery and development settings. *Adv. Drug Delivery Rev*., 23: 4-25.

[11] Kahn, C. M., Line, S. (2010). *Pharmacology. Merck Veterinary Manual*. New Jersey, USA: Merck Sharp & Dohme Corp.

In: Introduction to Drug Designing and Development
Editors: R. Kumar, A. Sharma and R. Kumar Tiwari
ISBN: 978-1-62948-556-0

Chapter 3

Pharmacodynamics

Rajnish Kumar*
Amity Institute of Biotechnology, AMITY University-Uttar Pradesh,
Lucknow, Uttar Pradesh, India

Abstract

The study of physiological and biochemical effects of drugs and their mechanisms of action is known as Pharmacodynamics. It is branch of pharmacology which deals with effect of drug on body. What the drug does to the body is studied under pharmacodynamics. Pharmacodynamic study covers mechanism of action of drugs, drug-receptor interaction, drug concentration-effect, factors that modify drug action and interactions etc. In this chapter we will explore various principles of pharmacodynamics in systematic manner.

Pharmacodynamics consist of two worlds: *Pharmakon* + *Dynamics*. Pharmacon means Drug and Dynamics means power. So, Pharmacodynamics is nothing but what the drug does to the body. Pharmacodynamics refers to the relationship between concentration of drug at the site of action and its effect. It also includes the time course and therapeutic intensity and adverse effects.

Drugs do not impart novel functions to cell, tissues, organ or body. However, they only modulate the pace of ongoing activity. Drug can work by stimulation, Depression, Irritation, replacement or cytotoxic action. By the process of stimulation drug selectively enhances the activity level of specialized cells, depression leads to decrease in the activity of specialized cells and mild irritation may lead to stimulation. Diseases due to deficiencies can be cured by the process of replacement of hormones (Insulin), natural metabolites (Levodopa) etc. Selective cytotoxicity helps in curing cancer cells and parasites etc. with no/minimal harm to

* Email address: 12.rajnish@gmail.com, rkumar2@lko.amity.edu.

the host cells. Drugs may act by physical action, chemical action or enzymatic activities. Majority of drugs act by binding to the specific molecule present into body (receptors).

However, number of drugs act by non-receptor mediated mechanism. Non-receptor effects by drugs are due to their particular physical and chemical properties. Drugs for example emollients have physical basis for their action. Antacids react with hydronium ion and act by chemical rather than receptor mediated activity as reactive proton has no permanent biological residence. Local anesthetics, general anesthetics, certain electrolytes etc are another example of non-receptor mediated type of drugs.

Now we will try to understand how drug molecules act. There are number of theories available to explain drug action.

Drug Receptor Theory

The receptive substance (receptor) should have structural requirement and chemical affinity for the drug. Receptor can be an intracellular constituent or a membrane that govern the spatial orientation of enzymes, compartmentalization of cytoplasm, contractile properties of subcellular structures, permeability of membranes or gene expression. In coupling system occupied receptor gives response. Example: neurotransmitters in central nervous system and acetylcholine couple with ion channels to elicit the response. Benzodiazepines receptors are coupled with gamma-aminobutyric acid (GABA) receptors. Receptor classification in general is based on differentiation between the subtypes of the receptors. Receptor subtypes are designated as Arabic or Greek alphabetical prefixes and numerical subscripts.

Occupation Theory

Law of mass action is principle to govern drug-receptor interactions. However, mass law concerns with the rate at which products formed or reagents disappear whereas receptor theory concerns with fraction of drug that bind to the receptor. The concept of occupational theory says that only when the receptor is actually occupied by the drug, it elicit functional response. In classical occupation theory, two parameters have prime importance: *affinity* and *intrinsic activity*. *Affinity* is measure of the equilibrium constant of drug receptor interaction. Intrinsic activity is ability of drug to induce conformational changes (positive change) to elicit biological response.

The mathematical equations of receptor theories are derived from chemical kinetics and law of mass action.

Assumptions:

1. It is assumed that intensity of effect is a direct linear function of the fraction of receptor occupied by drug. This is a theoretical assumption but it seems to be close enough to give useful approximation for drug-receptor interaction.
2. Drug –receptor interaction is at equilibrium.
3. Number of receptor molecules is very small (negligible) as compared to the drug molecules.

Above three assumptions really simplify the mathematical expression of drug receptor theory. Deviation from these assumptions may lead to significantly complicated equation.

First equation was derived by Clark [1].

$$K\,x^n = \frac{y}{100 - y} \tag{1}$$

where,

K is affinity constant.

x is concentration of drugs.

n is molecularity of reaction.

y is percentage of maximum response.

y was assumed as linear function of percentage of receptors occupied by drugs. Therefore, y could also be studied as percentage of occupied receptors. Rearrangement of equation (1) gives:

$$y = \frac{100K\,x^n}{1 + K\,x^n} \tag{2}$$

When equation (2) is put into *log* form

$$\log K + n \log x = \log \frac{y}{100 - y} \tag{3}$$

A plot of *logy/100-y* against *log x* yields straight line. Its slope can be depicted as *n*. Here *n* is theoretically number of molecules of drug that react with each molecule of receptor.

Limitations of occupational theory: The theory is unable to generate a realistic model of partial agonism and intrinsic activity. A rate theory, which says that intensity of response is proportional to the rate of drug-receptor interaction, was proposed later. However, it failed to give a mechanistic model of generation of response [2].

Mechanism of Drug Action

Drugs can act through physical action (e.g., Bulk laxatives, Kaolin, Charcoal, Mannitol etc), chemical action (e.g., Antacids [$Al(OH)_3$], Oxidizing agents [$KMnO_4$] etc.) enzymes (Acetazolamide on Carbonic anhydrase, Aspirin on Cyclooxygenase etc.) or receptors (Atropine on Muscarinic receptor, Hexamethonium on Nicotinic receptor etc.).

Drugs get distributed to almost all parts of body by circulatory system. However, they do not act everywhere. Drugs are more or less selective towards their binding to the specific proteins, lipoproteins, glycoproteins etc that are present in cell membrane, cytoplasm, nucleus or other organelles. Drugs that selectively bind and activate receptors to produce effect are referred as agonists. Drugs that block the normal effects of the respective endogenous substances are known as antagonists. Certain drugs stimulate or activate enzymes to elicit biological response but they are not useful as their responses are too widespread. In contrary, some drugs inhibit only one type of enzymes selectively to reduce the activity of enzyme to act on its normal biochemical substrate. In such cases the enzymes are drug receptors. In chapter 6 'Drug targets and validation techniques', we will see various drug targets in detail where drugs effectively bind to elicit biological response.

Difference between Drug Action and Drug Effect

Drug action and drug effect are not synonyms to each other. They are different and should not be used interchangeably. Drug action is initial interaction of drug with receptor and leads to change (in case of agonists)/prevention of change (in case of antagonists) in receptor conformation. Drug effect is consequence of drug action and it is ultimate change in biological function.

Factors that Influence Drug Action

Drug Type: Different drug impart different drug action. Each drug has its own time of response. Drugs are mostly weak acids or bases and their chemical nature of drug is vital in drug action.

Route of administration: Drug action largely depends upon its route of administration. Highly vascularized route of administration helps in faster action in comparison to less vascularized routes. Most of the drugs having oral route of administration have to undergo through first pass metabolism and part of drug get metabolized here. Parenteral route of administration such as intravenous, intra-arterial etc. have faster drug action as drugs through routes directly each to blood.

Table 1. Showing different species/races have different drug response

Species/ Race	Response
Rats and Mice	Resistant to Digitalis
Cats	Cats are less sensitive to Curare than rats
Rabbits	Resistant to Atropine
Human races: Blacks and Mangols	Mangols require less concentration of Ephedrine and Atropine for pupil dilation as compared to Blacks. β-blockers are more effective in Mangols as compared to Blacks (require higher concentration)
Human races: Indians and Whites	Thiacetazones are better tolerated by Indians than Whites.
Japanese and Indians	Japanese develop subcute myelooptic neuropathy (SMON) in treatment through Quiniodochlor. However, despite of extensive usage of Quiniodochlor no confirmed cases of SMON are found in India.

Drug dosage form: Drug dosage forms are vital in the process of drug action. Over 90% drugs are taken orally. Oral drugs have to pass through different biological barriers such as biological membranes; this delays the action of drug. Oral drugs in the form of liquid have comparatively faster action than solid oral dosage forms. Solid dosage forms first disintegrate, dissolve and then get absorbed in body. This takes more time in comparison to liquid dosage forms.

Species and race: Different species have different response for drugs. There are certain examples which show that drugs have different response in various species (Table 1) [3].

Genetics: Variations in drug response due to genetic differences is studied under Pharmacogenomics. Genetic differences lead to the variation in absorption, distribution, metabolism and excretion of drugs. The major contributing factor for variation is metabolism of drugs.

Gender: Gender based differences in drug action is largely dependent on hormonal fluctuations. Females require dosage from the lower side range in comparison to males. In women menstruation, pregnancy and lactation should be considered during the treatment of various diseases.

Body size: Body size is important while deciding the individual dose of drug. Concentration of drug attend at the site of action is dependent upon body size (equation 4).

$$Dose = \frac{BodyWeight\,(kg)}{70} * Average\ Adult\ Dose \tag{4}$$

It is believed that body surface area (BSA) gives more accurate dose calculation (equation 5).

$$Dose = \frac{BSA(m^2)}{1.7} * Average\ Adult\ Dose \tag{5}$$

It is important to note that dose calculation from BSA is only available for handful drugs including anticancer agents. For rest of the drugs body weight basis is used to calculate dose.

Age: Dose of drug is calculated on the basis of age (especially in case of child dose). There are two basic formulas available for calculation of dose on the basis of age (equation 6, 7).

1. Young's Formula

$$Child\ Dose = \frac{Age}{Age + 12} * Adult\ Dose \tag{6}$$

2. Dilling's Formula

$$Child\ Dose = \frac{Age}{20} * Adult\ Dose \tag{7}$$

There is a gradual decrease in various physiological functions in adults after the age of 30.

Pathological state: Type of diseases influence drug action. Liver diseases influence drug action by having high first pass metabolism and hence low bioavailability. In case of gastrointestinal diseases absorption can be increase or decrease. Congestive heart failure can influence pharmacokinetics of drug.

Psychological factors: Patient's attitude, belief and expectations play important role in treatment of diseases. Placebo is classical example which shows importance of psychological factors effecting drug action. Placebo is an inert substance with no medicinal agents. It is given to those patients who do not require any active agent in opinion of doctor. Patient believes that medicine is taken by him/her and this will cure the disease. Placebo works psychologically with no physiological responses.

Presence of other drugs: Drugs may change the effects of each other. Combined effects of drugs may have synergistic or antagonistic effects. Synergistic effects are further divided into two types; additive or supra-additive.

Additive effects: Effects of two or more drugs are in the same direction e.g., effect of Aspirin and effect of Paracetamol is equal to the combined effects of both drugs.

Supra-additive drugs: Combined effect of drugs is greater than the sum of individual effects e.g., combined effects of Acetylcholine and Physostigmine is greater than sum of individual effects of Acetylcholine and Physostigmine.

Antagonistic effect: When presence of one drug inhibits the effect of other drug, it is known as antagonism. Antagonism can further be divided into two types; competitive antagonism and non-competitive antagonism.

Competitive antagonism: In this type of antagonism both antagonists bind with the same receptor. They are chemically similar to each other and apparently reduce affinity/potency of each other e.g., Acetylcholine and Atropine.

Non-competitive antagonism: In this type of antagonism drugs bind to different locations of receptor. These drugs do not resemble but reduces intrinsic activity or efficacy of each other e.g., Bicuculline and Diazepam.

Environmental factors: Various environmental factors affect the drug action. Sedative and hypnotics that are taken in night are more effective in comparison to day time. Presence or absence of food in stomach in case of oral drugs may influence the drug absorption and hence drug action.

Tolerance: It is adoptive biological phenomenon which leads to requirement of higher dose to impart given response. Different types of tolerance include natural/innate tolerance, acquired/Chronic tolerance, Metabolic / dispositional tolerance, acute tolerance and cross tolerance etc.

Natural/Innate tolerance: It is due to inborn ability to be less sensitive to certain drugs e.g., rabbits are naturally tolerant to Atropine.

Acquired/Chronic tolerance: It happens due to continuous and repeated use of the drug. Person has responses to the drug initially and the due to acquired tolerance response to the drug decreases e.g., acquired tolerance to the sedative action of Chlorpromazine.

Metabolic / dispositional tolerance: It is due to accelerated drug clearance.

Acute tolerance: It is quick alteration in functional sensitivity during a single drug exposure.

Table 2. Classes of drugs that misused

S. No.	Class of drug	Examples
1	Opioids	Diamorphine, Heroin
2	Sedatives	Benzodiazepines: Diazepam, Temazepam
3	Stimulants	Cocaine
4	Hallucinogens	Lysergic acid diethylamide (LSD)
5	Miscellaneous	Cannabis, Tetrahydrocannabinol

Cross tolerance: It develops due to use of pharmacologically related drugs. Closer drugs have tendency to develop higher degree of cross tolerance e.g., Barbiturates and general anesthetics are more prone to develop cross tolerance to alcoholic patients.

Dependence: It occurs due to use of repeated high dose of drug. In the beginning it appears to be functional normally but abrupt stopping of drug leads to the withdrawal effect. Drug dependence is considered a multi-factorial health disorder that often follows the course of a relapsing and remitting chronic disease. Drug dependence could be considered a "self-acquired disease", based on individual free choice leading to the initial experimentation with illicit drugs [4].

There is no single physiological explanation for dependence of drugs. There are five classes of compounds which come under drug misuse and cause dependence.

There are five classes of drugs that induce drug abuse and frequent dependence (Table2).

Mechanism of Action of Various Drugs

Acetylcholine: It is generally co-transmitted with peptide neurotransmitters. Acetylcholine acts on muscarinic and nicotinic receptors. Muscarinic receptors are G- protein coupled receptors whereas nicotinic receptors are receptor operated cation channels.

Diuretics: Thiazide diuretics inhibit sodium reabsorption in distal nephron. Spironolactone inhibits aldosteron. Aldosteron is responsible for sodium reabsorption. Amiloride is another drug in this class, which blocks sodium-hydrogen transporters. Furosemide is loop diuretic. It prevents sodium and chloride reabsorption from loop of Henle.

Beta-Blockers: Mechanism of action of β-blocker antihypertensive is poorly understood. β-blockers possibly block the effect of catecholamines and hence reduces the cardiac output and heart rate e.g., propranolol, atenolol. β-blockers can reduce release of rennin from kidneys (rennin is responsible for the synthesis of angiotensin II). β-blockers are also used in case of acute arrhythmias and prophylaxis of angina.

Antihypertensive agents: Nifedipine causes arterial vasodilation by preventing L-type voltage gated calcium ion channels. Nifedipine can be used in angina, while verapamil is used for antiarrhythmic activity.

Heart failure: Diuretics e.g., frusemide (promotes renal excretion of sodium and reduces blood volume), vasodilators e.g., glyceryl trinitrate (reduces preload by venodilation and after load by arterial vasodilation), positive inotrope infusions e.g., dobutamine are used in heart failure treatment.

Lipid lowering drugs: Anion-exchange resins such as cholestyramine binds with bile acids in intestine and prevent their reabsorption. It leads to conversion of bile acids from cholesterol in liver. Fibrates such as bezafibrate stimulate lipoprotein lipase. Lipoprotein lipase converts very low density lipoproteins (VLDLs) to low density proteins (LDLs). It also enhances the clearance of LDLs from systemic circulation by liver. Another lipid lowering compound is Nicotinic acid (Vitamin). It inhibits the production of VLDLs which intern reduces the total cholesterol concentration. Hydroxy-methyl-glutaryl-coenzyme-A (HMG-CoA) reductase inhibitors such as simvastatin catalyses the rate limiting step for de novo synthesis of cholesterol.

Antipsychotic (Neuroleptic) drugs: Antipsychotic drugs like haloperidol have antagonistic activity to dopamine. They partially relieve symptoms of schizophrenics. Some other drugs used as antipsychotics are chlorpromazine, thioridazine, trifluoperazine, droperidol, flupenthixol, clozapine, sulpiride, respiridone etc.

Antidepressant drugs: Older tricyclic antidepressants prevent the presynaptic reuptake of noradrenaline serotonin. This activity potentiates the neurotransmitters effect. Apart from tricyclics, monoamine oxidase inhibitors, lithium (in manic-depressive psychosis) etc. are also used for antidepressant activity.

Sedatives and hypnotics: Benzodiazepines are common sedatives. They act on separate site of $GABA_A$ receptors. No endogenous agonist at benzodiazepine binding site has been discovered yet. $GABA_B$ agonists such as baclofen works as muscle relaxants. They are use in muscle spasticity.

Nonsteroidal anti-inflammatory drugs (NSAIDs): These drugs are used in mild pain, rheumatoid arthritis, pyrexia, anti-platelet action etc. NSAIDs are cyclooxygenase inhibitors. They prevent prostaglandins, prostacyclin and thromboxanes. Paracetamol, ibuprofen, diclofenac, piroxicam, indomethacin etc are potent NSAIDs.

Opioid analgesics: These classes of drugs have agonistic activity to cellular opioid receptors. They reduce the membrane calcium conductance, increase potassium conductance and inhibit the Cyclic adenosine monophosphate (cAMP) synthesis. This causes hyperpolarization of nerve cells. It leads to decrease the excitement of nerve cells and pain is relieved. Morphine, diamorphine, codein, pethidine, methadone etc. are used as opioid analgesics.

General anesthetics: General anesthetics bind to the specific receptor operated ion channels and hence inhibit synaptic transmission. Propofol, etomidate and ketamine are some potential general anesthetics.

Local anesthetic agents: Local anesthetics such as lignocain inhibit action potential initiation and conductance. They act on ion channels and plug them to inhibit conductance through voltage sensitive sodium channels. Bupivacaine (marcaine), prilocaine, cocaine and procaine are some of the frequently used local anesthetics.

Neuromuscular blocking agents: These agents act on nicotinic cholinergic receptors, which are located on skeletal neuromuscular junction. suxamethonium, vecuronium, atracurium, tubocurarine etc. are some potent neuromuscular blocking agents.

Antiepileptic agents: Mechanism of antiepileptic agents is not clear. They probably inhibit the conduction of action potential away from epileptic focus. Antiepileptic agents act by voltage dependent sodium channel e.g., carbamazepine or by increasing the effects of GABA neurotransmitters e.g., sodium valproate, vigabatrin etc.

Anti-Parkinson's disease drugs: Anti-Parkinson's disease drugs mainly act by two mechanisms: (a) antagonizing excitatory action of acetylcholine with anti-muscarinic activity. (b) replacing/mimicking the dopamine action.

Some drugs used in Parkinsonism are L- Dopa, carbidopa, selegilin, amantadine, benzhexol, bromocriptine etc.

Anti-migraine drugs: Anti-migraine drugs like sumatriptan is agonist for 5-HT receptor present in cranial vessels. Apart from this, pizotifen, propranolol, amitriptyline are other drugs used in prophylaxis of migraine. Ergotamine is used in acute treatment of migraine.

Bronchodilators: Salbutamol which is also known as ventolin has agonistic activity to β_2 – adrenoceptors. It causes relaxation of bronchial smooth muscle and bronchodilation. Glucocorticoids such as beclomethasone are strong anti-inflammatory agents and used through inhalers in acute asthma attacks. Ipratropium bromide (muscarinic receptor antagonists), Methylxanthines (adenosine receptor antagonists) etc. are other drugs used as bronchodilators.

Drugs used in Peptic ulcer: Cimetidine is histamine H_2-receptor antagonist and selectively inhibits acid secretion. Omeprazole is proton pump inhibitor. It inhibits the gastric acid secretion by blocking active transport of hydrogen-potassium on parileta cells. Antacids such as alluminium hydroxide and magnesium hydroxide are used to chemically neutralize gastric acids.

Anti-diabetes drugs: Oral hypoglycemics such as glicazide stimulates pancreatic insulin. Insulin is used in case of insulin deficiency as supplement. It acts at receptors that are membrane bound. Insulin as supplement is used in type 1 diabetes as type 1 diabetes is due to the deficiency of insulin (usually occurs in younger age group). Glicazide is used in type 2 diabetes in elderly people. Type 2 diabetes is due to the deficiency or resistance for insulin leading to hyperglycemia.

Oral contraceptives: Combination of ethinyloestradiol with norethisterone is frequently used oral contraceptive. These steroidal hormones act on intracellular receptors to regulate gene transcription.

Drugs used in rheumatoid arthritis: Sulphasalazine is used to scavenge the destructive oxygen free radicals which are generated at the site of inflammation. other anti-rheumatoid drugs are also used that modify inflammatory conditions but their mechanism is poorly understood.

Drugs used in skin disease: Drugs used in eczema are topical steroids (e.g., hydrocortisone), immunosuppressives (e.g., cyclosporin), calamine lotion etc. Hydrocortisone acts as anti inflammatory agent, cyclosporine inhibits interleukin-2 synthesis by T- cells and calamine lotion works as antipruritic agent. In case of psoriasis, calcipotriol (reduces epidermal cell proliferation), dithranol (prevents DNA synthesis), methotrexate (prevents DNA synthesis) etc. are used.

Anti-glaucoma and mydriatics: β-blockers such as timolol reduce the secretion of aqueous humor by acting on β-receptors of ciliary body cell linings. Pupil constriction occurs due to acetylcholine from parasympathetic terminal. Drugs such as atropine which are muscarinic antagonists are used in mydriatic conditions.

Anticoagulants: Heparin is secreted from liver. It potentiates antithrombin III. Antithrombin III inhibits the functioning of six protease enzymes in coagulation process. It makes an irreversible complex with these factors to inhibit clot formation. Warfarin blocks vitamin K epoxide reductase. It leads to the inhibition of formation of coagulation factors.

Antibiotics: Penicillin (β-lactams) and its derivatives inhibit the bacterial cell wall synthesis by blocking transpeptidase enzyme. Transpeptidase enzyme cross-links the N-acetylmuramic acid and N-acetylglucosamine. Penicillin and cephalosporines irreversibly bind to transpetidase to prevent cross-linking between polymers. Macrolides act on 50S ribosomal subunit of bacteria to prevent the movement of nascent peptide chain on ribosome. Tetracyclines act on 30S bacterial ribosomal subunits to stop the t-RNA attachment to the A site (here amino acids are added to nascent peptides). Chloramphenicol binds to the 50S of ribosomal subunitnear a site to prevent translation. Metronidazole (damages DNA) and quinolones (blocks DNA gyrase) inhibit bacterial DNA.

Anticancer drugs: Cytotoxic drugs block DNA replication and cell division. However, these drugs can cure only 5% of total types of cancer. Alkylating agents such as cyclophosphamide covalently cross-link DNA strands. Methotrexate inhibits folate synthesis which leads to prevention of nucleic acid synthesis. Vincristine prevents microtubule formation. Tamoxifen is used as oestrogen receptor antagonist in the treatment of breast cancer.

References

[1] Clarck, A. J. (1926). The reaction between acetyl choline and muscle cells. *J. Physiol.* 61, 547-556.

[2] Hanson, G. R., White, H. S. (2000). Pharmacodynamics. pp 1053-1175. In, Remington: The science and practice of pharmacy. 20th ed. Philadelphia: Lippincott Williams and Wilkins.

[3] Tripathi, K. D. (2003). *Essentials of medical pharmacology*, edition 5, pp 3. New Delhi: Jaypee brothers medical publishers Ltd. New Delhi.

[4] WHO. (2008). United Nations office on drugs and crime, 1-32. [URL: https://unodc.org/documents/drug-treatment/UNODC-WHO-Principles-of-Drug-Dependence-Treatment-March08.pdf]

In: Introduction to Drug Designing and Development
Editors: R. Kumar, A. Sharma and R. Kumar Tiwari
ISBN: 978-1-62948-556-0

Chapter 4

Plants As a Source of Lead Molecules

***Mala Trivedi*[1], *Anju Sharma*[1,*] *and Suresh Kumar Yadav*[1]**

[1]Amity Institute of Biotechnology, AMITY University-Uttar Pradesh, Lucknow, Uttar Pradesh, India

Abstract

According to the World Health Organization (WHO, 1977) "a medicinal plant" is a plant that contains properties or compounds which can be used for therapeutic purposes or those that synthesize metabolites to produce useful drugs. Medicinal plants constitute an important component of the flora of the world. Plant selection for drug discovery can be achieved by various means: through phytochemical screening, by conducting bioassays on experimental models, from ethnobotanical evidence or from the biological activity report of the plant. Despite the benefits derived from plants, some of them have unpleasant side effects which may be related to overdoses or other factors. This definition distinguishes those plants whose therapeutic properties and constituents have been established scientifically and plants that are regarded as medicinal but which have not yet been subjected to a thorough investigation.

1. Introduction

Traditional medicinal plants are a vast therapeutic resource, either in crude form or as starting materials of drugs. Plants have provided us variety of drugs such as analgesics (Morphine), antihypertensives (Reserpine), antimalarials (Quinine and Artemisinin), anticancerous (Taxol) etc. Medicinal plants and their extracts have been used for therapeutic purposes since time immemorial or since the inception of human civilization. With the development of civilization, uses of herbs became more sophisticated and are still used today without any documented evidence of adverse effects. In the beginning herbal plants were used

* E-mail: anjusharma.online@gmail.com, asharma3@lko.amity.edu.

in crude form as tinctures, powders etc. followed by proper formulations and lastly as pure compounds. Historically, knowledge about which plant or part of the plant is to be used for a particular ailment, its application etc., was passed on orally from one generation to another. Later proper documentation of medicinal plants and their usage was done. The earliest record of any medical document dated back to 4000-year-old Sumerian clay tablet which contains detailed information of plant remedies for various illnesses. The Egyptian Ebers papyrus compiled approximately 3500 years ago is another record which contains a list of hundreds of remedies. Shen-nung, China's legendary emperor, 4500 years ago complied a database named "Pun-Tsao" listing out thousands of herbal cures. Indian system of medicine 'Ayurveda' is the most ancient system amongst all. Its origin is lost in prehistoric antiquity, later its characteristics matured between 2500 and 5000 BCE in ancient India. Badianus Manuscript reports traditional medical knowledge of the Aztecs. Interest in herbal drugs and natural medicine is undergoing a renaissance at the present time [1]. Approximately 80% of the world's population still relies on traditional medicines for primary health care, the rest 20% are effectively using medicinal plants as therapeutic agents [2]. The medicinal plants, in crude or purified form, have been used significantly in drugs of traditional systems of medicine (TSM) and serve as lead compounds for drugs of the modern system of medicine. As a result many modern drugs have been isolated from natural plants. Quality crude drugs from plants are obtained by expert collection/isolation techniques, proper processing followed by drying, packaging and correct storage. Isolation of active compounds is done by variety of separation techniques, afterwards chemical and structural characteristics are determined on the basis of which structure activity relationship (SAR) is established. The identification of active principles of medicinal plants leads to use, misuse and abuse of substances. The use may be therapeutic (e.g., aspirin, reserpine) or narcotic abuse (cocaine, morphine etc.). Plant derived medicines has more benefits as compared to synthetic alternatives. They are safer, cheaper and provide profound therapeutic benefits [3].

2. System of Medicines

Traditional medicine constitute: Ayurveda (India), Acupuncture (China), Unani (Arabic countries), mental healer's medicine, traditional birth attendant's medicine, herbal medicine and various forms of indigenous medicine. It is a compilation of knowledge, beliefs, experiences, practices, skills, theories adopted by different cultures for prevention and cure of ailment, improvement of physical and mental illness and maintenance of health. Traditional medicine has maintained its popularity and effectives in all parts of the world.

Treatment in traditional medicine is carried out by:

(i) Using medicinal plant, minerals, animal material
(ii) Therapies like acupuncture and yoga

Alternative medicine or Complimentary medicine refers to practices that are not inherent to one's own tradition and not included into the dominant health care system i.e., herbal treatment, manual, spiritual and dietary treatments [4]. Homeopathy and chiropathy are relatively new one, around 200 years old. Modern science has exploited the traditional knowledge of medicines to a large extent. Advances in instrumentation, drug designing and computational biology have opened new horizons for usage of traditional knowledge in the drug development process. But with the advancement, we are facing huge threat of depletion of vital resources. Destruction of the forests, the erosion of tribal cultures, development and usage of fully synthetic drugs are a major threat to herbal practices. It is hoped that more investigations/ advancement not only protect the plant kingdom but will also add new medicinal plants to the world's pharmacopoeia before they are lost forever.

2.1. Traditional Indian Medicine

Ayurveda is an offshoot of Atharva Veda which was written 3000 thousand years ago. '*Ayur*' meaning life and '*Veda*' meaning knowledge, therefore Ayurveda means '*the science of life*'. The basic philosophy of Ayurveda is that man is an inseparable part of the universe. The human body, mind and spirit continuum is an integral whole and the individual is linked to the family, society, the environment and ultimately the universe. The definition of health is that "It is a state of complete psychosomatic equilibrium. It does not mean only absence of diseases but a state in which the mind, senses and spirit are pleasant and active". That agrees with the definition of WHO "Health is a state of complete physical, mental and social well being and not merely the absence of disease or infirmity" [5]. According to Ayurveda, the primary cause of disease is an undesirable effect on body and/or mind due to external factors or intrinsic causes. Disease is the consequence of an imbalance between various elements (earth, fire, water, air and space). Ayurvedic treatment combines the salubrious use of drugs, diet and certain practices while targeting patient as an organic whole with an aim to restore the balance between different elements. Ayurveda is the most ancient of all medical traditions, its characteristic concepts appear to have matured between 2500 and 500 BCE in ancient India. The earliest references to drugs and diseases can be found in the Rigveda and Atharvaveda, dating back to 2000 BCE. Atharvaveda, comprised of 6599 hymns and 700 prose lines, is considered as the forerunner of Ayurveda. The 'Samhitas,' or encyclopedia of medicine, were written during the postvedic era, and include 'Charak Samhita' (900 BCE), 'Sushruta Samhita' (600 BCE) and 'Ashtang Hridaya'(1000 CE). Later on, many more treatises were prepared and the use of medicinal plants is described in 'Nighantu Granthas' between the 7th and 16th centuries. [6, 7].

2.2. Traditional Chinese Medicine

Chinese Medicine history is amongst the ancient science and believed to be 5000 years old. Traditional Chinese medicines are based on two theories ; first theory deals with natural laws that govern good health and long life, namely 'Ying and Yang' while a second theory deals with five elements (earth, metal, water, wood and fire), namely 'Wu Xing'. Each element is linked to main organs of the body- spleen, lungs, kidney, liver, heart. According to Chinese medicine, disease is caused due to an unbalanced diet, improper lifestyle or environment. Therefore the treatment aims to restore health by identifying and removing the prime cause of the ailment, correct abnormal functioning caused due to imbalance, oppose the imbalance and normalize the flow of energy. China is the leading country for incorporating traditional herbal medicine into a modern health care system; this resulted in a blend of herbal medicine, acupuncture.

Table 1. List of few medical plants found in India along with their local names

SNo.	Plant Species	Local Name	SNo.	Plant Species	Local Name
1	Achillea millefolium	Gandana, Millfoil	37	Evolvulus alsinoides	Shankhpushpi
2	Achyranthes aspera	Aandhijhara	38	Gentanella moorcroftiana	Tikta
3	Adhathoda vasica	Ardusta	39	Gymnema sysvestre	Gudmar
4	Aegle marmelos	Bael	40	Hamidesmus indicus	Anantmool
5	Ajaquemontii Kibber	Konche, Pharna La Darcha	41	Helicteres ispara	Marorphali
6	Allangium salvifolium	Aankol	42	Heracleum condicans	Heypomo Padara
7	Allium carolinianum	Laot, Jangli Lahasun	43	Holarrhena antidysenterica	Indrajo
8	Aloe barbadensis	Gwarpatha	44	Hyoscyamus niger	Khurasani ajwain, Henbane
9	Andrographis paniculata	Kalmegh	45	Hyssopus officinallis	Tengu, Juffa
10	Arnebia euchroma	Khamet, Ratanjot	46	Jatropha curcas	Ratanjot
11	Artemisia brevifolia	Nurcha, Seinki	47	Juniperus communis	Hauber, Dhuppi
12	Asparagus racemosus	Satavari	48	Juniperus macropoda	Dhup, Dhoop
13	Azadirachta indica	Neem	49	Malva rotundifolia	Khubasi
14	Balanites aegyptiaca	Hingot	50	Mucuna prutita	Konch
15	Barleria cacrulea	Bajrandantis	51	Ocimum americanum	Bapchii
16	Barleria cristata	Badradantip	52	Onoma hispidum	Ratanjot, Gaojaban
17	Barleria prinoitis	Bajradantip	53	Oroxylum indicum	Shyonaka
18	Bergenia stracheyi	Gatikpa, Pashand bhed	54	Pedalium murex	Badagokhru
19	Betula jaquemontii	Bhojpatra, Bhuj	55	Physochlaina praealta	Laltang
20	Boerhaavia diffusa	Santhi	56	Plantago ovata	Isabgol

SNo.	Plant Species	Local Name	SNo.	Plant Species	Local Name
21	Butea monosperma	Palas	57	Plumbago zeylanicum	Chitrak
22	Caesalpinnia bonducella	Tas	58	Rhododendron anthopogon	Talis, Talispatra
SNo.	Plant Species	Local Name	SNo.	Plant Species	Local Name
23	Carum carvi	Shingu, Dru, Mawo	59	Sida cordifolia	Bala
24	Cassia fistula	Amaltas	60	Solanum surattense	Kantkari
25	Cassia occidentalis	Kasaundi	61	Soymida febrifuga	Rohan
26	Centella asiatica	Brahmibuti	62	Tamarindus indica	Imli
27	Chlorophytum arundinaceum	Safed musli	63	Taraxacum officinale	Khurmang, Dandelion
28	Colocynthes vulgaris	Indrayan	64	Terminalia arjuna	Arjuna
29	Convolvulus arvensis	Haranpadi	65	Terminalia bellerica	Baheda
30	Corydalis govaniana	Bhutjata	66	Tinospora cordifolia	Nimgiloy
31	Curculigo orchioides	Kali Musali	67	Tribulus terrestris	Gokhru
32	Curcuma aromatica	Vanhaldi	68	Urginea indica	Kolikanda
33	Dactylorrhiza hatagirea	Angbolaghp, Panja,Salampanja	69	Vitex negundo	Negad
34	Datura metel	Dhatura	70	Withania somnifera	Ashwagandha
35	Dyerophytum indicum	Chhitral	71	Woodfordia fruticosa	Dhavri
36	Eclipta alba	Bhringraj	72	Ephedra gerardiana	Som, Chha,Chhedang

Chinese prescriptions are filled with a large amount of specific herbs rather than with pills or ointments.Various documentation is available for traditional Chinese medicine; *Yellow Emperor's Inner Classic* (Hung Di Nei Jing; ~200 BCE to 100 CE), *Divine Husbandman's Classic of Materia Medica* (Shen Nong Ben Cao Jing; 25-220 AD) and cold-induced disorders (Shang Han Lun; 220 AD). The complete reference to Chinese herbal prescriptions is *Chinese Materia Medica*, published in 1977. It lists nearly 6000 drugs, of which 480 are of plant origin.

Chinas most important medicinal plants are *Angelica polymorpha* var. *sinensis, Artemesia annua, Ephedra Sinica, Paeonia lactiflora, Panax ginseng, Rheum palmatum* and *Peuraria lobata* [8, 9].

2.3. Traditional Egyptian Medicine

Egyptian medicine dates back from 3000 BCE. Greek physician Hippocrates (460-377 BCE) believed that disease is caused due to natural reasons. He used various herbal remedies to cure ailments and sufferings. Dioscoride's compiled a document, namely *De Materia Medica*, containing information about more than 600 species of plants along with their medicinal value. Dioscorides' work remained the standard medical reference in most of Europe for the next 1500 years.

Many herbal remedies used by the Greeks and Romans were effective and have been incorporated into modern medicine (e.g., willow bark tea, the precursor to aspirin). Subsequent naturalists like Theophrastus (~300 BCE) and the pharmacist Galen (130–200 CE) also recorded the use of medicinal plants. Egyptian literature gives in insight of most common herbs/ plants used in treatment ex. *Ricinus communis* seeds, *Citrilus colocynthes, Senna alexandrina* and *Prunica granatum* roots [10].

2.4. Traditional Arabic Medicine

The Babylonians, Assyrians and Sumerians comprised one of the oldest civilizations and several plants were explored and used during this early period. Several medicinal plants were named in civil laws which were carved on stone walls and commissioned by the King of Babylon (1700 BCE).

The Arabs established drugstores in the eighth century, and the Persian pharmacist Avicenna described all Greco-Roman medicine in his book *Canon of Medicine*. This text forms the basis of the distinct Islamic healing system known today as Unani-Tibb. *Papaver somniferum* was known to the Sumerians in 4000 BCE as *Hul Gil* (joy plant). The most frequently used medicinal plants in the Middle East are: *Allium cepa, Astracantha gummifera, Carthamus tinctorius, Carum carvi, Ferula asafoetida, Lawsonia inermis, Papaver somniferum, Peganum harmala, Prunus dulcis, Prunica granatum, Salvadora persica, Senna alexandrina, Sesamum indicum, Trachyspermum ammi, Trigonella foenum-graecum* and *Vitisvinifera* [11, 12].

2.5. European, African and other Traditional Systems of Medicine

South American countries have rich flora and fauna and diverse healing cultures. However due to lack of proper documentation, information regarding the use of medicinal plants is sparse. The famous medicinal plants from this region are *Cinchona pubescens, Erythroxylum coca, Ilex paraguariensis, Paullinia cupana, Spilanthes acmella* and *Uncarina tomentosa*.

The European medicine is believed to have originated with Hippocrates (460–377 BCE) and Aristotle (384–322 BCE). The philosophy was based on the belief that the body is composed of earth, wind, fire and water, similar to that of the Indian system. The use of herbal teas and decoctions is still very popular in Europe, e.g., teas prepared from *Humulus lupulus, Rosmarinum officinalis, Hypericum perforum* and *Valeriana officinalis* [9].

African medicine is also the oldest medicines and perhaps the most diverse of all healthcare systems [11]. Traditional African medicine involves both body and mind. Famous African medicinal plants include *Acaccia Senegal* (source of gum Arabic), *Aloe ferox, Aloe Vera, Artemisia Afra, Asplanthus linearis, Boswellia sacra,Catha edulis, Commiphora myrrha, Harpagophytum procumbens, Catharanthus roseus*, etc.

2.6. Modern Prescription Drugs

The remedies provided by traditional medicine systems played a crucial role in developing modern drugs. In traditional medicine system, treatment began with known remedies followed by extraction, isolation and purification of pharmacologically active compounds.

On the contrary modern drug design process begins by examining the root cause of disease, determining its physiological state and then design a molecule to cure the ailment. Nineteenth century witnessed advancement in the field of pharmacology and instrumentation leading to the development of synthetic drugs based on natural products. Scientists identified and purified active extracts from medicinal plants (e.g., isolation of morphine from the opium poppy).

Salicylic acid, a '*lead*' molecule for development of aspirin, was identified in 1839 as an active component in plants known for their pain-relieving qualities and was synthesized in 1853. It is estimated at present 25% of prescriptions are based on plant-derived ingredients and an even greater percentage are based on semi-synthetic or wholly synthetic ingredients originally isolated from plants. 75% to 90% of the rural population of the rest world still rely on herbal medicine as their only health care.

3. Plant Metabolites

Medicinal plants exert their beneficial effects through additive or synergistic activity of several chemical compounds, carried out at single or multiple sites [13]. These compounds are called as biologically active compounds and are found in different organs of plants, like seeds, fruits, herbs etc.

They possess variable composition, property and activities. Biologically active compounds play crucial role in (i) physiological and ecological state of the plant, (ii) in treatment and prevention of diseases. Biologically active components of plants are divided into two groups:

a) Products resulting from primary metabolism
   Primary metabolism is directly related to survival, growth and reproduction of organisms. Primary metabolites are produced during primary processes like photosynthesis. Products obtained from primary metabolism are glucides, lipids, and amino acid derivations.
b) Products resulting from secondary metabolism

Products derived from the precursors produced in primary metabolic processes are called as secondary metabolites. They are important active components, though they do not play a direct role in processes like photosynthesis and other metabolic process but are synthesized to provide defense or adaptation to species. Secondary metabolites are classified into different groups depending on their basic chemical structure and distribution in the plant world.
Primary metabolites are found throughout the plant kingdom, while secondary metabolites are found in related plant species or group of species.

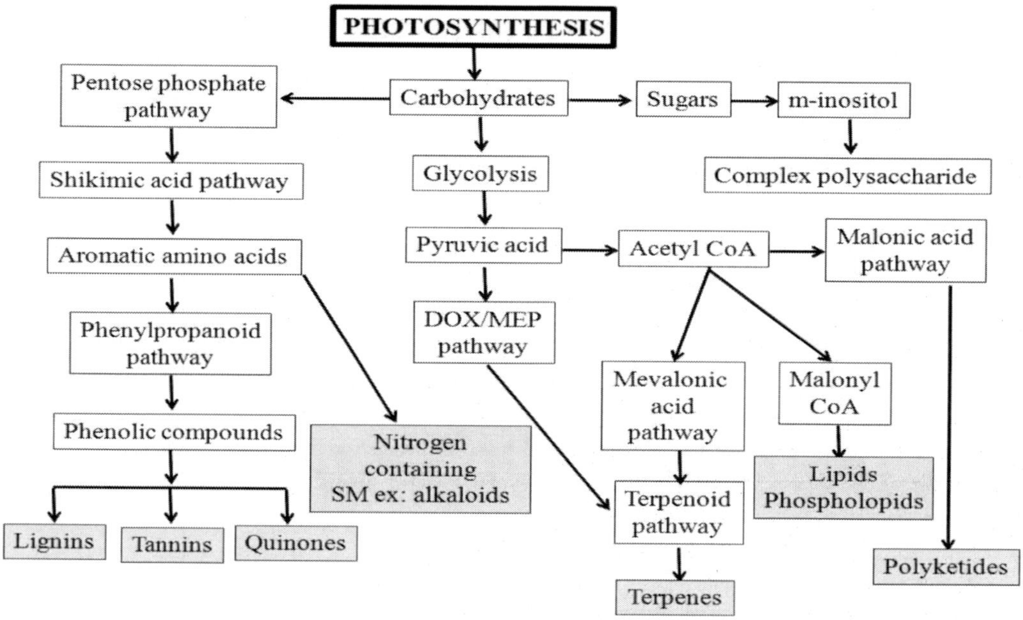

Figure 1. Principal biosynthetic pathways leading to synthesis of secondary metabolites.

3.1. Secondary Metabolites

Secondary metabolites are chemical compounds which are formed during normal metabolic processes in a variety of plants. All plants produce secondary metabolites. They can change or modify the functions of human and animal systems. Being end products of metabolic processes they are observed through color, taste, odor and different chemical properties [2].

Development and quality of secondary metabolites mainly depend on physical environment which includes light, temperature, type of soil etc. A typical feature of secondary metabolites is they are stored in large concentrations, as complex mixtures, in organs of plants which do not even produce them. Both physiological and biochemical properties of secondary metabolites are directly related to its function. More than 100,000 secondary metabolites are known [14]. A list of secondary metabolites is given in Table 2.

4. Classification of Secondary Metabolites

Secondary metabolites are classified into four major groups: heterosides, polyphenols, terpenoids, and alkaloids.

Heterosides: Anthraquinones, cardiac glycosides, cyanogenics, coumarins, phenols, flavonics,

ranunculosides, saponosides, sulphurides.

Polyphenoles: Phenolic acids, cumarins, flavonoids, lignans, tannins, quinones.

Terpenoids: Essential oils, iridoids, lactones, diterpones, saponins.

Alkaloids

Table 2. Numbers of secondary metabolites reported from higher plants by M. Wink [14]

Type of secondary metabolite	Approximate numbers*
Nitrogen-containing secondary metabolites	
Alkaloids	21000
Non-protein amino acids (NPAAs)	700
Amines	100
Cyanogenic glycosides	60
Glucosinolates	100
Alkamides	150
Lectins, peptides, polypeptides	2000
Secondary metabolites without nitrogen	
Monoterpenes including iridoids (C10)**	2500
Sesquiterpenes (C15)**	5000
Diterpenes (C20)**	2500
Triterpenes, steroids, saponins (C30, C27)**	5000
Tetraterpenes (C40)**	500
Flavonoids, tannins	5000
Phenylpropanoids, lignin, coumarins, lignans	2000
Polyacetylenes, fattyacids, waxes	1500
Anthraquinones and other polyketides	750
Carbohydrates, organic acids	200

*The approximate number of known structures; **total number of terepenoids exceeds 22000 at present.

4.1. Heterosides

Heterosides or glycosides have a divergent metabolic origin; as a result they possess different chemical structures and show different physiological effect. They are produced by the condensation of two components: one is of the sugar moiety (e.g., glucose) and the other is of non sugar moiety also known as active component (called aglycones or aglucones). The bond between the two components involves a hydroxyl group, thereby resulting in O-glycoside, C-glycosides, N-glycoside or S-glycoside. The non-sugar or active component is essentially responsible for the pharmacological activity as well as categorization.

4.1.1. Anthraquinones Heterosides

Anthraquinones also known as anthracenedione or dioxoanthracene are yellow crystalline powder with molecular formula $C_{14}H_8O_2$ (figure 2).

They are insoluble in the water. The non-sugar part consists of two or more phenols linked by a quinine ring. Most abundant anthraquinones are O-glycosides or C-glycosides. They are primarily used in the manufacturing of dyes. They have shown considerable therapeutic property thereby used as laxatives and purgatives.

Table 3. Classification of Glycosides

Type	Properties	Species
Anthraquinones	Purgatives	Holy peel, Sen
Cardiac glycoside	Diuretic, Heart tonic	Digital
Cyanogenics	Anaesthetics, Antispasmodic, Hypo-tenser	Cherry tree, Almond tree
Coumarine	Antibacterial, Anticoagulant, Protection from the sun.	Oats
Phenol	Antipyretic and febrifugues	Pear tree, willow
Flavonoids	Weak capillaries, Vitamin C	Sunflower, rude
Ranunculosides	Irritation of the skin	Berry plants
Saponins	Hemolytic anemia. Emolients. Dermatitis	Fir tree, Maize, Liquorice, Saponaria, Violet
Sulphurates	Antibiotics	Garlic, Onion, Radish

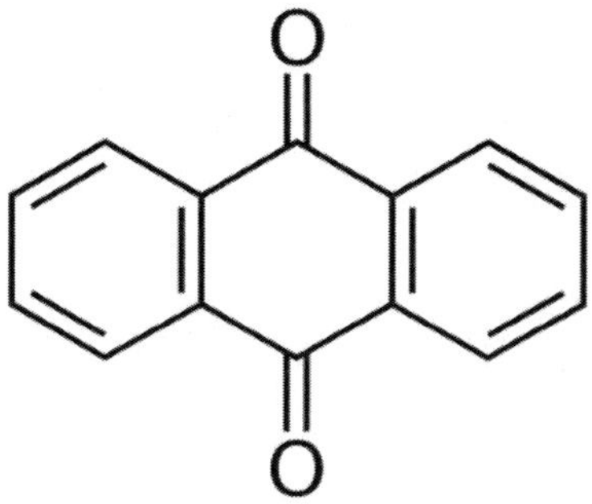

Figure 2. Structure of Anthraquinone.

Anthraquinones are found in following plants:

- Aloes (aloe juice, especially liliacs)
- Rhubarb (rhizomes from Rheum especially F. Polygonaciae)
- Senna (leaves and pods of Cassia, especially F. Caesalpinaceae leguminous plants)

- Buckthorns (bark of the Rhamnus catharticus and R. Frangula. F. Rhamnaceae)
- Cascara sagrada (bark of the Rhamnus Pursiana. F. Rhamnaceae)

4.1.2. Cardiac Glycosides

Cardioactive glycosides contain a steroid molecule as active component. Active group in cardioactive glycosides influences the contraction of heart muscles and thus exert a therapeutic effect on congestive cardiac insufficiency, if given in proper doses. They are strong neurotoxins as they cause death through cardiac and respiratory arrest. Cardiac heterosides are also known as *digoxin*, which is a derivative of glycosides in *Digitalis purpurea* and *D. Ianata.* Cardioactive glycosides are found in following plants:

- Digitalis purpurea and D.lanata (F. Scrophulariaceae).
- Adonis vernalis (F. Ranunculae).
- Urginea maritima (F. Liliaceae).
- Nerium oleander (F. Apocynaceae).
- Strophanthus (F. Apocynaceae). Its
- Digital: Dried leaf of Digitalis purpurea
- Strophant: seeds of two different types of the species, Strophantus gratus and Strophantus kombe (Apocinaceae).
- Escila: Dried scales of bulbs of Urginea maritime or Scilla maritime.

4.1.3. Cyanogenic Heterosides

Cyanogenic heterosides release cyanide (HCN) when it is broken. The most abundant cyanogenic glycosides are amygdalin and prunasin. Amygdalin is found in seeds, pits, bark of members of the rose family and pits of apricots. Prunasin is found in wild cherry laurel (*Prunus serotina*). They are used in controversial cancer treatment; HCN is released in the presence of tumor cells and selectively destroys them. If a wound caused by pathogens or herbivore decompose tissues, then β-glucosidase comes in contact with cyanogenic glucosides. As a result they are split into sugar and nitrile components which are further hydrolyzed to hydrocyanic acid (HCN) and aldehyde. Cyanogenic heterosides causes lethal poisoning in most animals because HCN binds to cytochrome oxidase and effectively blocks mitochondrial respiration as a result adenosine triphosphate (ATP) is blocked [15]. It is also used as an antispasmodic, to stimulate breathing, as distilled water and as an aromatic.

Cyanogenic heterosides are found in more than 2000 plant species. Few plants are listed below:

- Rosaceae.
- Fabaceae (leguminous plants)
- Caprifoliaceae
- Linaceae
- Lamiaceae
- Passifloraceae
- Sapindaceae
- Juncaginaceae

- Ranunculaceae
- Euforbiaceae.
- Poaceae less common gramineae.

Organs include:

- Roots: manioc (Manihot utilissimo,) belonging to Euforbiaceae, gives starch and tapioca.
- Bark: the wild cherry laurel.
- Leaves: elder (Sambucus nigra).
- Seeds: bitter almonds (Prunus dulcis) and the kernel of apricot, peaches and plums.

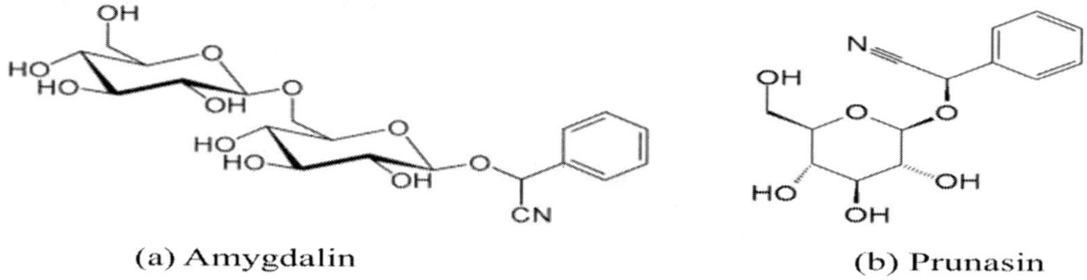

Figure 3. Structure of Cyanogenic Heterosides (a) Amygdalin, (b) Prunasin.

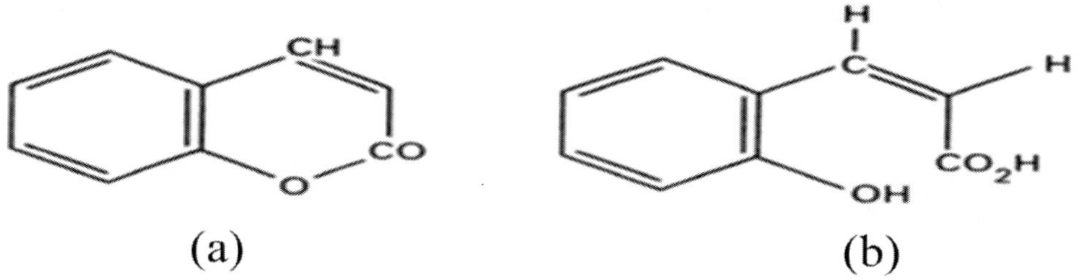

Figure 4. Structure of (a) Coumarin, (b) Coumarinic acid.

4.1.4. Coumarinic Heterosides

Coumarinic is a colorless crystalline substance whose lactone is coumarin. Coumarin is an anticoagulant as well aromatic. It is widely used in: (i) medicine because of anticoagulant property, (ii) flavoring of food due to aromaticity. Some coumarins have sedative as well as hypnotic properties such as angelican. They are often used to treat kidneys and bladder because of their diuretic, anti-rheumatic and anti-arthritic properties. Coumarinic heterosides also protect from capillary weakness and act as a tonic for veins.

Coumarinic heteroside is found in many plants, example:

- Bark of Indian chestnut
- Ash leaves Fraxinus excelsior (Fraxina)
- *Tonka bean* (Dipteryx odorata
- Vanilla grass *(Anthoxanthum odoratum)*

- *Sweet woodruff* (Galium odoratum)
- *Mullein* (Verbascum spp.)
- *Sweet grass* (Hierochloe odorata)
- *Cassia cinnamon* (Cinnamomum aromaticum)
- *Melilot/sweet clover* (Melilotus ssp.)
- Deer's tongue (*Panicum clandestinum*)

4.1.5. Ranunculosides

Ranunculosides are known as volatile lactones. On hydrolysis they split up into ranunculine and glucose. Ranunculine is further converted into an unsaturated lactone: protoanemonine, which is toxic but its derivatives are non toxic. These are used as poultices, liniments, and ointments etc. as remedies for neuralgia, sciatica, arthritic joint pain and similar problems.

Apart from the beneficial aspect they are also recognized as dangerous neurotoxins producing tingling, numbness on contact with skin and irritation on contact with mucous membranes. Plants containing ranunculosides are:

- Chrishmas rose (*Helleborus niger*)
- Marsh marigold (*Calatha palustris*)
- Clematis (*Clematis recta*)
- Wood anemone (*Anemone nemorosa*)
- Hepatica (*Hepatica nobilis*)
- Field buttercup (*Ranunculus acris*)
- Globe flower (*Trollius europaeus,*)
- Pasque flower (*Pulsatilla vulgaris*)

4.1.6. Saponosides

Saponosides, is a Latin word where '*sapo'* means soap. Saponins are glycosides of both triterpenes and steroids, characterized by their bitter or astringent taste, foaming property, haemolytic effect on red blood cells and cholesterol binding properties [15]. Saponins possess both beneficial (lowering cholesterol) and deleterious (highly toxic when injected into the blood and permeabilization of intestinal epithelium) properties. Their toxicity is less when taken orally. In medicine, it is used to some extent as an expectorant and an emulsifying agent [16].

Steroid saponins are typically found in monocots, especially for *Dioscoreaceae, Liliaceae, Agavaceae, Asparagaceae, Poaceae, Smilacaceae etc.* Triterpene saponins are found in *Caryophyllaceae, Styracaceae, Rosaceae, Sapotaceae, Cucurbitaceae, Araliaceae, Polygalacdeae etc.* They are absent in gymnosperms. Saponins are also stored as *bidesmosidic c*ompounds in the vacuole, which are cleaved to active monodesmosidic compounds by β-glucosidase on wounding-induced decompartmentation. *Monodesmosidic* saponins are amphiphilic compounds which bind to glycolipids and glycoproteins with their sugar side chain thereby leads to severe tension in biomembrane and leakage. Some saponins have additional functional groups, such as cardiac glycosides, which inhibits Na^+-, K^- -ATPase resulting in inhibition of transport activities of cell as well as neuron signaling.

Cucurbitacis, steroidal glycoside is highly cytotoxic as it interferes spindle formation during mitosis [14].

Saponsides are found in following plants:

- Seed of the Indian chestnut
- Liquorice *(Glycyrrhiza glabra)*
- Asian centella (*Centella asiatica*)
- Ginseng (*Panax ginseng*)
- Ruscus (*Ruscus aculeatus*)
- Agave *(Agave sisalana)*
- Dioscorea (*Dioscorea).*

4.1.7. Glucosinolates

Glucosinolates function as prefabricated vacuolar defense compounds. It exhibits antimicrobial effect; being a precursor for mustard oil. Mustard oil disrupts the fluidity of biomembranes and bind to various enzymes, receptors or macromolecules (DNA). They are found prominently in seeds, leaves and roots of Brassicales.

4.2. Polyphenols

Polyphenols are aromatic compounds, characterized by the presence of hydroxyl (OH) group attached to an aromatic ring. Polyphenols usually combine with sugars to form heterosides. Polyphenols possess antioxidant characteristic.

They tackle problems caused by oxidative stress to the walls of arteries, creates heart-healthy environment by reducing the oxidation of LDL cholesterol. It also relieves chronic pain, as seen in rheumatoid arthritis, due to their anti-inflammatory properties. Polyphenols are also used in the prevention of cardiovascular diseases, cancers, and osteoporosis and plays a vital role in the prevention of neurodegenerative diseases and diabetes mellitus [17]. Polyphenols interferes with the development of malignant tumors and play a role in inactivating carcinogens and inhibiting the expression of mutagens [18, 19]. The health effects of polyphenols depend on the amount consumed and on their bioavailability. Phenols also exhibit potential toxicity to the growth and development of pathogens [18]. Polyphenols are further categorized into different components ranging from very simple compound to very complex ones. Different categories of phenol are phenolic acids or phenols, cumarines, flavonoids, lignanes, tannins and quinines.

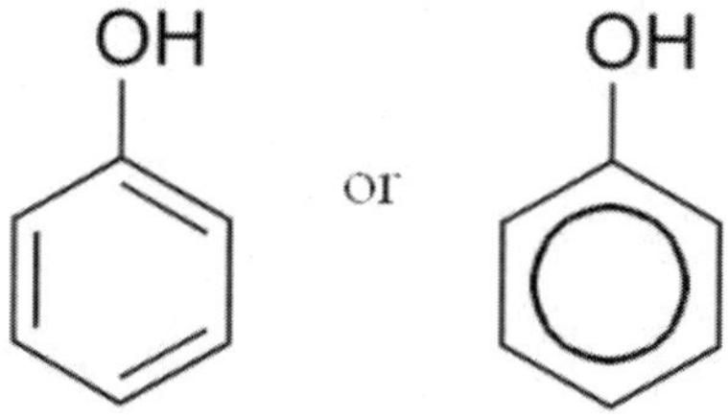

Figure 5. Phenol.

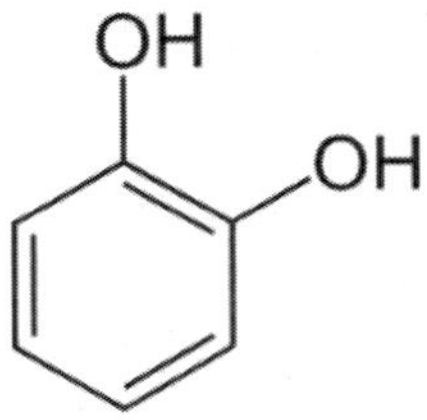

Figure 6. Catechol.

4.2.1. Phenolics

Simple phenolics have at least one hydroxyl group attached to an aromatic ring, e.g., catechol (Figure 6).

In phenolic compounds C6C1 carbon skeleton, usually containing the carbonyl group, is attached to the aromatic ring [20].

Phenolics occur in plants as:

- Soluble compounds, which can be extracted with water (garlic acid esters) or with methanol and aqueous acetone (proanthocyanidins, flavonols, flavonolglycosides)
- Non-extractable compounds.

Phenolic compounds are mostly synthesized via the shikimate pathway (Figure 7) and polyketide pathway. The shikimate pathway starts with phosphoenol pyruvate and erythrose-4-phosphate and terminates with the formation of chorismate [1, 21]. Chorismate act as a substrate for all subsequent products (Figure 7) [22] which further produce a variety of phenolic compounds e.g., phenylalanine is a common precursor for C6C3 and C6C3C6 compounds, and their polymers such as tannins and lignins [23].

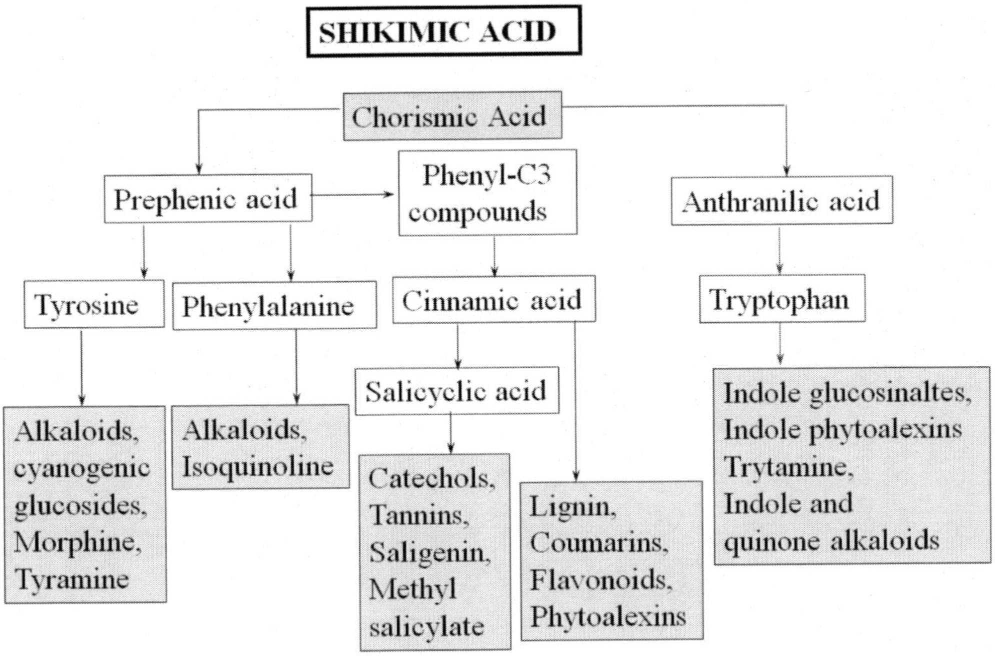

Figure 7. Biosynthesis of diverse phenolic compounds in shikimic acid pathway [23].

A phenyl group containing three carbon side chains is known as a phenylpropanoid, such as hydroxycoumarins, phenylpropenes. Simple phenylpropanoids are the secondary metabolites derived from phenylalanine e.g., cinnamic acid, *o*-coumaric acid, *p*-coumaric acid, caffeic acid and ferulic acid [24]. The phenylpropenes are important components of many essential oils, e.g., eugenol in clove oil (*Syzygium aromaticum*) and anethole and myristicin in nutmeg (*Myristica fragrans*) [25].

Phenolic compounds have various pharmacological properties like anti-oxidant, analgesics, choleretic. For example, Eugenol is an antiseptic as well local anesthetic used in dentistry.

4.2.2. Cumarines

Cumarines are benzo - α pyrones. It is a large group of phenolic active components which share a chemical structure 2H-1-benzopiran-2-on known as cumarin. Cumarines may range from very simple to complex ones depending upon the chemical nature of the substituent. Practically all cumarins, with the exception of cumarin itself, have a hydroxilic substitute (OH) at number 7, be it free or in combination (methyl, sugars, etc.).

Cumarines are mainly known for their aroma. They are responsible for the typical smell of hay in the dried grass. Cumarin and its derivatives are used for medicinal purposes like warfarin, phenprocoumon in accordance with high-risk individuals. Cumarines are also used as *rodenticides* to control rats, as it causes fatal internal bleeding in rats. Certain derivatives exhibit fluorescence, therefore used as effective dyes in lasers and optical brighteners. Cumarin are also used in sun creams as they enhance melanin production (photodynamic), example essence of bergamot (*Citrus bergamia).*

In plants coumarin is partially glycosidically bound to sugars and is released by cleavage caused due to injury or wilting of the plant. Coumarin is found in following plants:

- *Cumarin*, found in extracts of the melilotus *(Melilotus oficinalis),* which is used to treat venolymphatic insufficiency.
- *Esculoside,* found in Indian chestnuts *(Aesculus hippocastanum).* It is both a tonic for the veins and a protector of the cell wall.
- *Visnadine,* is a dilator of the blood vessels found in the *fruit of the visnaga, Amni visnaga.*
- *Dicumarol* is an anti-coagulant *which forms in melilotuses* when conditions for conservation are bad.
- *Furanocumarins* are photosensitizing and are used to treat psoriasis.

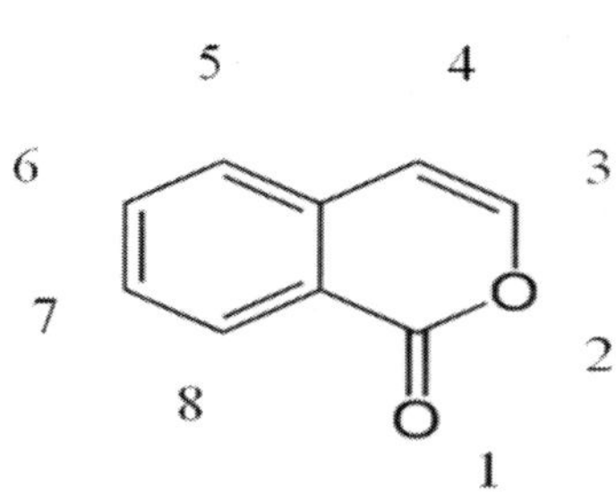

Figure 8. Couramin structure.

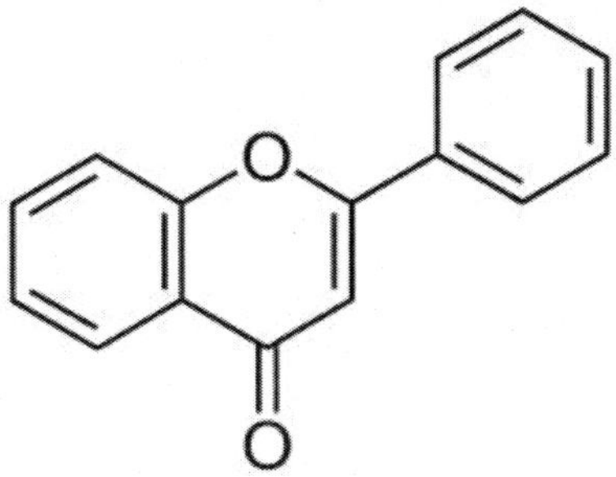

Figure 9. Structure of Flavone ($C_{15}H_{10}O_2$).

4.2.3. Flavonoids

Falvonoids are 15-carbon compounds present in majority of plants as yellow pigment. Its molecular structure is C6-C3-C6.

Flavonoids are responsible for the color of flowers, leaves, fruits etc. They are water soluble, good anti-oxidants and protect plants from microbes as well as UV radiation. Falvonoids are secreted by plants in response to microbial infection and have been found *in vitro* to be effective against a wide array of microorganisms [16]. Flavonoids are categorized into: flavones, flavonols, flavones and their correspondent heterosides / anthocyanosides. Anthocyanosides are the red and blue pigments in flowers, having special characteristics and are highly soluble in water. Example: cranberry *Vaccinium mirtyllus* (Ericaceas) and blackcurrant *Ribes nigrum* (Saxifragaceas). Flavones exhibits fitoestrogenic properties and are used to treat menopausal symptoms (e.g., soya). Flavonoids prevent oxidative cell damage by trapping free radicals. They are often used to treat cancers because they inhibit the initiation of cancer/ tumors and suppress its promotion as well as progression. Flavonoids in the body are known to reduce the risk of heart diseases [18, 26]. They are found to be important dietary cancer chemo-protective agents [27, 28]. Plants whose activity are similar to that of flavonoid are:

- Passion flower (Passiflora incarnate)
- Roman camomile (Chamaemelum glabra)
- Aquilea (Achillea millefolium)
- Liquorice (Glycyrrhiza glabra)
- Ginkgo (Ginkgo biloba)
- Marian thistle (Sylibum marianum)
- White thorn (Crataegus).

4.2.4. Lignanes

Lignanes are polyphenolic compounds which are formed by dimerization of two units of phenile propane (C6-C3). Dimerization takes place in the presence of oxidative enzymes and is controlled by proteins which dictate the stereochemistry of newly synthesized compounds i.e., *dirigent* proteins.

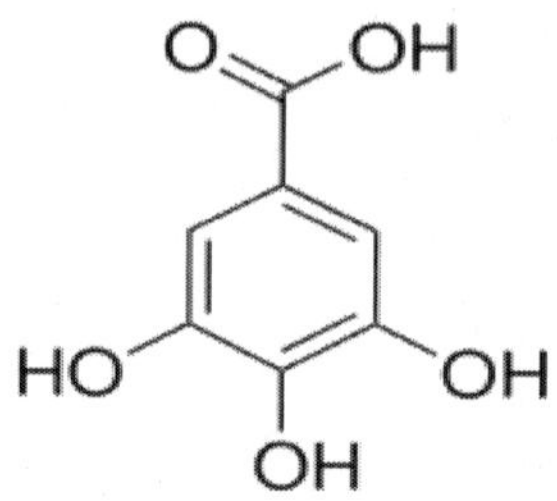

Figure 10. Structure of Tannin.

Lignans bind to estrogen receptor, thereby preventing estrogen to cause cancer in breast tissues. They are also found to be super anti-oxidants and free radical scavengers. Lignans are most commonly found in flax and sesame seeds, cereals, soybeans and vegetables like cabbage and broccoli.

4.2.5. Tannins

Tannins are non-nitrogenous polymeric/ phenolic substance. Molecular weight of tannins lies between 500-3000. They are water soluble and can be condensed easily.

Tannins are classified into two groups:

- Hydrolyzable tannins
  Hydrolyzed or hydrolyzable tannins are formed by multiple esterification of D-glucose.
- Condensed tannins
  Condensed tannins are made up of flavonoid monomers. They are also known as proanthocyanides.

Tannins stimulate phagocytic cells, host mediated tumor activity and possess a wide range of anti-infective action [29]. Properties of tannins are:

- Astringent
- Precipitate gelatine, alkaloid salts, heavy metals from solutions
- Tanning leather (capable of forming hydrogen bonds with fibres of collagen)
- Treat hemorrhages (constriction of blood vessels), burns, ulcers, frostbites
- Antibacterial
- Antiseptic
- Anti-diarrhea
- Antidote to intoxication
- Unpleasant taste

Tannins are most commonly found in roots, leaves and barks of some plants like:

- Ericaciae
- Rosaceae
- Salicaceae
- Legume

4.2.6. Quinones

Quinones are aromatic compounds that are formed by the oxidization of phenols. Quinones are natural pigments having color from pale yellow to almost black. Quinones act as intermediate in the melanin production pathway in humans. On cutting fruits or vegetables become brown in color due to the presence of quinines. Quinones exhibits pharmacological properties like antimicrobial, antidepressant, antiviral, antifungal, antibiotic and are also used as laxatives and purgatives. There are more than 450 types of quinines [16]. Each type has different properties and characteristics. Different types of quinines along with their pharmacological activities are listed in table 4.

5. Terpenoids

Terpenes are hydrocarbon based natural products found in plants. They are made up of repeating units of isoprene (C5) (Figure 11). Terpenes are essential oils and posses various pharmacological properties. Depending upon the number of isoprene units they are further classified as monoterpenes, sesquiterpenes, diterpenes, treterpenes, carptenes, polyterpenes. Mono-, sesqui-, di-, triterpenes are highly hydrophobic compounds and are usually found in resin ducts, oil cells and glandular trichomes of plants [14]. They readily react with membrane proteins; however, this reactivity is membrane specific.

Table 4. Types of quinines and their activity

Name	Class	Activity
Anthraquinones	Anthracene derivative	Laxative or purgatives
Anthracicflaxnes	Naphtacene derivative	Antibiotic
Napthaquinones	Napthalene derivative	Anti-bacterial and anti-fungal
Para-benzoquinone	Benzene derivative	Anti-microbial and antifungal

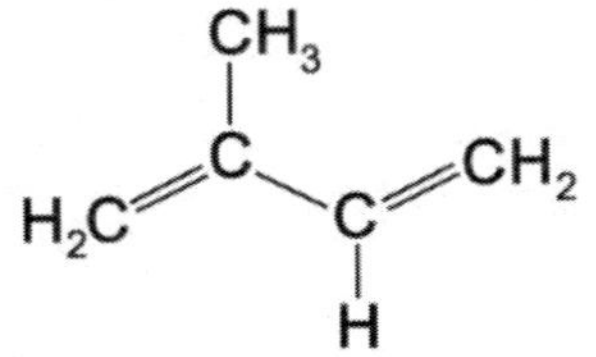

Figure 11. Structure of Isoprene; basic structural unit of terpenes.

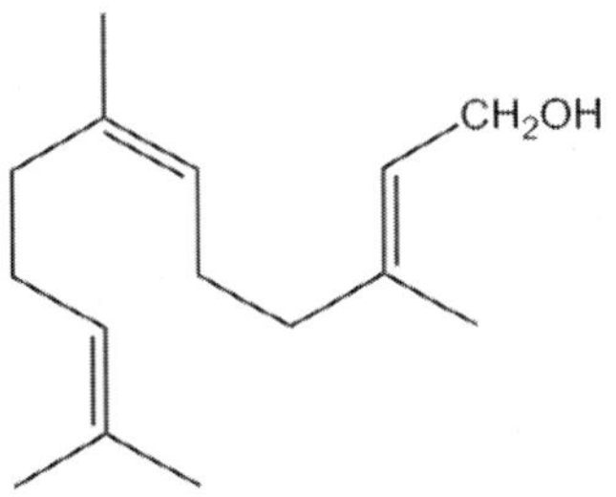

Figure 12. Structure of Farnesol.

They increase the fluidity of membranes, which causes uncontrolled efflux of ions and metabolites, cell leakage thereby causing cell death. Terpenes are cytotoxic against variety of organisms.

- ***Monoterpenes***
  Monoterpenes contains two units of isoprene (C10). It exists as cyclic as well as acyclic compound. Monoterpenes are major components of various essential oils. Its major characteristics are strong odor therefore monterpenes are mostly used in perfumes and fragrances. Examples are camphor, menthol, myrcene, linalool etc.
- ***Sesquiterpenes***
  Sesquiterpenes contains three units of isoprene (C15). It exists in aliphatic bicyclic and tricyclic framework. Sesquiterpenes lactones are pharmacologically active, they binds to protein with –SH group. Sesquiterpenes and its derivatives have shown anti-malarial activity (ex. *Arteether derived from artemisinin*). Farnesol, a sesquiterpenes, plays important role in terpenoid biosynthesis. Sesquiterpenes and its lactones are common in *Asteraceae, ferns, Lauraceae, Apiaceae.*
- ***Diterpenes***
  Diterpenes contains four units of isoprene (C20). Like other types of terpenes they are not considered as oils. They have a high boiling point and are found as components of plant resin. Several diterpenes are toxic in nature. Example:
  - Phorbol ester common in *Euphorbiaceae* and *Thymelaeaceae*. It causes severe inflammation by activating protein kinase C
  - Andromedotoxin common in *Ericaceae* is strong neurotoxic as it inhibits sodium channels
- ***Triterpenes***
  Triterpenes contains six units of isoprene (C30). They are colorless, optically active and crystalline compounds having very high melting points. They occur in plants as a component of resins, cork and waxy coating of leaves. They are often used for repelling insects and microbial attacks in plants (Azadirachtin from seeds of *Azadirachta indica*). Another application of triterpenes is as potent insect steroid hormone antagonist (Limonins and Cucurbitacins). Important triterpenes are Saponins, steroids and cardiac glycosides. Steroids are modified triterpenes and have importance as of hormones, coenzymes and provitamins.
- ***Other terpenes***
  Carotenes contain eight units of isoprene (C40). Terpenes containing multiple units or higher number of isoprene units are termed as polyterpenes (Cn units).

Terpenes have shown additional characteristics because they posses structure similarity to variety of hormones and neurotransmitters [13, 14, 22].

5.1. Essential Oils

Essential oils are made up of a mixture of terpenes and terpene derivatives, mostly monoterpenes and sesquiterpenes. They are volatile in nature and evaporate even at room temperature leaving behind a strong odor, due to the combined effect of all constituents present in it. They are insoluble in water and usually extracted by steam distillation process, expression, or solvent extraction from plants. Oils are present in specialized cells/glands or organelles of plants which may be present anywhere depending upon the morphology and physiology of the plant. Sometime it may be on leaves, flowers, stems, roots, bark or wood. A strong aroma or smell is released when these glands are pressed, rubbed or ruptured. List of essential oils found in India are listed in table 5. *The parts of plants yielding essential oils:*

Flowers: Jasmine, Rose, Violet, Hyacinth etc.
Leaves: Lavender, Rosemary, Eucalyptus, peppermint etc.
Fruits: Lemon, Oranges, Bergamot, Bursera etc.
Barks: Cinnamon, Casia, Camella etc.
Stem: Citronella, Geranium, Patchouli etc.
Wood: Sandal, Cedar, Bursera.
Rhizome: Ginger, Calamus.
Roots: Vetiver

Essential oils are used in perfumery, aromatherapy, cosmetics, incense, medicine, household insect repellent cleaning products, and for flavouring food and drink [30]. *Uses of essential oils:*

- *Medicinal use:* Oils may be used directly either in isolation or in formulations. Formulations may contain single or a mixture of oils. Oils have been used as anti-microbial, analgesic, antiseptic, anti-inflammatory, astringent, sedative, antispasmodic, expectorant, diuretic, stress and brain relaxant, inhalants and for bathing/ massage purposes.
- *Cosmetic use:* Oils have been used for facial and hair care purposes for decades.
  - *Skin care:* As skin creams, face packs, gels, astringents, scrub etc. Examples: jasmine, lavender, lemon, rose, etc.
  - *Hair care:* Treat dandruff, hair loss in form of tonics, shampoos, oils, conditioners etc. Examples: Basil, eucalyptus, lavender, lemon, mints etc.

Table 5. Essential Oils in India [30]

S.No.	Common Name	Botanical Name	Constituents
1	Ajowan oil	*Trachyspermum ammi*	Thymol, carvacrol. ρ-cymene
2	Basil oil	*Ocimum sanctum, O. basilicum* *O kilmanandaschricum*	Eugenol, linalool methyl chavicol camphor, 1,8-cineole
3	Champor oil	*Cinnamomum camphora*	Camphor
4	Carway oil	*Carum carvi*	Carvone ,limonene
5	Cardamomum oil	*Elettaria cardamomum*	1,8-cineole, Terpenyl acetate,
6	Celery seed oil	*Apium graveolens*	Limonene

Table 5. (Continued)

S.No.	Common Name	Botanical Name	Constituents
7	Chamomil oil (German)	*Matricaria chamomila*	Azzulenes
8	Cinnomomum oil	*Cinnomomum zeylanicum*	Cinnamaldehyde
9	Citronella oil	*Cymbopogan winteranius*	Citronellol, citronellal, Geraniol
10	Clary sage oil	*Salvia sclarea*	Linolool, linalyl acetate
11	Corriender oil	*Corindrum sativum*	Linolool, linalyl acetate
12	Clove oil	*Syzygium aromaticum*	Eugenol
13	Eucalyptus oil	*Eucalyptus globulus* *Eucalyptus citriodora*	1,8-cneole Citronellol. citronellal
14	Geranium oil	*Pelargonium graveolens*	Geraniol. citronellol
15	Ginger oil	*Zingiber officinale*	Sesquiterpenes
16	Haldi leaves	*Curcuma longa*	Terpinoline,virdifloral
17	Lavender oil	*Lavendula offecinalis*	Linolool, linalyl acetate
18	Lemongrass oil	*Cymbopogan flexiosus*	Citral a, citral b
19	Mint oils	*Mentha arvensis, Mentha piperita* *Mentha spicata, Mentha cardica* *Mentha citrata*	Menthol, menthone, menthyl acetate, carvone, Linalool ,linalyl acetate
20	Patchauli oil	*Ppogestemone patachauli*	Patachauli alcohol
21	Palmarosa oil	*Cymbopogan martini*	Geraniol, geranyl acetate
22	Rose oil	*Rosa damecena*	Citronellol, Geraniol, nerol
23	Rosemary	*Rosmarinus officinalis*	1,8-cineole

5.2. Iridoids

Iridoids represents a large group of cyclopenta[c]pyran monoterpenoids. Iridiods are widespread in nature. The basic structure of iridoids has a cyclopentane ring fused with oxygen containing heterocyclic ring. They are mainly found in dicotyledonous plant families like *Apocynaceae, Scrophulariaceae, Diervillaceae, Lamiaceae, Loganiaceae and Rubiaceae.*

Iridoids exhibit a wide range of bioactivity, such as neuroprotective, antinflammatory and immunomodulator, hepatoprotective and cardioprotective effects. Iridoids have also shown anticancer, antioxidant, antimicrobial, hypoglycemic, hypolipidemic, choleretic, antispasmodic and purgative properties. [31]

5.3. Lactones

Lactones are cyclic esters of hydroxy carboxylic acids, containing a 1-oxacycloalkan-2-one structure. Sesquiterpene lactones are found in large and diverse group of *biologically active* plant. Most abundantly they are found in the *Composite, Lauraceae* and *Magnoliaceae* families. *Composite* family solely contains 3000 different structures. Sesquiterpene lactones are responsible for the toxicity of several livestock poisons. It is also present as one of the constituents of natural products used in the flavors and fragrance industry. Lactones are bitter in taste and exhibit antioxidant, antimicrobial, anticancer, antifungal activity.

Table 6. Common essential oils and their Therapeutic properties [30]

S. No.	Therapeutic properties	Oils	Botanical name
1.	Sedatives	Sandal wood, Lavender, Bergamot, Chamomile, Sweet marjoram	*Santalum album, Lavandula officinalis, Cirus bergamia, Matricaria chamomilla Majorana hortensis*
2.	CNS stimulant	Basil, Clove, Jasmine, Peppermint, Ylang Ylang, Chamomile, Achillea, Cajuput	*Ocimum basilicum, Syzgium aromaticum Jasminum officnale, Mentha piperita Cananga odorata, Matricaria chamomilla, Achillea millefolium Melaeeuca leucadendron*
3.	Adaptogen	Geranium, Ylang Ylang	*Pelargonium graveolens Cananga odorata*
4.	Bronchitis	Eucalyptus, Angelica, Ginger, Black pepper, Pumilio pine	*Eucalyptus globules, Angelica archangelica, Zingiber officinale Piper nigrum, Pinus mugo*
5.	Antiseptic	Geranium, Sandal wood, Thyme	*Pelargonium graveolens, Santalum album, Thymus vulgaris*
6.	Antistress	Cedarwood, Borneol, Lemon, Patchouli	*Cedrus deodara, Drybalanops aromatica Citrus lemon, Pogestmone patchouli*
7.	Muscle relaxant	All spice	*Pimento dioica*
8.	Carminative	Dill, Spearmint, Peppermint, Chamomile, Ajowan, Caraway, Fennel, Thyme	*Anethum graveolens, Mentha spicata, Mentha piperita, Matricaria chamomilla Trachyspermum ammi, Carum carvi Foeniculum vulgare, Thymus vulgaris*
9.	Haemostatic	Achillea	*Achillea millefolium*
10.	Antispasmodic	Clove, Thyme	*Syzgium aromaticum, Thymus vulgaris*
11.	Analgesic	Clove	*Syzgium aromaticum*
12.	Prostaglandin inhibitor	Nutmeg	*Myristica fragrans*

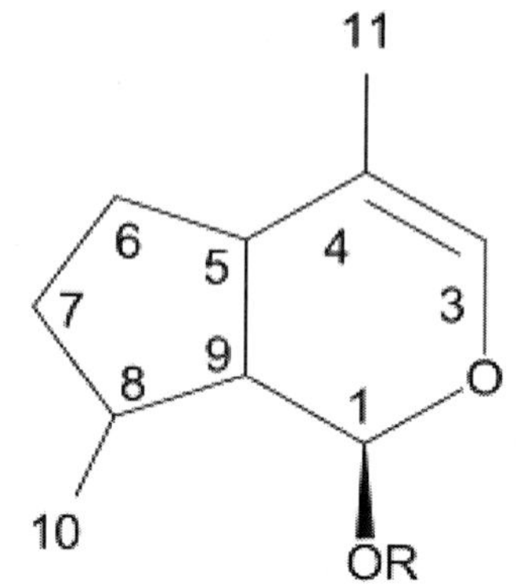

Figure 13. Basic structure of Iridiods.

5.4. Saponins

Saponins are glycosides of triterpenes and steroids. The name saponin is derived from the Latin word "*sapo*" meaning soap. Saponins produces foam in water and are bitter in taste. Steroid saponins are found in monocots especially *Dioscoreaceae, Melanthiaceae, Agavaceae, Ruscaceae, Liliaceae, Poaceae, Zingiberaceae, Alliaceae, Smilacaceae*. They are less found in dicots. Triterpene saponins are present in large amount in *Caryophyllaceae, Ranunculaceae, Styracaceae, Primulaceae, Theaceae, Apiaceae, Aquifoliaceae, Sapotaceae, Chenopodiaceae* and *Hippocastanaceaae*. Triterpene saponins are absent in gymnosperms. Monodesmosidic saponins are amphiphilic in nature. They can complex cholesterol in biomembranes with their lipophilic terpenoid moiety and bind to the surface of glycoproteins and glycolipids with their sugar side chain. This leads to severe tension of the biomembrane and leakage. Saponins are used as anti-infecting agents [14]. Saponins are naturally tenso-active and possess both beneficial (lowers cholesterol) and deleterious (cytotoxic and permeabilize intestinal epithelium) characteristics. They are less toxic when taken orally but highly toxic when injected into the blood [15, 16].

6. Alkaloids

Alkaloids are a huge and diverse group of low molecular weight nitrogen-containing compounds. These are usually colorless, bitter in taste; often optically active substances which are mostly are crystalline at room temperature with very few exceptions. These are generally secondary metabolites which are secreted by plants, microbes or animals. These are the largest class of plant secondary metabolites which contain one or more Nitrogen atom. This nitrogen is usually present as a part of a heterocyclic structure [16] which provides a basic nature to the compound. Due to its 'alkali like' nature, the term *Alkaloid* was coined by W. Meibner, a German pharmacist. Morphine, was first alkaloid to be isolated from the latex of opium poppy, by F.W. Serturner in 1806. Its structure was confirmed 1952 [32]. In 1886, Ladenburg synthesized the first alkaloid quinine.

In plants, alkaloids are generally present as salts of organic acids like oxalic acid, acetic acid, citric acid, malic acid, tartaric acid, lactic acid etc. Some weak alkaloids like nicotine is present freely in nature. Some 12,000 different types of alkaloids are known to be present in about 150 families. Some important families are Papaveraceae, Apocynaceae, Solanaceae, Fabaceae, Ranunculaceae, etc. and some fungi (ergot alkaloids). Few alkaloids also occur as glycosides of sugar like alkaloids of the solanum group (solanine), as amides (piperine), and as esters (atropine, cocaine) of organic acids [24]. Alkaloids may be present throughout the plant, or may be localized in specific parts like roots (belladonna, aconite), stem bark (pomegranate, cinchona) and seeds (*Areca*, nux vomica). The occurrence of alkaloids is more in dicots when compared to the monocots.

Alkaloids are light and heat sensitive. They can be stabilized using inorganic acids. They are usually insoluble in extraction solvents due to their polarity. They undergo racemisation (atropine and hiosciamin) and isomerisation (lysergic and isolysergic acid).Alkaloid production is a characteristic of almost all plants. Most of the alkaloids have a potential to show pharmacological effects. Isolated and purified plant alkaloids or their synthetic derivatives are used as medicinal agents as they show bactericidal, antispasmodic and analgesic effects [33]. Their most prominent physiological and/or psychological actions can be seen on the nervous system [15, 16] due these physiological activities they are widely used in drug development. The main difference between an alkaloid acting like a medicine or showing a toxic effect is mostly the matter of dosage. Many exhibits marked physiological activity when administered to animals [29].

According to Pelletier [34] "an alkaloid is a cyclic organic compound containing nitrogen in a negative oxidation state which is of limited distribution among living organisms". Earlier term alkaloid was implied to pharmacologically active compounds mostly bases, derived from plants, but now the definition has been widened and now it contains the majority of nitrogen containing compounds with exception of proteins, amino acids and aminoglycosidic compounds.

However sometimes it is very difficult to differentiate true alkaloids from certain plant bases.

Some plant bases, like methylamine, trimethylamine and other alkyl amines having straight chains, are not considered to be alkaloids. Polyamines like putrescine, spermine, spermidine; phenylalkylamines, dopamine, ephedrine, mescaline and tryptamineare are also not considered as alkaloids. Similarly, purine-based compounds like caffeine, theophilline, theobromine are also not included in the class of alkaloids by some workers, as they are not a derivative of amino acids. A few more compounds like betaines, choline and muscarine are also not kept in the class of alkaloids by some experts. It is so because their nitrogen is not involved in the heterocyclic system thus these compounds are categorized as biological amines as and these are synthesized from amino acids.

Similarly vitamin B1 is not categorized as an alkaloid although it contains heterocyclic nitrogen and shows physiological activity. While neutral compounds like colchicines, having nitrogen as part of amide group are considered as alkaloids owing to their medicinal properties and its localization into the plants. Few more examples of neutral compounds considered as alkaloids are piperine from black pepper, indicine-n-oxide, di-n-oxide trilupine, betaines, trigonelline etc [35].

Alkaloids are of different types, based on the type of molecule from which they are formed.

They can be tropane, quinoleine or isoquinoleine.

a) *Tropane* alkaloids are a class of alkaloids that contain a tropane ring (pyrrolidine and a piperidine ring sharing a common nitrogen atom and 2 carbon atoms) in their chemical structure. Tropane alkaloids occur naturally in many members of the plant family *Solanaceae.*

   Tropane alkaloids can be categorized into two classes i.e., anticholinergics and stimulants.

   An *anticholinergic* alkaloid is a substance which blocks the acetylcholine (neurotransmitter) in the central nervous system and the peripheral nervous system. Anticholinergic checks the parasympathetic nerve impulse conduction by blocking the binding of the acetylcholine to its receptor in nerve cells. A *Stimulant* (sometimes known as *psychostimulants*) alkaloid is a substance which induces temporary improvements in either physical or mental functions or both.

   In nature Tropane does not in the free form. It is found as part of esters in plant species. Most of the tropane based drugs are natural or semi-synthetic esters. Tropane moiety is used in the drugs having antispasmodics, anesthetics, antiemetic and bronchodilators properties. [36]

b) *Quinolines* are a class of alkaloids which have a heterocyclic aromatic organic compound. Quinolines are benzopyridines, which are comprised of a benzene ring which is fused to a pyridine ring. It is a colorless and hygroscopic liquid having a strong odor. It is sparingly soluble in cold water but completely dissolves in hot water and most organic solvents.

   Quinoline has very limited applications, but its derivatives have broader applications. For e.g., quinine, which is found naturally in plants are involved in antibiotic resistance. Quinoline is used in the production of dyes. It is also used as organic solvent for resins.

c) *Isoquinolines* are structural isomers of quinoline. Isoquinoline is the structural backbone in naturally occurring alkaloids including papaverine. It is also colorless hygroscopic liquid at room temperature. It is slightly soluble in water but readily soluble in organic solvents like acetone, diethyl ether, carbon disulphide etc. Isoquinoline derivatives are used in anesthetics, antifungal agents, disinfectant, vasodilators, anti-hypertension agents etc.

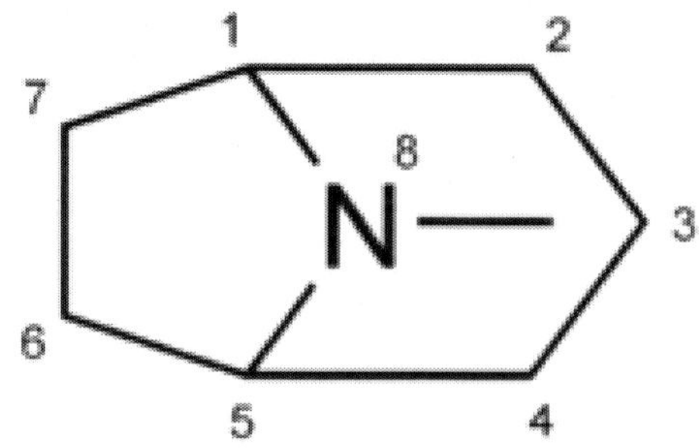

Figure 14. Tropane Nucleus.

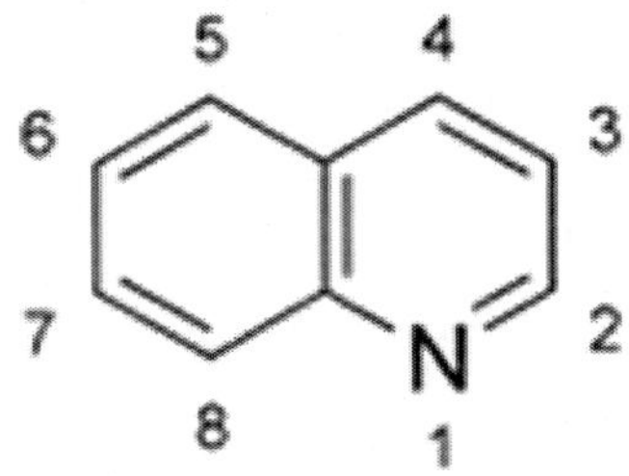

Figure 15. Quinoline derivative.

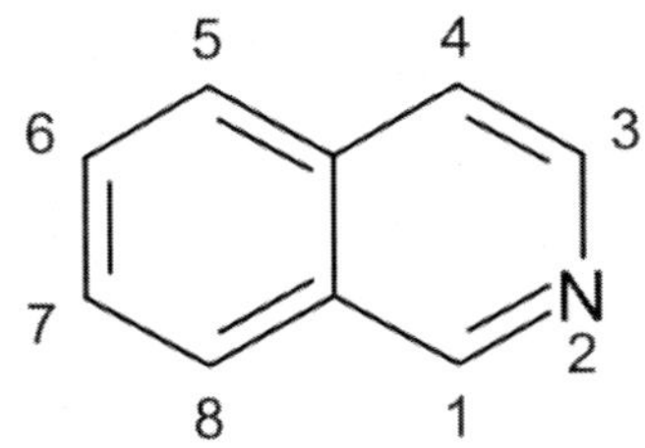

Figure 16. Isoquinoline nucleus.

Table 7. List of few drugs obtained from Alkaloids

Drugs	Plant	Plant part	Function
Tropane			
Cocaine	*Erythroxylum coca*	Leaves	Local anesthetic
Atropine	*Atropa belladonna*	Leaves, flowers	Treat colitis, spastic bladder, diverticulitis, infant colic, renal and biliary colic, peptic ulcer, and irritable bowel. Used in emergencies involving the heart, and to treat certain heart disorders,
Lysergic acid	*Claviceps purpurea* (fungus)	Seeds, Erot fungus	Used in psychedelic drugs (LSD)
Caffeine	Coffee tree	Seed	Improve mental alertness, central nervous system stimulant reduces redness and itching in dermatitis,
Hiosciamin	*Hyoscyamus niger*	Leaves	It is used to treat Parkinson's disease.
Quinoleine (derivatives)			
Quinine	*Cinchona*	Dried bark of the trunks and branches, roots	Anti-malarial
Isoquinoleine			
Opium	*Papaver somniferum*	Dried latex	Analgesic, useful against persistent, acute pains.

7. Non-Protein Amino Acids (NPAA's)

Non-protein amino acids are structural analogues of 20 amino acids. There are about 700 NPAA's out of which 250 are derived from plants [37]. They are produced as intermediates during the synthesis and catabolism of the protein amino acids. Three probable mechanisms of NPAA' formation are:

- Modification of existing amino acid
- Modification of existing pathways
- Development of novel pathways.

NPAAs act by blocking the uptake and transport of amino acids. They often disturb biosynthetic feedback regulation of amino acids. Due to their structural similarity to amino acids, they are not recognized by transfer ribonucleic acid (tRNA) and thus incorporated into proteins during translation process, thereby resulting in defective or malfunctioning protein. Many non-protein amino acids act as defensive agents.

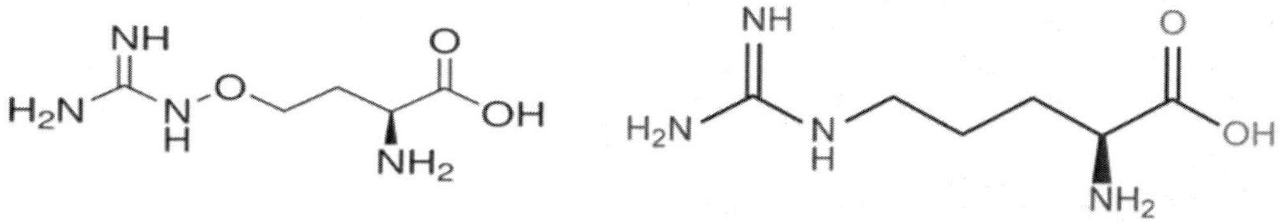

Canavanine Arginine

Figure 17. Structure of Non-protein amino acids.

Examples of NPAA's are L-canavanine and L-canaline (Figure 17) [38, 39].

L-canavanine, the 2-amino-4-(guanidinooxy) butyric acid is structural analog of L-arginine. It accumulates in the seeds of many legumes. It protects plants against predation and also serves as a nitrogen seed storage reserve which can be rapidly mobilized during seed germination.

L-Canaline (L-2-amino-4-(aminooxy) butyric acid) is a structural analog of L-ornithine and acts as lysine antagonist.

NPAA's are found in seeds, leaves roots of legumes (Fabaceae) and in some monocots (Alliaceae, Hyacinthaceae etc.), but also occur in Cucurbitaceae, euphorbiaceaee, Resedaceae, Sapindaceae and Cycadaceae [14].

8. Polyketides

Polyketides are secondary metabolites from bacteria, fungi, plants, and animals. Polyketides are usually biosynthesized through the decarboxylative condensation of malonyl-CoA derived extender units in a similar process to fatty acid synthesis (a Claisen condensation). Polyketides include anthraquinones, hydro- and naphthoquinones.

Polyketides exhibits a vast array of biological and pharmacological activities such as antibacterial, antifungal, anticholesterol, antiparasitic, anticancer, and immunosuppressive properties [40], example anthraquinones:

- Produce severe diarrhea
- Intercalate DNA; mutagenic
- Interfere with adenylyl cyclase

Table 8. Types of polyketides and their occurrence

Type	Occurrence
Anthraquinones	*Polygonaceae, Rhamnaceae, Fabaceae, Asphodelaceae, Hypericaceae, Rubiaceae*
Hydroquinones	*Ericaceae*
Napthoquinones	*Droseraceae, Iridaceae, Bignoniaceae, Juglandaceae, Balsaminaceae*

9. Polyacetylenes

Polyacetylenes are secondary metabolites, made up of repeating units of $(C_2H_2)_n$. Polyacetylene consists of a long chain of carbon atoms joined by alternating single and double bonds. It is a highly reactive compound because of presence alternate bonds. They are activated by light and interact with proteins and membranes. They possess anti-microbial activity and are cyto- and neurotoxic in nature. Polyacetylenes are found in plants like Dahlia, Eclipta, Tagetes, Flaveria, Rudbeckia, Tessaria and Porophyllum [14].

Conclusion

The pharmacological potential of plants has been well recognized by different systems of medicines. Plants are reservoirs of active chemical compounds which are used in various therapies. Some of the most common secondary metabolites are reported in table 9. One fourth of drugs approved by drug regulatory authorities during 1981-2002 was either plant products or based on plant products [41]. Plant based drugs are comparatively cheaper and safe as compared to synthetic drugs. Efforts should be carried out to create biosphere reserves to protect economically and therapeutically valuable species of plants from extinction. More extensive exploratory studies should be carried with an aim to increase valuable information to plant resources of different regions and their properties. There is a need to improve existing technology to speed up the process of isolation of active compounds for evaluation and testing purposes.

Table 9. Selected secondary metabolites of medicinal and aromatic plants [13]

Class	Characteristics	Use	Action
Alkaloids	Bitter taste, colorless, Nitrogen containing bases, crystalline or liquid at room temperature	Raw material for the synthesis of useful drugs	Analgesic, antispasmodic, bactericidal effect
Phenols	Weakly acidic, Hydroxyl group attached directly to an aromatic ring	Disinfection	Antiseptic, anti-inflammatory, antimicrobial, anti-tumor
Flavonoids	Water soluble, super antioxidant and free radical scavenger	In prevention of oxidative cell damage, allergies free radicals, micrfobes	Antioxidant, anti-carcinogens, antimicrobial, antitumor
Saponins	Bitter taste, foaming property, hemolytic effect on red blood cells.	Emulsifying agent	Expectorant, cough suppressant, hemolytic activity
Essential oil	Distinctive scent, aroma and fragrance	In perfumes, flavorings and medicines	Medicating, soothing relief
Tannins	Unpleasant taste, tans leather	In the production of leather and ink; in treating wounds, varicose ulcers, hemorrhoids, frostbite and burns	Soothing relief, regenerates skin, anti-inflammatory, Diuretics

References

[1] Ramawat, K. G., Das, S., Mathur, M. (2009). The chemical diversity of bioactive molecules and therapeutic potential of medicinal plants. Herbal Drugs: Ethnomedicine to Modern Medicine. Springer-Verlag Berlon Heidelberg.

[2] Mathe, A. Medicinal and aromatic plants. Soils, Plant growth and crop production-vol 2.

[3] Ramawat, K. G., Goyal, S. (2008). The Indian herbal drugs scenario in global perspectives. In: Ramawat K. G., Merillon J. M. (eds) *Bioactive Molecules and Medicinal Plants.* Springer, Berlin Heidelberg New York, pp 323.

[4] Iwu, M. M. (1993). Handbook of African Medicinal Plants. CRC Press inc, Florida.

[5] Kumar, A. Ayurvedic Medicines: Some Potential Plants for Medicine from India. http://geb.uni-giessen.de/geb/volltexte/2003/1240/pdf/FestschriftNeumann_09.pdf

[6] Ramawat, K. G., Sonie, K. C., Sharma, M. C. (2004). Therapeutic potential of medicinal plants: an introduction. In: Ramawat KG (ed) Biotechnology of Medicinal Plants: Vitalizer and Therapeutic. Science Publishers, Enfield, CT, pp 1.

[7] Dev, S. (2006). Selection of Prime Ayurvedic Plant Drugs Ancient-Modern Concordance. Anamaya, New Delhi.

[8] Zhang, L., Zia, W. (2007). Chinese herbal drug industry: past, present and future. In: Ramawat K. G., Merillon J. M. (eds) Biotechnology: Secondary Metabolites: Plants and Microbes, 2nd edn. Science Publishers, Enfield, CT, pp 417.

[9] Chevallier, A. (1996). The Encyclopaedia of Medicinal Plants. Dorling Kindersley, London, pp 17.

[10] Heinrich, M., Barnes, J., Gibbons, S., Williamson, E.M. (2004). Fundamentals of Pharmacognosy and Phytotherapy. Churchill Livingstone, Elsevier, UK.

[11] Gurib-Fakim, A. (2006). Medicinal plants: Tradition of yesterday and drugs of tomorrow. Review article. *Mol. Aspects Med.*, 27(1): 1-93.

[12] Theis, N., Lerdau, M. (2003). The evolution of function in plant secondary metabolites. *Int. J. Plant Sci.,* 164(suppl): S93–S102.

[13] Okigbo, R. N., Anuagas, C. L., Amadi, J. E. (2009). Advances in selected medicinal and aromatic plants indigenous to Africa. *Journal of Medicinal Plants Research,* 3(2): 86-95.

[14] Wink. M. Occurrence and functions of natural products in plants. Phytochemistry and Pharmacognosy. Encyclopedia of Life Support Systems.

[15] Okwu, D. E. (2005). Phytochemicals, Vitamins and Mineral contents of two Nigeria Medicinal plants. *Int. J. Mol. Med. Adv. Sci.*, 1(4): 375-381.

[16] Harborne, J. B. (1973). Phytochemical Methods: A Guide to Modern Techniques of plant analysis. Chapman and Hall Ltd, London. p. 279.

[17] Scalbert, A., Manach, C., Morand, C., Rémésy, C., Jiménez, L. (2005). Dietary polyphenols and the prevention of diseases. *Crit. Rev. Food Sci. Nutr.,* 45(4): 287-306.

[18] Okwu, D. E. (2004). Phytochemicals and vitamin content of indigenous spices of South Eastern Nigeria. *J. Sustain. Agric. Environ.,* 6: 30-34.

[19] Urquiaga, I., Leighton, F. (2000). Plant polyphenol, antioxidants and Oxidative stress. *Biol. Res.,* 33:159-165.

[20] Dewick, P. M. (2002). Medicinal Natural Products. Wiley, West Sussex, UK.

[21] Herrmann, K. M., Weaver, L. M. (1999). The Shikimate Pathway. *Annu. Rev. Plant Physiol. Mol. Biol.,* 50:473-503.

[22] Mustafa, N. R., Verpoorte, R. (2005). Chorismate derived C6C1 compounds in plants.

[23] *Planta,* 222:1-5.

[24] Bennett, R. N., Wallsgrove, R. M. (1994). Secondary metabolites in plant defense mechanisms. *New Phytol.*, 127:617-633.

[25] Wink, M. (2000). Biochemistry of Plant Secondary Metabolism: Annual Plant Review, Vol 2. Academic, Sheffield, UK, p 151.

[26] Archer A. W. (1988). Determination of safrole and myristicin in nutmeg and mace by high-performance liquid *chromatography*. *J. Chromatogr.,* 438:117.

[27] Urquiaga, I., Leighton, F. (2000). Plant polyphenol, antioxidants and Oxidative stress. *Biol. Res.*, 33:159-165.

[28] Hertog, M. G., Feskeen, E. J., Hollman, P. C., Katan, M. B., Kromhoit, D. (1993). Dietary antioxidant flavonoids and Risk of Coronary Heart Disease: the Zutphen Elderly Study. *Lancet,* 342(8878):1007-11.

[29] Elangevan, V., Sekar, N., Godndasamy, S. (1994). Chemopreventive Potential of Dietary Bioflavonoids against 20- Methylchofanthrene induced tumoringenesis. *Cancer Lett.,* 87: 102-113.

[30] Okwu, D. E., Okwu, M. E. (2004). Chemical composition of *Spondias mombin* Linn. Plant parts. *J. Sustain. Agric. Environ.,* 6 (2): 140-147.

[31] Singh, A. K. Essential oils: Their importance for mankind http://www.vigyanprasar.gov.in/chemistry_application_2011/briefs/Essential_Oils.pdf

[32] Tundis, R., Loizzo, M. R., Menichini, F., Statti, G. A., Menichini, F. (2008). Biological and pharmacological activities of iridoids: recent developments. *Mini Rev. Med. Chem.*, 8(4): 399-420.

[33] Facchini, P. J. (2001). Alkaloid Biosynthesis In Plants: Biochemistry, Cell Biology, Molecular Regulation, and Metabolic Engineering Applications. *Annu. Rev. Plant Physiol. Plant Mol. Biol.*, 52:29-66.

[34] Stary, F. (1998). The Natrural Guide to Medicinal Herbs, and Plants. Tiger Books International, London. pp. 12-16.

[35] Pelletier, S. W. (1982). The nature and definition of an alkaloid. In: Pelletier SW(ed) Alkaloids: Chemical and Biological Perspectives. Wiley, New York.

[36] Ramawat, K. G. (2007). Secondary metabolites in nature. In: Ramawat K. G., Merillon J. M. (eds) Biotechnology: Secondary Metabolites. Science Publishers, Enfield, CT, p 21.

[37] Grynkiewicz, G., Gadzikowska, M. (2008). Tropane alkaloids as medicinally useful natural products and their synthetic derivatives as new drugs. *Acta. Pol. Pharm – Drug Res.*, 60: 439-463.

[38] Swain, T. (1977). Secondary compounds as protective agents. *Annu. Rev. Plant Physiol.*, 28: 479-501.

[39] Rosenthal, G. A. (1982). Plant nonprotein amino and imino acids. Biological, Biochemical and Toxicological Properties. Academic Press, New York.

[40] Rosenthal, G. A. (1990). Metabolism of L-canavanine and L-canaline in leguminous plants. *Plant Physiol.*, 94: 1-3.

[41] Yolande, A. C., Podevels, A. M., Kevany, B. M., Thomas, A. G. (2009). Biosynthesis of Polyketide Synthase Extender Units, *Nat. Prod. Rep.*, 26(1): 90-114.

[42] Newmann, D. J., Cragg, G. M., Snader, K. M. (2003). Natural products as sources of new drugs over the period 1981-2002. *J. Nat. Prod.*, 66: 1022.

In: Introduction to Drug Designing and Development
Editors: R. Kumar, A. Sharma and R. Kumar Tiwari
ISBN: 978-1-62948-556-0

Chapter 5

Animals As a Source of Lead Molecules

***Gunjan Pandey*[1,2] *and J. K. Srivastava*[1,*]**
[1]Amity Institute of Biotechnology, Amity University Uttar Pradesh, Lucknow, India
[2]Current Address: Nanoscience Centre, University of Jyväskylä, Finland

Abstract

Lead molecules are the first step in the long ladder of drug discovery. These are further identified, extracted, purified, analyzed, optimized, tested and implemented as successful pharmaceutical candidates. Since traditional times, animals have been serving impeccably for this cause. Zoo therapy uses animals as fodder for drug industries. Here, we get acquainted with the vast diversity of the Animal Kingdom. They form a strong foundation on which relies the proper nourishment of human ailment therapy.

Introduction

From the breakfast every morning to energy supplementing capsules for hectic daily schedules animals and their products provide for most of our nutritional, aesthetic as well as recreational needs. Both terrestrial and marine organisms are intriguing sources for the perennial flow of derived products. Sundry recipes in traditional pharmacopeias are filled with animals as basic ingredients. Gigantic numbers of mammals, aves, reptiles, fishes etc. have been and are still being used all over especially in the developing countries. These countries cater to 80% of the world population [1].

They are used both internally and externally as ointments, powders, snuffs, charms, amulets and in a plethora of other forms [2]. As reported by Mahavar and Jaroli in their review that Indian natives themselves utilize 109 species at present for the cure ranging from tuberculosis to paralytic attacks to muscular pains. Ancient medical practices of Ayurveda, Susrut Samhita and Charak Samhita have elaborated on zootherapeutics quite vividly.

* E-mail: jksrivastava@lko.amity.edu.

Mammals are utilized in most of the concoctions prepared [1]. Although, modernization has played its part in reducing the hunting of animals as healing agents but the strong roots coupled with negligible expenditure accounts for the strong inclination of masses towards it. Pigs, cows, horses, snakes, sponges, echinoderms compose the major classes actively employed in the production of a broad spectrum of pills (i.e., painkillers, anti-diabetic, anti-cancerous, anti-paralytic, auto-immune disease curing agents etc.).

Every coin has two sides and so does the animals' role in pharmacology. The extensive inclusion of certain species (Tiger, Rhinoceros, Sun Bear, Water Buffalo, Chinese Alligator, Grevy's Zebra, Asian Elephant, Musk Deer, Hawkbill Sea Turtle as reported by Stromberg and Zielinski article) by Chinese, African, Latin American and several other indigenous healing systems have caused poaching at accelerated rates [27]. To exemplify the situation musk used in perfumes can be extracted from Musk Deers without harming them but just for the ease traders kill them [10]. Such callous actions have led to devastating effects on species either eliminating them from the face of the planet or tagging them with the label of endangered ones. Although, several symposiums on endangered species used in traditional medicine by WWF, IUCN (International Council for Conservation of Nature) etc. with the local activists have led to few reforms but still much needs to be done. As documented in a Jill Robinson's report traditional Chinese system has started using pigs instead of beer for bile, chrysanthemum in place of antelope's horn and is further researching to minimize the toll on endangered species. Black market and illicit trade of innocent animals is functional in soiling these steps. Irrespective of these persistent erosions it's time to roll up our sleeves and hit the ground running.

Henceforth we elaborate on the multifarious benevolent creatures both on land and sea helping us lead a healthy life with exponentially increased life expectancy.

Terrestrial Animals as Drug Resource

The earliest use of animals as a drug source dates back to the beginning of the twentieth century when the insulin derived from the pancreas of pigs and cows cured diabetes by reducing the amount of blood sugar. This discovery made by Canadian surgeon Frederick Banting and his assistant Charles Best earned them the highest honor of Nobel Prize [4]. Since then, several hormones, amino acids, venoms, toxins as well as organs have been extracted and analyzed for their pharmacodynamics.

Adrenal extract is prepared from the glands of pigs and cats. It is administered orally to reduce varied states of stress, management of blood pressure and sugar, also to cure asthma, eczema, psoriasis and rheumatoid arthritis. Intravenous injections are supposed to be functional in the maintenance of potassium levels in blood, ulcerative colitis, and for healthy fetus development by production of adrenaline and cortisol hormones mimicking normal body state [5].

Hypothyroidism is cured by desiccated thyroid gland extract made from a mixture of beef and pork called porcine. The product is commercially available as Armour Thyroid. It consists of both Thyroxine and Triiodothyronine also known as T4 and T3 respectively. One grain (about 60 mg) of desiccated thyroid contains about 38 mcg of T4 and 9 mcg of T3 which helps in regulating thyroid levels [6]. Synthetically synthesized Levothyroxine has replaced this extract to a great extent.

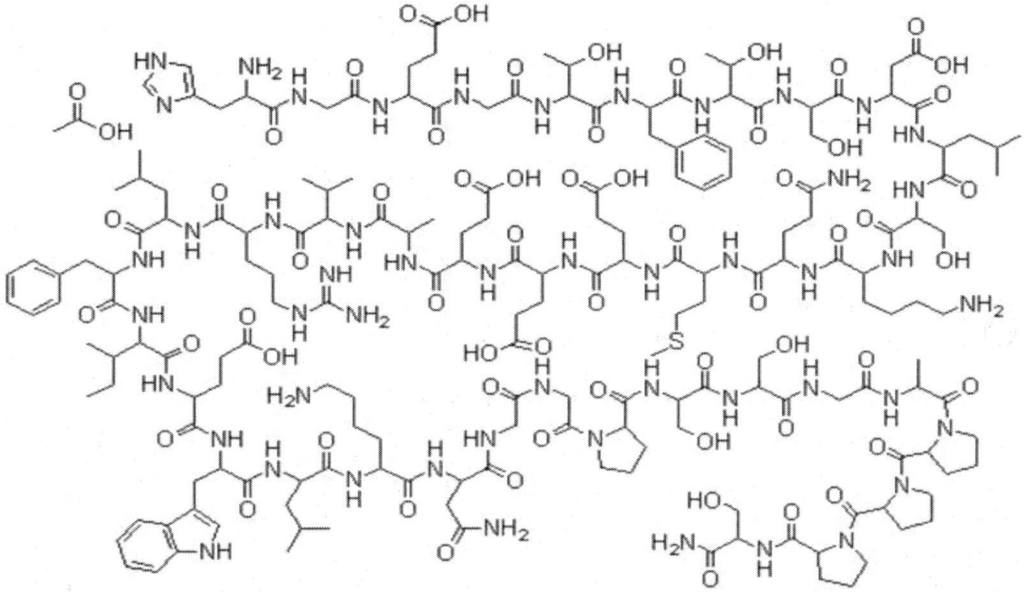

His-Gly-Glu-Gly-Thr-Phe-Thr-Ser-Asp-Leu-Ser-Lys-Gln-Met-Glu-Glu-Glu-Ala-Val-Arg-Leu-Phe-Ile-Glu-Trp-Leu-Lys-Asn-Gly-Gly-Pro-Ser-Ser-Gly-Ala-Pro-Pro-Pro-Ser-NH_2

[Courtesy: Lookchem: look for chemicals http://www.lookchem.com/cas-141/141732-76-5.html].

Figure 1. Exenatide Structure.

Since 1921, the discovery of Insulin has saved more than 15 Million people from Diabetes. It is a 3,500 year old identified medical condition [4, 7]. Insulin is a polypeptide consisting of two chains – A and B, linked by two interchain disulfide bridges that connect A7 to B7 and A20 to B19. A third inter-chain disulfide bridge connects residues 6 and 11 of the A chain.

Human insulin has a total of 51 amino acids, out of which 21 form ‘A’ chain while the remaining 30 make up the ‘B’ chain. Substitutions can occur at many positions without affecting the bioactivity and are particularly common at positions 8, 9, 10 of the A chain. The only kind of insulin available before the advent of recombinant technology and fine amino acid structure elucidation techniques was porcine and bovine extracted . Former (procine) differs from human insulin by one amino acid and the latter(bovine) by three. Several fishes including sharks were also used for the purpose of insulin extraction. Exenatide ($C_{184}H_{282}N_{50}O_{60}S$), a drug manufactured by Eli Lily from the saliva of the Gila monster (large venomous lizard) (figure 1).

Subcutaneous administration of the drug was approved by the FDA in 2005 for those who do not respond to other combinations. Its trade name is Byetta [4]. Insulin is synthesized as prohormone which is then directed to Endoplasmic Reticulum (ER). In the ER, proinsulin is formed which contains an amino terminal- B Chain, connecting C peptide and A chain. A series of site specific cleavage in the proinsulin molecule results in the formation of mature insulin and C peptide (figure2).

Among the hypertension monitoring drugs snakes play a vital role. Peptide of *Bothrops jararaca* a Brazilian pit viper's venom is used for synthesis of the drug i.e., Teprotide ($C_{53}H_{76}N_{14}O_{12}$) (figure 3). Sergio Ferreira (1965), reported its anti-hypertensive property for the first time.

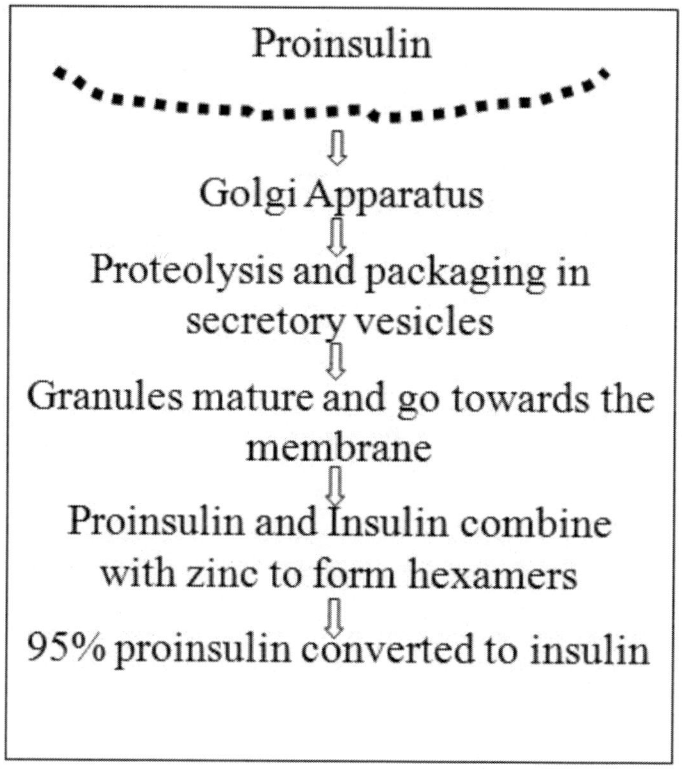

Figure 2. Conversion of Proinsulin into Insulin.

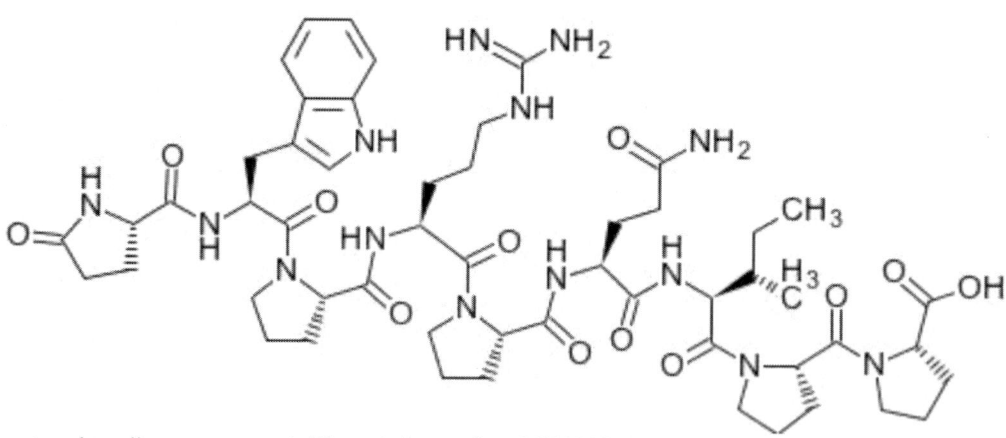

[Courtesy:http://www.genome.jp/dbget-in/www_bget?C11712+D06076].

Figure 3. Teprotide Structure.

Its ACE (Angiotensin-Converting Enzyme) Inhibitor property blocks the conversion of angiotensin I to angiotensin II thus rendering it with the vasodilatation and inhibition of some renal function activities.

Antiplatelet drugs include Eptifibatide (figure 4) isolated from *Sistrurus miliarius barbouri* (South Eastern Pygmy Rattle Snake) and Tirofiban from *Echis carinatus.* They efficiently block Glycoprotein IIb/IIIa receptor thus preventing platelet aggregation. Its injection is helpful in lowering the instances of Acute Cardiac Ischemic events in patients with cardiovascular risks. Ancrod (*Agkistrodon rhodostoma*) and Batroxobin (*Bothrops moojeni*) are classified as defibrinogenating and thrombin and prothrombin inhibiting agents respectively. Atroxase, Lebetase from rattle snake and viper belong to fibrinogenolytic enzymes. *Agkistrodon contotrix* produces Protac which works as protein C activator [9].

Wings of Asian sulfur butterflies and the legs of Stag beetle from Taiwan are used in the development of drugs against cancer [10]. *Bothus martens* (scorpion) extracted peptide has shown its efficacy against S-180 fibrosarcoma cells. Traditional uses of the sting and whole body extracts of scorpions include mitigation of pain. It is induced by secretion of bradykinin and prostaglandins. This activity has been helping in ailing several neural afflictions such as epilepsy, facial paralysis, apoplexy etc. [11]. Spider venom from *Agelenopsis aperta* can be used to increment the agonist tail flick anti-nociception [12].

Batrachotoxins and Histrionicotoxin (figure 5) isolated from frogs are alkaloids. The former acts as both the cardiotoxin and neurotoxin steroidal alkaloid activating sodium ion channels, whereas the latter is pieprdine alkaloid inhibiting nicotine receptors. It was reported in the 1960s that golden Phyllobates terribilis and multicolored Phyllobates bicolor are the sources of batrachotoxin and homobatrachotoxin. They are among the most toxic substance known, more toxic than curare or the tetrodotoxin, found in puffer fish, whose poison is over 1000 times more poisonous than cyanide [13, 14].

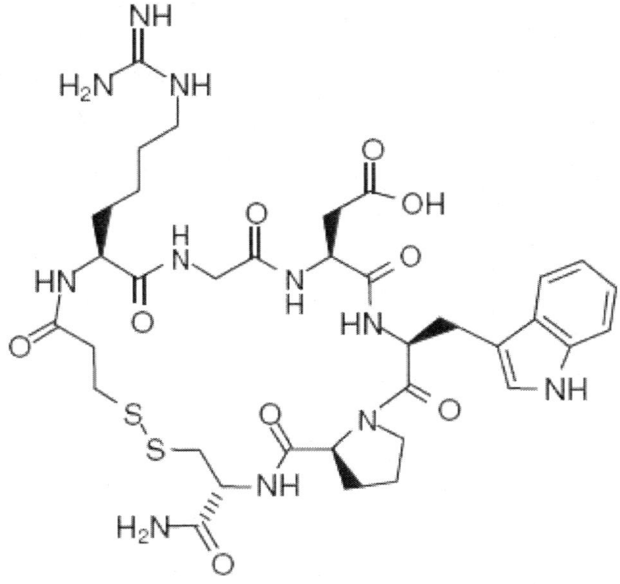

[Courtesy: http:// dailymed.nlm.nih.gov/dailymed/archives/ fdaDrugInfo.cfm?archiveid=9876].

Figure 4. Eptifibatide.

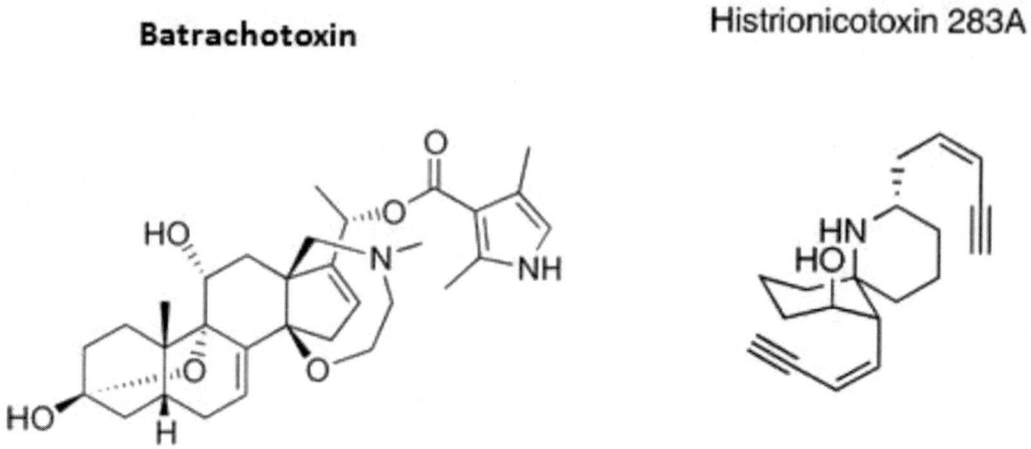

[Courtesy: http://www.chm.bris.ac.uk/motm/batrachotoxin/batrah.htm and http://www.rsc.org/ejga/NP/2007/ b604203c-ga.gif].

Figure 5. Structure of Batrachotoxins and Histrionicotoxin.

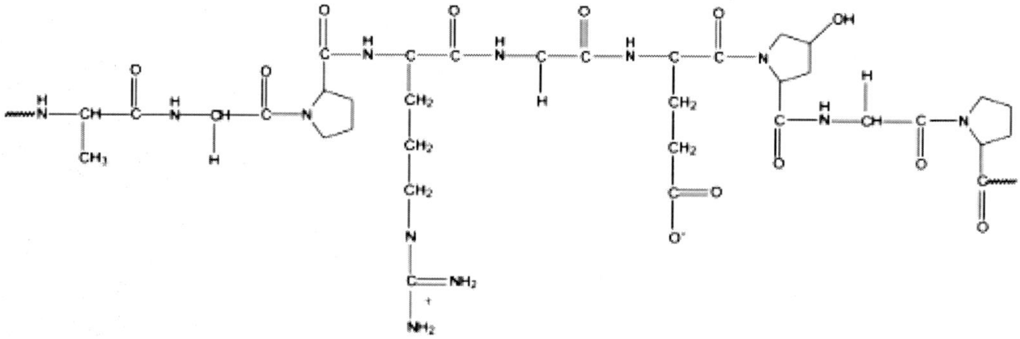

[http://www.madehow.com/Volume-5/Gelatin.html#b].

Figure 6. Structure of Gelatin.

Scientists are using these molecules to identify the way in which nerve impulses are transmitted in animals. They are being studied for possible applications in areas like heart drugs and anesthetics.

Gelling property of gelatine makes it the backbone of the food industry. The pharmaceutical industry utilizes it as a base agent for (emergency medicine) blood plasma expanders used for replacing lost blood; and to make drug capsules. Pork skins are majorly used in gelatine production along with cattle hides and bones [15, 16].

Gelatin is derived from collagen, a natural protein present in the ligaments and tendons of mammals. Cows and pigs are the main resources for gelatin production, their connective tissues, bones and skin are boiled to make the product. Gelatin has a property to form strong, transparent gels and flexible films .These films can be easily dissolved in hot water. The steps involved in gelatin production are depicted in figure 7.

Premarin also known as "conjugated equine estrogens" (CEE), is isolated from pregnant mare’s urine and is used as hormone replacement therapy. Estrogen components in Premarin are estrone (>50%), equilin (15-25%) and equilenin (figure 8).

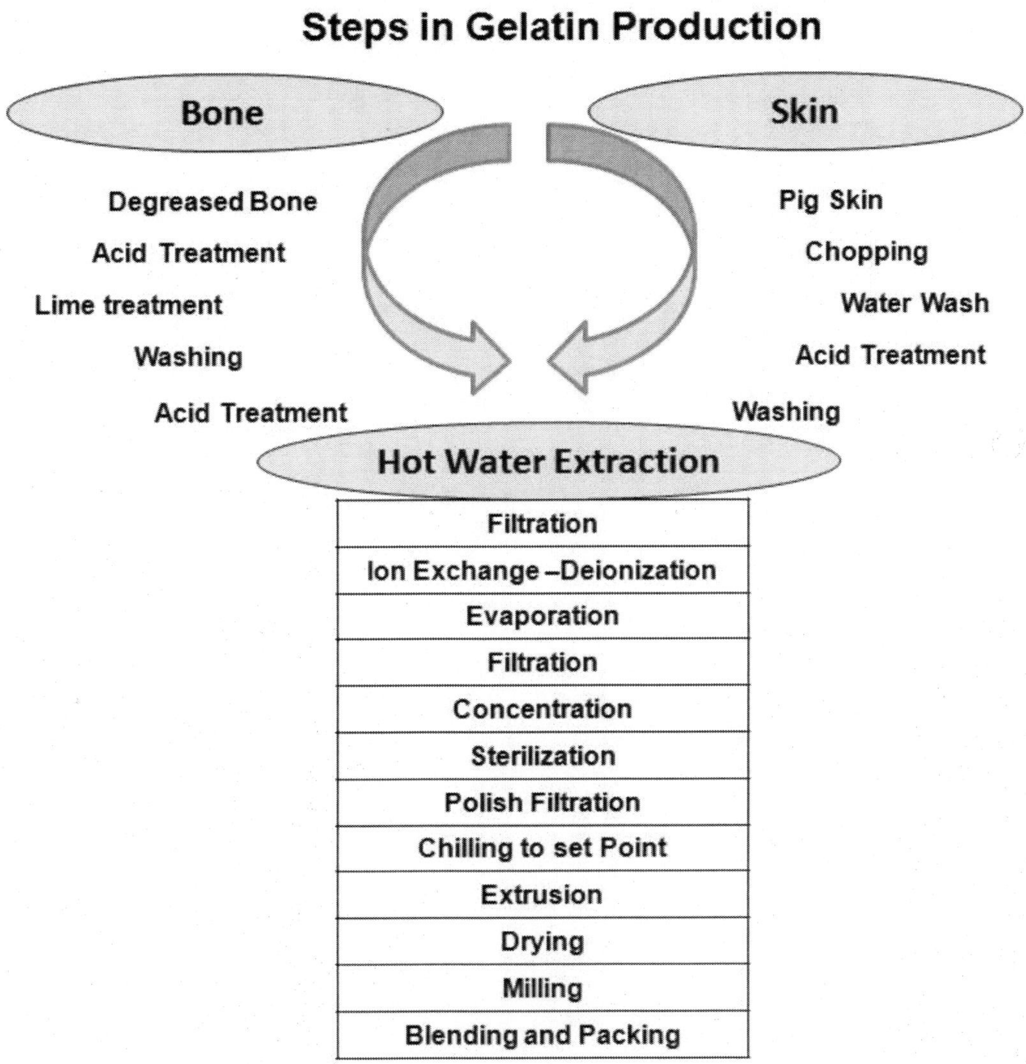

Figure 7. Flow diagram showing production of Gelatin.

The estrogen molecules are generally present with hydrophilic side-groups attached such as sulfate.

Estrone sulfate is easily absorbed into the blood after Premarin pills are taken by women. Estrone sulfate is converted to estradiol, an active estrogen normally found in women. Intake of the drug by post menopausal women who have had a hysterectomy is done to treat hot flashes, burning, itching, and dryness of the vaginal areas. The side effects associated with it are vaginal yeast infections, spotting/bleeding, painful menses, and cramping of the legs [17].

Catgut suture is the first absorbable suture. They are made up by writhing together purified collagen strands from the serosal or submucosal layer of the small intestine of cattle, sheep, goats.

Sometimes beef tendons are also utilized in the process. At present, due to infection risks they are being replaced by cotton sutures. Carmine (figure 9) is a red dye produced by boiling of insects and then treating the solution with alum [18].

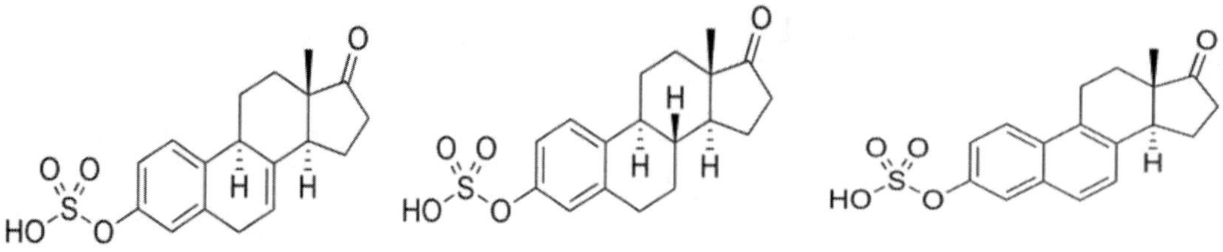

Equilin Sulfate Estrone Sulfate Equilenin Sulfate

[http://www.fda.gov/Safety/MedWatch/SafetyInformation/SafetyRelatedDrugLabelingChanges/ucm121062.htm].

Figure 8. Structure of Equilin Sulfate, Estrogen Sulfate and Equilenin Sulfate.

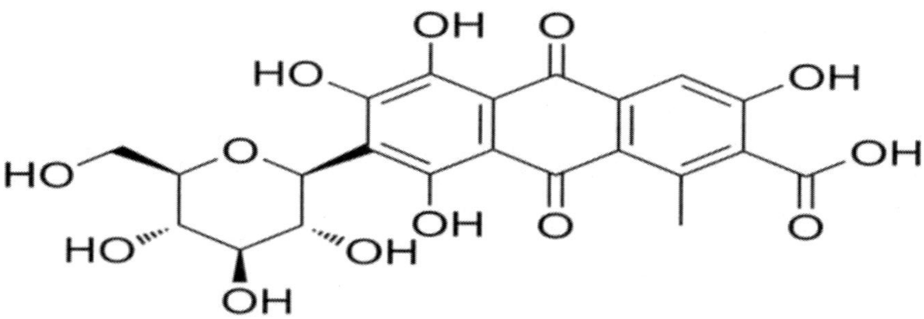

[Courtesy: Allevi, P. et al.].

Figure 9. Structure of Carminic acid.

Considering the importance of human health, extensive researches were conducted on lower to higher animals and a number of species were identified as potential source for the production of therapeutic molecules listed the Table 1 below.

Marine Organism as Drug Resource

Covering almost three-fourth of the Earth's surface, oceans form an infinite reserve engendering potential for development of chemical compounds which can be used as a remedy for a myriad of maladies.

Fish are commonly available and comprehensively studied marine organisms for drug development. Omega -3 fatty acid extracted from fishes, squids and krill are utilized as anti-oxidant agents, in reducing chances of myocardial infarction and dementia (figure 10).

Fish oil as a source for the compound is also used for treating ADHD (Attention deficit hyperactivity disorder) related characteristics [19]. In addition to that Squalamine (figure 11) extracted from sharks (*Squalus acanthias*) are being evaluated in phase-II trials against oncological conditions [20]. The serendipitous discovery of spongouridine and spongothymidine (figure 12) from *Cryptotheca crypta* a Caribbean sponge led to an extensive exploration of their therapeutic activities.

Table 1. Summary of Terrestrial Animal Sources as lead molecules

Compounds	Source	Use
Epinephrin/ adrenalin	Adrenal Gland of Pig and Cat	Heart diseases, Asthma
Thyroxin	Thyroid gland Extract	Hypothyroidism
Insulin	Pancreatic gland of pigs and cats.	Diabetes
Teprotide	Poison of Bothrops jararaca (Brazilian Viper)	Anti-hypertensive agent
Eptifibatide	*Sistrurus miliarius barbouri* (South Eastern Pygmy Rattle Snake) from	Platelet aggregation Inhibitor
Tirofiban	*Echis carinatus* (West African saw scaled viper)	Glycoprotein IIb/IIIa Inhibitor
Ancrod	*Agkistrodon rhodotoma* (Malayan pit viper)	Fibrinogen Inhibitor
Batroxobin	*Bothrops moojeni* (Brazilian Lancehead snake)	Thrombin and Prothrombin Inhibitor
Atroxase Fibrolase Lebetase	*Crotalus atrox*(Western Diamond Back Rattlesnake) *Agkistrodon contotrix* (Copperhead/Moccasin) *Vipera lebetina* (Blunt-nosed viper)	Fibrinogenolytic Enzymes
Protac	*Agkistrodon contotrix* (Copperhead/Moccasin)	Protein C Activator
Antitumor, Analgesic peptide	*Bothus martense* (Scorpion)	Painkiller, Tumor killing activity
Neurotoxins (Coagatoxin)	*Agelenopsis asperta* (Spider)	Antinociception agent
Batrachotoxins	Phyllobates genus of Frogs	Causes Na^+ Ion channel selectivity alteration
Histrionicotoxin	Dendrobatidae family of Frogs	Nicotine receptor Inhibitors
Anti-neoplastic compounds	*Catopsilia crocale cram* (Asian sulfur butterfly) and *Allomyrina dichotoma* (Stag Beetle)	Anti-carcinogenic agents
Gelatin	Skin and bones of cattle	Used in pharmaceuticals and vitamins as a stabilizer.
Carmine (Red Dye)	Insects / beetles	Red pigment used in medicines and syrups
Catgut	Intestine of horses and sheep	Surgical sutures
Estradiol	Pregnant mare Urine	Birth control pills
Melittin Hyaluronidase	*Apis sp.* (Honey Bee)	Antitumor, anti-viral activity Membrane permeability, anti-tumor activity
Cantharidin	*Cantharis vesicatorea* (Blister Beetles)	Potent anti-tumor activity, cure for cutaneous leishmaniasis in animal models
Recombinant Hirudin	Leeches	Intravenous anticoagulant
Samandarine	*Salamandra maculosa* (Salamander)	Potent local anesthetic activity

Figure 10. Flow of Omega-3 Fatty acid through Marine Channel.

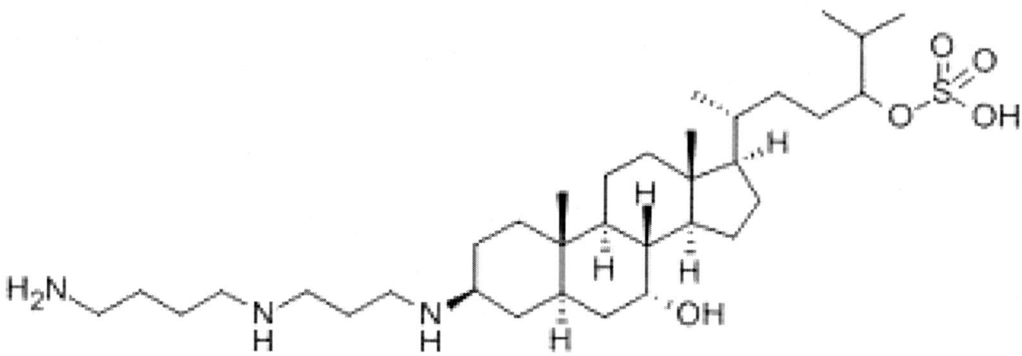

[Courtesy: http://www.marinebiotech.org/squalamine.html].

Figure 11. Structure of Squalamine.

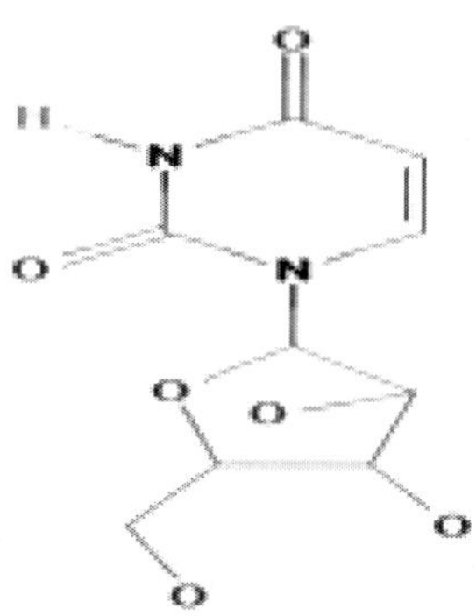

Spongouridine

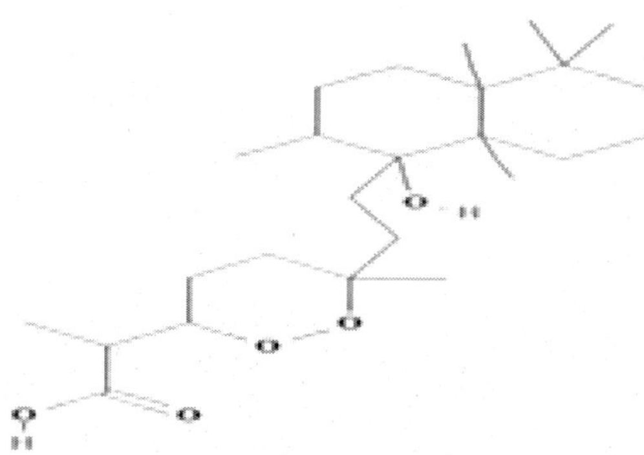

Spongothymidine

Figure 12. Structure of Spongouridine and Spongothymidine.

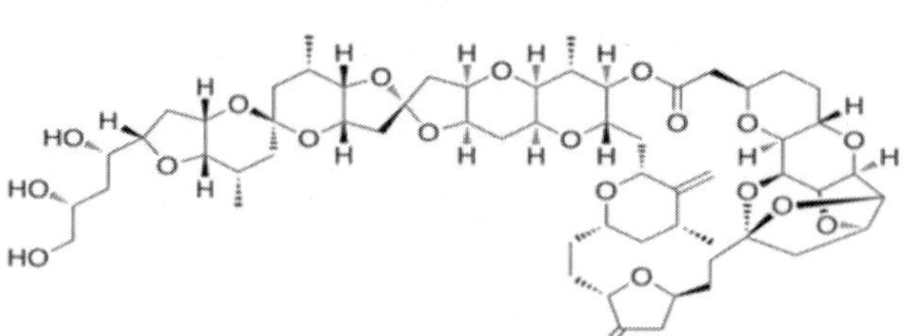

Halichondrin B

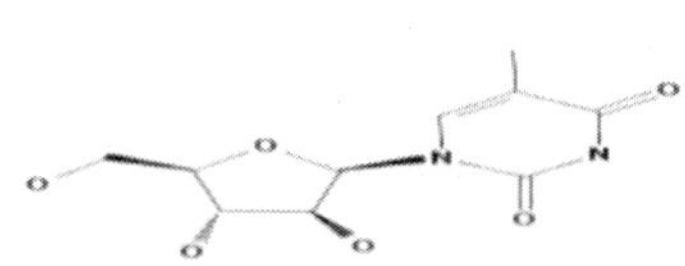

Mycaperoxide B

Figure 13. Structure of Halichondrin B and Mycaperoxide B.

Halichondrin B and Mycaperoxide B (figure 13) from Hawaiian and Thailand species have shown anti-neoplastic activities whereas Australian sponges are effective in curing nematode infection via Dithiocyanates found in them [20]. The Anti-Asthmatic compound Contignasterol is a sponge papue product from New Guinea. *Cymbastella sp., Jaspis sp., Mycale hentscheli, Heliclona sp.* produce Hemiasterlin, Agelasphin and Bengamide derivative along with Laulimalide, Discodermolide, Peloruside, Salicylhalimides. They are either in phase I or preclinical trial stage as potential anti-cancerous agents [20, 23]. *Petrosia contignata* isolated IPL-512602 and IPL-576092 form phase II experimental drugs for inflammation and psoriasis [20]. Manoalide (Sesquiterpenoide from *Luffareilla variabilis*) is another agent being tested for its psoriasis treating efficacy [21].

Tunicates are chordates commonly known as sea squirts, sea pork or sea tulips. Ecteinascidin-743 (ET-743) (figure 14) from them possesses the potential to annihilate tumors of soft tissue sarcoma, metastatic breast cancer and osteosarcoma in their phase I clinical trial studies [20]. Blocking the P-glycoprotein constitution in tumors refers to its property that can prevent tumors from getting drug resistant after all.

Aplidine and Dehydrodidemnin B (figure 15) were isolated from the Mediterranean tunicate *Aplidium albicans* and also reflect similar properties. Other preclinical phase tunicate species encompass *Diazona angulata* and *Didemnum cucliferum* which produces Diazonamide reported to be active against colon cancer cells similarly Vitilevuamide, a bicyclic 13 amino acid peptide, was isolated from two marine ascidians, *Didemnum cuculiferum and Polysyncranton lithostrotum.*

Vitilevuamide was cytotoxic in several human tumor cell lines, Cyclodidemniserinol trisulfate and Lamellarina 20 sulfate from Palau andAustralian tunicates respectively shows anti-viral capacity. They are being tested against HIV [20].

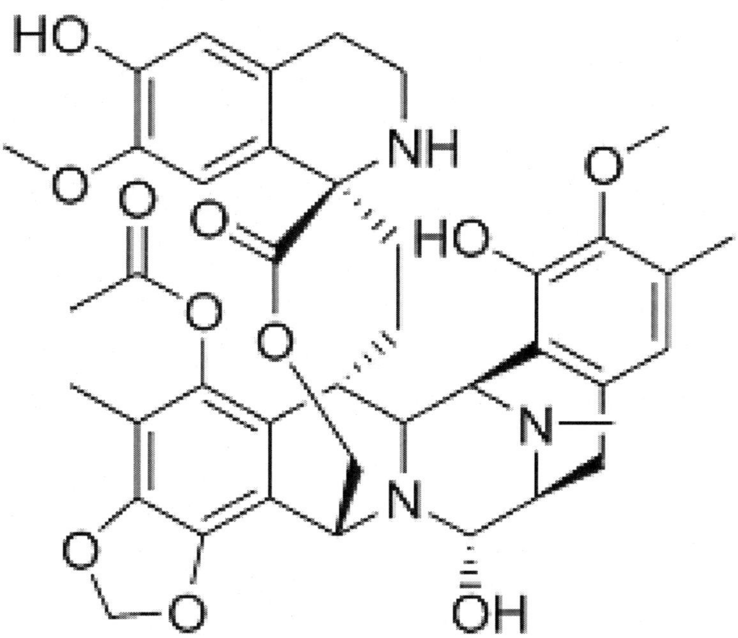

[Courtesy: http://onlinelibrary.wiley.com/doi/10.1002/cjoc.201180450/references].

Figure 14. Structure of Ecteinascidin 743.

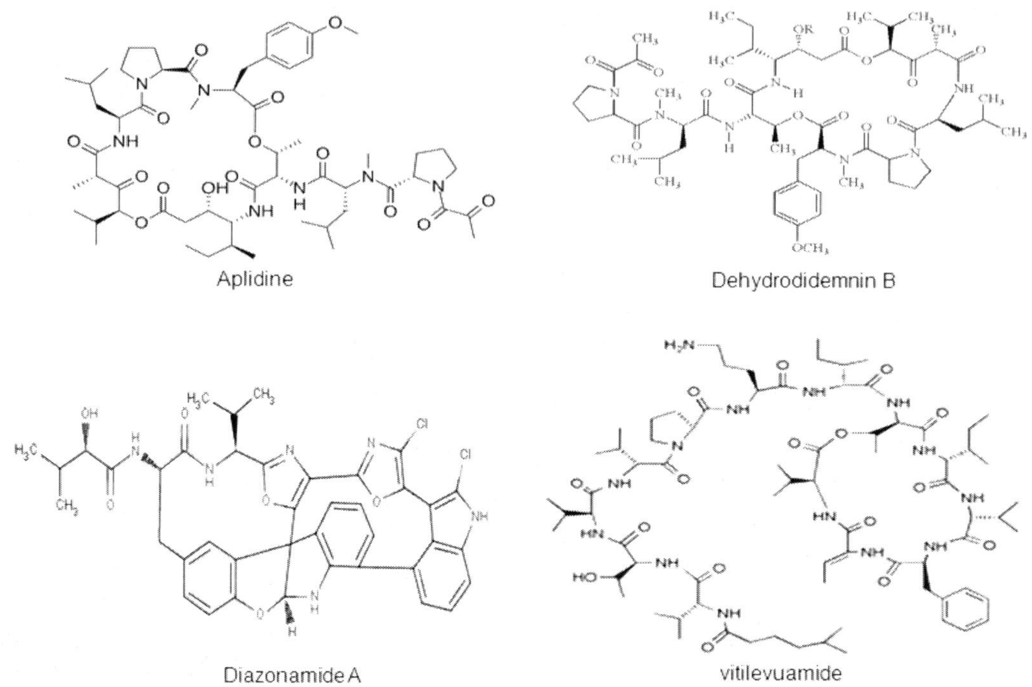

[Courtesy: http://www.chemspider.com/ and d)Marinebiotech.org http://www.marinebiotech.org /diazonamidea.html d),Marinebiotech.org http://www.marinebiotech.org/diazonamidea.html, http:// www.sciencedirect.com/science/article/pii/S000629520100898X].

Figure 15. Structure of Aplidine, Dehydrodidemnin-B, Diazonamide-A and Vitilevumide.

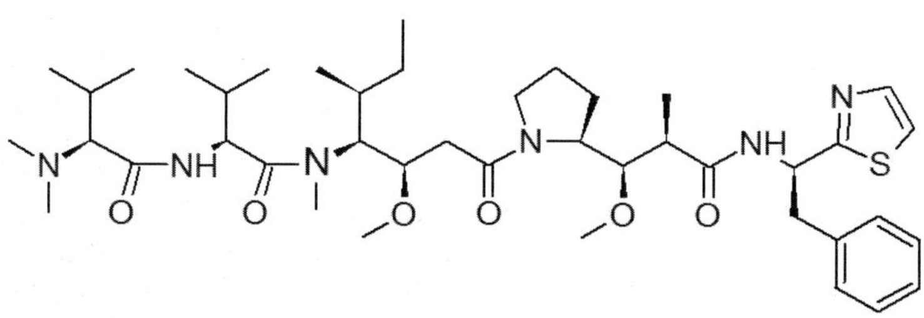

[Courtesy: http://naturalproductforum.org/tag/dolastatins/].

Figure 16. Structure of Dolostatin-10.

Mollusca phylum provides for edible delicacies as well as bioactive peptides effective against cancer andpain killers. Kahalalide F extracted from Hawaiian *Elysia reufedcens* showed anti-tumor activity against prostate cancer cell lines. Its peculiar apoptosis instigating procedure by disrupting lysosome membrane and forming large vacuoles tends to increase acidity. It is subjected to phase I clinical trials [20]. *Conus magnus* releases a twenty five amino acid Ziconitide (Conotoxin MVIIV) (figure 17) in its venom. This is commercially available as Prialt and is used as a painkiller. It blocks the pain fibers to receive signals from the spinal cord by obstructing the neurotransmitter release. Inhibition of presynaptic calcium channels by its addition is considered the base s property [20]. Dolastatin-10 (figure 16) from Dolabella *auricularia* commonly known as Indian Sea Hare is a linear peptide with striking in vitro anti-neoplastic activity.

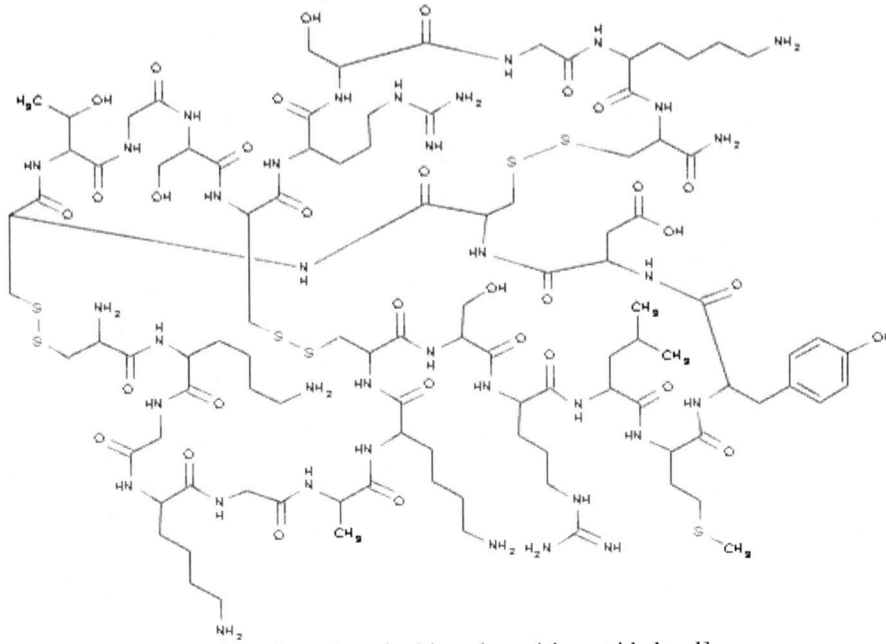

[Courtesy:Marinebiotech.org http://www.marinebiotech.org/ziconotide.html].

Figure 17. Structure of Ziconotide.

Monomethylauristatin E (MMAE) derivative of the compound is being coupled with monoclonal antibodies to function against cancer cell specific antigen [22]. A bryozoa -- *Bugula neritina,* is used for the production of Bryostatin I. It is used for amplifying the chemotherapeutic activities of cisplatin andTaxol used in the treatment of breast, ovarian and lung cancers. It functions by binding with protein kinase C [20]. It is also used for memory enhancing agent [24].

Other marine species with anti-cancerous compounds include Australian soft corals (*Eleutherobia Sp.*). They produce Eleuthrobin (figure 18) which is a diterpene but due to its low production source not much research has been done on it. Isididae, a coral family's skeleton is used for bone grafting purposes [35]. The skeletal structure of these corals is similar to that of bone. Anti-inflammatory and analgesic effects are reflected by the tricyclic diterpenes glycosides distilled from *Pseudoptergorgia elisabethae* (Carrabian Sea Whip). These glycosides are also known as pseudopterosins [20]. Fluoroscent marine compounds from squid, jellyfishes etc are used in illuminating the empirical process. They help in curbing the need to process the middle steps requiring cumbersome computing and other biochemical analysis. Marine animal identified as sources of lead molecules are listed in table 2.

Impact of Indiscreet Animal Application for Medicinal Purposes

Global modernization has increased life expectancy along with the variety of diseases afflicting populations. As a result of which people try to find inexpensive traditional ways of cure.

Table 2. Summary of Marine Animals as a Source of lead molecules

Compounds	Sources	Use
Omega -3 fatty acid	Fishes, Squids and Krill	Anti-oxidant agents, in reducing chances of myocardial infarction, treating ADHD
Squalamine	*Squalus acanthias*(shark)	Potent anti-cancer compound
Halichondrin B, Mycaperoxide B Discodermolide Hemiasterlin derivative Bengamide derivative Agelasphin derivative Laulimalide Peloruside Salicylhalimides Dithiocyanates Contignasterol IPL-576092 Manoalide IPL-512602 IPL-550260	Sponges Sponge Papue *Petrosia contignata* *Luffareilla variabilis* *Petrosia contignata* *Petrosia contignata*	Potent anti-cancer compound Nematode infection Asthma treatment Potent for psoriasis treatment Potent for asthma treatment and as an anti-inflammatory Potent anti-inflammatory agent
Ecteinascidin 743 Vitilevuamide Diazonamide Dehydrodidemnin B Cyclodidemniserinol trisulfate Lamellarina 20 sulfate	Tunicates	Potent anti-cancer compounds Potent anti-viral compounds (HIV)
Dolastatin 10 Kahalilade F ES-285(spisulosine) Ziconotide	Mollusks	Potent anti-cancer compounds Neuropathic pain killer
Bryostatin I	Bryozoans (*Bugula neritina*)	Potent anti-cancer compound
Eleuthrobin diterpene	Corals (*Eleutherobia Sp.*)	Potent anti-cancer compound
Pseudopterosins	Gorgonians	Potent analgesics and anti-inflammatory agents

These native healing methods heavily rely on animal consumption in all forms; exacerbating the already present conditions of animal extinction due to habitat loss, population explosion and hunting.

Exponentially exceeding killing rates has led the situation close enough to the Sixth Mass Extinction as reported by Stromberg and Zielinski. All these factors end up incrementing the size of IUCN's threatened species' list. The following is the table representing most popular hunted species [26, 27]:

Table 3. Endangered Animals Used as Medicine

Animal	Parts used in medicine	Uses
Panthera tigris	Bones	Arthritis
Rhinoceros	Horn	Fever, convulsions, delirium
Bear	Bile	Liver ailments and headaches
Musk deer	Musk Gland	Skin infection, abdominal pain, perfume synthesis
Seahorse (hippocampus)	Whole Animal	Kidney and circulatory Problems
Water Buffalo	Whole Animal	As an alternative to Rhinoceros (fever to convulsions)
Asian Elephant	Meat, hide, tusks, foot and other body parts	Hernia and other diseases.
Chinese Alligator	Meat	Common Cold, Cancer
Sun Bear	Gall bladders	For bile stock
Grevy's Zebra	Meat. Fat and skin	Tuberculosis
Banteng	Horns, meat	Hunting trophies, edible value
Hawksbill Sea Turtle	Whole animal, shells	Animal oil, as delicacy. Aesthetic value

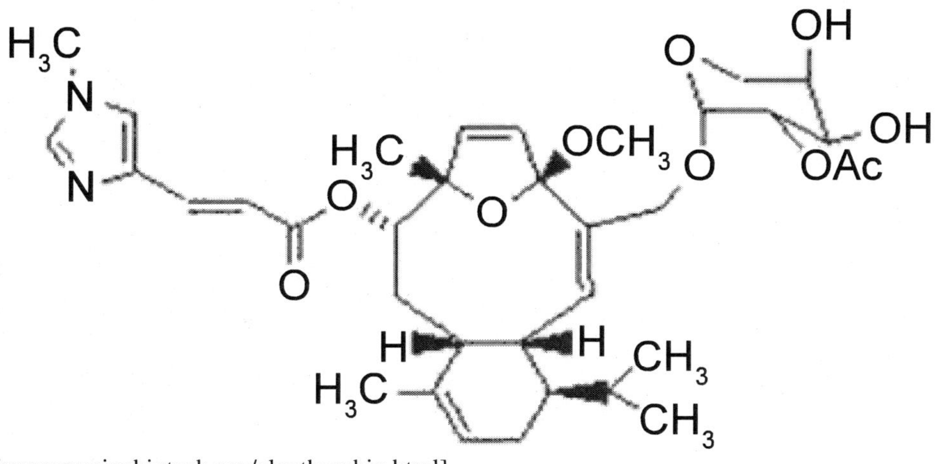

[http://www.marinebiotech.org/eleutherobin.html].

Figure 18. Structure of Eleuthrobin.

Future of Animals as Drug Resource

Animals form an integral part of human life especially in the field of medicinal treatments. Due to the lack of proper measures, the poaching of certain animals has caused havoc in their lives. Unfortunately, complete dependence on synthetic medicines still can't be attained due to the long production spans coupled with numerous expenses. All these factors are incurred in the cost price marked on the medicine. On the other hand, the positive feedback of fellow community members and lower costs lure the commoners towards native remedies. Thus, alternate methods such as animal farming and cloning can be fruitful in mitigating the circumstances.

References

[1] Mahawar M. M. and Jaroli D. P. (2008). Traditional zootherapeutic studies in India: a review, *J. Ethnobiol. Ethnomed.*,4:17.

[2] Alves R. R. N. and Alves H. N. (2011).The faunal drugstore: Animal-based remedies used in traditional medicines in Latin America, *J. Ethnobiol. Ethnomed.*, 7: 9.

[3] Robinson J. (2009). Healing without harm Working to replace the use of animals in traditional Chinese medicine. Animal Asia Foundation.

[4] Animal derived drugs (2011) http://www.docstoc.com/docs/72839292/Animal-Derived-Drugs.

[5] WebMed. Adrenal Extract (2013) http://www.webmd.com/vitamins ingredientmono-941-ADRENAL%20EXTRACT.aspx?activeIngredientId= 941andactiveIngredientName=ADRENAL%20EXTRACT

[6] Gilbert J. Central Hypothyroiidism (2013) https://online.epocrates.com/u/293136/ Central+hypothyroidism/Diagnosis/Approach

[7] Barr D., The history of Insulin, http://www.med.uni-giessen.de/itr/history/inshist.html

[8] Ferreira S. H. (1965). A bradykinin potentiating factor (BPF) present in the venom of Bothrops jaraca, *Brit. J. Pharmacol.*, 24,163-164.

[9] Gibson J. L. and Georgia M. Over-the-Counter Use of Neuroactive Peptides for the Treatment of Chronic Pain, (2010). http://www.uspharmacist.com/ continuing_education/ceviewtest/lessonid/107115/

[10] Ref for butterfly: Maiti P. K. and Maiti P. (2011) Biodeversity: perception, peril and preservation: Biodiversity conservation(2011). New Delhi: PHI learning private limited.

[11] Dorcas M. E. Animal toxin: hidden cures (2011) http://www.bio.davidson.edu/ people/midorcas/animalphysiology/websites/2010/Baldeon/Scorpion%20Toxin.html

[12] De Lima M. E., Borges M. H., Verano B. T. et al. Some arachnidan peptides with potential medical application, (2010). http://www.scielo.br/scielo.php?pid=S1678-91992010000100004andscript=sci_arttext

[13] Feeding dart frogs (2010) http://www.reptileforums.co.uk/forums/amphibian-articles/580733-feeding-dart-frogs.html

[14] Rapier C., Wonnacott S., Lunt G. G. et al., The neurotoxin histrionicotoxin interacts with the putative ion channel of the nicotinic acetylcholine receptors in the central nervous system (1987) http://www.sciencedirect.com/science 0014579387813637

[15] Gelita-improving quality of life. Gelatine a gelling agent for numerous applications (2013) http://www.gelita.com/solutions-and-products/gelatine-gelling-agent-numerous-applications

[16] Gelatin Manufacturers Institute of America. Gelatin Handbook (2012) http://www.gelatin-gmia.com/gelatinhandbook.html

[17] Premarin.org. The beginning of the end? (2003) http://premarin.org/

[18] Demetech-a trusted name in medicine, Plain Catgut Suture (2013) http://www.demetech.us/plain_catgut_suture.php

[19] Wold Fitness Notebook, The story of omega-3s (2012) http://woldfitness.com/2012/03/the-story-of-omega-3s/

[20] Chin Y. W., Balunas M. J., Chai H. B. et.al. (2006). Drug discovery from natural sources, *The AAPS Journal,* 8:2.

[21] Epstein P. E., Taiolas D. M.,Motti C. A. et al., Production of manoalide and its analogues by the sponge Luffariella variabilis is hardwired (2008) http://www.deepdyve.com/lp/springer-journals/production-of-manoalide-and-its-analogues-by-the-sponge-luffariella-RD3mRCWNqN

[22] Natural Product Forum, The story of the dolastatins (2012) http://naturalproductforum.org/tag/dolastatins/

[23] Jain R., Sonawane S., Mandrekar N. (2008). Marine organisms: Potential source for drug discovery, *Current Science*, 94:9.

[24] Kuzirian A. M., Epstein H. T., Gagliardi C. J. et al. 2006. Bryostatin enhancement of memory in Hermissenda. *Biol. Bull.*, 210 (3): 201–14.

[25] Iptechex pharmalicensing. Natural source for eleutherobin and anti mitotic analogues: a source for the anti-mitotic eleutherobin, a potential cancer therapeutic (2013) http://pharmalicensing.com/public/outlicensing/view/12121/natural-source-for-eleutherobin-and-anti-mitotic-analogues-a-source-for-the-anti-mitotic-eleutherobin-a-potential-cancer-therapeutic

[26] Stromberg J. and Zielinski S., Ten Threatened and Endangered Species Used in Traditional Medicine (2011) http://www.smithsonianmag.com/science-nature/Ten-Threatened-and-Endangered-Species-Used-in-Traditional-Medicine.html

[27] Traditional Chinese medicine and endangered species (2007). http://advocacy.britannica.com/blog/advocacy/2007/10/traditional-chinese-medicine-and-endangered-animals/

In: Introduction to Drug Designing and Development
Editors: R. Kumar, A. Sharma and R. Kumar Tiwari
ISBN: 978-1-62948-556-0

Chapter 6

Drug Targets and Validation Techniques

Rajnish Kumar*

Amity Institute of Biotechnology, AMITY University-Uttar Pradesh,
Lucknow, Uttar Pradesh, India

Abstract

Drug target identification is vital for modern drug discovery. Due to advancements in the development of molecular docking, potential drug candidates can be obtained and in this process knowledge of drug target plays a very important role. In this chapter, various drug targets are discussed. In addition, drug targets identification methods and their validation are also introduced.

Until the year 1997, when 100,000 protein-coding sequences were hypothesized to exist in the human genome, Drews and Ryser estimated the number of molecular targets 'hit' by all marketed drug substances to be only 482 [1]. By the year 2000, the total number of potential drug targets remain confined around 500 [2]. In 2002, after the sequencing of the human genome, others arrived at ~8,000 targets of pharmacological interest, of which nearly 5,000 could be potentially hit by traditional drug substances, nearly 2,400 by antibodies and ~800 by protein pharmaceuticals [3]. On the basis of ligand-binding studies, 399 molecular targets were identified belonging to 130 protein families, and ~3,000 targets for small-molecule drugs were predicted to exist by extrapolations from the number of currently identified such targets in the human genome [4].

* Email address:12.rajnish@gmail.com, rkumar2@lko.amity.edu.

What Are Drug Targets?

When a drug molecule enters the body, it binds to the specific site of the body which leads to biological activity.

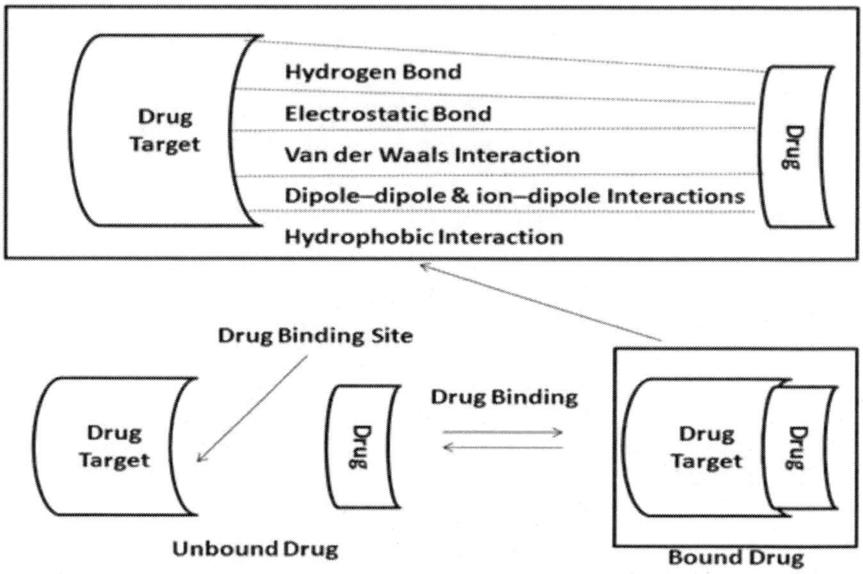

Figure 1. Drug binding to the target at the molecular level.

This specific site is known as drug targets. Drug binding to the target at molecular level is illustrated in figure 1.

Characteristics of Drug Targets

I. Drug target is a relative concept. For beginners, a drug target is, just like other biological molecules, such as a biological molecule involved in transduction pathway. The contrast between the two is their location and role in transduction pathway.
II. There can be a number of drug targets for a disease and they may not equally contribute to the pathogenesis of disease.
III. The discovery of a drug target depends upon the knowledge and understanding of disease. At times drug targets tend to change with the development of insights into biological molecules and their role in pathogenesis of certain diseases.
IV. Same drug targets can be targeted by many drugs and one drug can act on many targets.
V. More specific drug for a given target may lead to disturb the homeostasis of body, e.g., Rofecoxib is a specific COX-2 inhibitor in comparison to Aspirin. However, Rofecoxib increases cardiovascular risks.

Classification of Drug Targets

1. Receptors
2. Enzymes
3. Transporter Proteins
4. Deoxyribonucleic acids (DNAs)
5. Ribonucleic acids (RNAs)
6. Other Drug Targets

1. Receptors

A) G Protein-Coupled Receptors

G-protein coupled receptors (GPCRs) are widely expressed proteins that span the cell membrane 7 times and respond to a variety of stimuli including peptides, proteins, small organic compounds, lipids, amino acids and cations. Recent estimates predict that humans have approximately 800 GPCRs which can be grouped into five major phylogenetic families: Rhodopsin, Secretin, Adhesion, Glutamate and Frizzled/Taste2 families [5]. GPCRs from every family are highly attractive targets for pharmacological manipulation by recombinant proteins, small molecule compounds, allosteric ligands or antibodies. There are currently 46 GPCRs that serves as drug targets for the treatment of a multitude of conditions including hypertension, pain, ulcers, allergies, alcoholism, obesity, glaucoma, psychotic disorders and HIV. However, this leaves several hundreds of GPCRs as potential drug targets and among those approximately 150 are still considered orphan receptors (receptors for which the endogenous ligand has yet to be identified) [6]. One major impediment to increasing the repertoire of pharmacologically useful GPCRs is our general lack of knowledge regarding the association of a putative GPCR with a precise physiological function or disease condition. Therefore, as scientists embark on the journey of elucidating the pathophysiology of complex and poorly treatable diseases, one beneficial approach may be to identify GPCRs associated with the condition, because they may eventually translate into effective drug targets [7].

B) Ligand-Gated Ion Channels

Ion channels are important drug targets because they play a crucial role in controlling a very wide spectrum of physiological processes [8] and because their dysfunction can lead to pathophysiology [9]. Given the strong historical precedent that exists for discovering and commercializing successful drugs that modulate the activity of voltage-gated sodium, calcium, or potassium channels, or ligand-gated ion channels, new generations of therapeutic agents are expected to result from targeting this protein family. Early ion channel drug discovery used classical pharmacological approaches, in which profiling in animal models, designed to simulate human disease states, and was used to optimize compound activity, even if the nature of the molecular target was unclear. Serendipity, insight, and brute force effort drove these drug discovery efforts and resulted in a number of notable successes including successful therapies and discovery of research tools that have been invaluable in mapping out signalling pathways, purifying channel proteins, and characterizing gating mechanisms, all of which has sustained the present era of ion channel drug discovery [10, 11].

C) Receptor Tyrosine Kinases

Receptor tyrosine kinases (RTKs) are the main mediators of the signalling network that transmit extracellular signals into the cell, and control cellular differentiation and proliferation. Recent and rapid advances in our understanding of cellular signalling by receptor tyrosine kinases, in normal and malignant cells, have brought to light the potential of RTKs as selective anti-cancer targets. Their activity is normally tightly controlled and regulated. Overexpression of RTK proteins or functional alterations caused by mutations in the corresponding genes or abnormal stimulation by an autocrine growth factor loops contribute to constitutive RTK signalling, resulting in deregulated cell growth and cancer [12].

D) Immunoglobulin Like Receptors

The main receptors in the immune system are pattern recognition receptors (PRRs), Toll-like receptors (TLRs), killer activated and killer inhibitory receptors (KARs and KIRs), complement receptors, Fc receptors, B cell receptors and T cell receptors [13].

E) Nuclear Receptors

Nuclear receptors (NRs) are a large superfamily of transcription factors involved in important physiological functions such as control of embryonic development, organ physiology, cell differentiation and homeostasis. Apart from the normal physiology, nuclear receptors have been identified to play a role in many pathological processes, such as cancer, diabetes, rheumatoid arthritis, asthma or hormone resistance syndromes. Therefore, despite their already long history, these transcriptional regulators are still of great interest in modern biomedical research and drug discovery [14]. NRs are ideal targets for drug discovery. Not only do they control a myriad of biological and disease processes, but they are also regulated by small lipophilic molecules that can be easily exchanged with a drug of choice. All 48 of the NR genes in the human genome have been identified, many of their structures have been solved and their ligands identified. Their mechanism of action has been elucidated and many of their target genes have been identified [15].

2. Enzymes

Enzymes offer unique opportunities for drug design that are not available to cell surface receptors, nuclear hormone receptors, ion channels, transporters, and DNA [16]. New drugs are the products of a long drug development process, the first step of which is often the discovery of a new enzyme inhibitor. In the past the only way to discover these new inhibitors was by trial and error: screening huge libraries of compounds against a target enzyme and hoping that some useful leads would emerge.

This brute force approach is still successful and has even been extended by combinatorial chemistry approaches that quickly produce large numbers of novel compounds and high-throughput screening technology to rapidly screen these huge chemical libraries for useful inhibitors [17]. Examples of enzymes as drug targets and their corresponding common therapeutic actions are as follows [18]:

a) Oxidoreducreses	Anti-inflammatory and Antineoplastic etc.
b) Transferase	Antineoplastic and Bisphosphonate etc.
c) Hydrolases	Antihypertensive and Vasodilator etc.
d) Lyase	Antihypertensive and Diuretics etc.
e) Isomerases	Antineoplastic and Immunosuppressive etc.
f) Ligases	Antineoplastic and Antifibrinolytic etc.
g) Multiple EC groups	Antineoplastic and Antiadrenal etc.

3. Transporter Proteins

Ions and small organic molecules are often too polar to penetrate the cellular membrane on their own, and require a transport protein. Trans-membrane solute transporters may be divided into channels that function as selective pores opening in response to a chemical or electrophysiological stimulus, thus allowing movement of a solute down an electrochemical gradient, and active carrier proteins which use an energy-producing process to translocate a substrate against a concentration gradient [19]. Transporter proteins have a recognition site making them specific for a particular solute. The human genome contains many different transporters, including those responsible for the transport of glucose and amino acids into cells, transport of ions and organic molecules by the renal tubules, transport of Ca 2+ and Na + out of cells, uptake of neurotransmitters and neurotransmitter precursors into nerve terminals and vesicles, and transporters involved in multidrug resistance. Drugs may exert their effect by binding to transporters and either inhibiting transport of the solute or functioning as a false substrate for the transport process. Examples of such drugs include the antidepressant drugs that inhibit the neuronal transporters for noradrenaline and serotonin [20, 21], probenecid which inhibits the weak acid transporter protein in the renal tubule [22], loop diuretics inhibiting the Na +/K+/2Cl– co-transporter of the loop of Henle [23], and the irreversible inhibitor of the H+/K+ ATPase (proton pump) of the gastric mucosa, omeprazole [24]. Examples of Transporter Proteins are voltage-gated ion channels, solute carriers, active transporters, auxiliary transport units etc.

4. Deoxyribonucleic Acids (DNAs)

DNA can be targeted via various means like intercalation of drug into double helical structure, alkylation, cleavage etc.

Intercalation

The DNA double helix model has major and minor groove. The major and minor groove binders are found to be settled in between the helix, thereby destroying the molecule and stopping DNA replication phenomenon.

Example: Proflavine intercalates in DNA forming electrostatic bonds with oxygen of a phosphate group and Van der Waal forces with nitrogenous base (figure 1).

Alkylation

Drugs lead to alkylation of DNA strands (proton loving) and ultimately inhibit the transcription. Such drugs are known as alkylating agents (electron loving).

Alkylation may lead to mono-alkylation, Intra-strand cross linking or Inter-strand cross linking of DNA (figure 2).

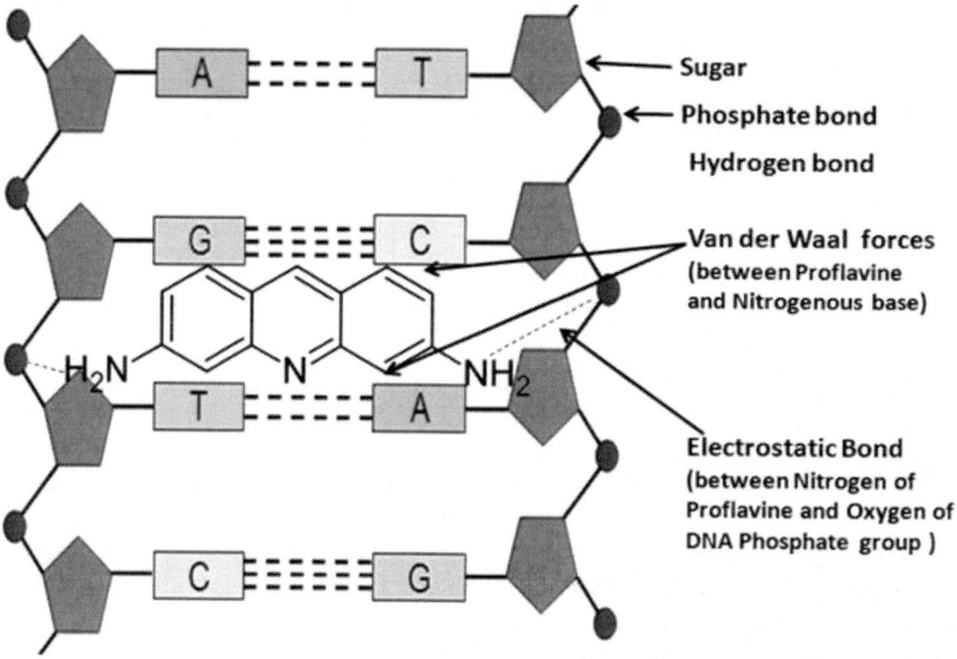

Figure 1. Intercalation of Proflavine with DNA by means of Electrostatic bond (between Nitrogen of Proflavine and Oxygen of DNA Phosphate group) and Van der Waal forces (between Proflavine and Nitrogenous base).

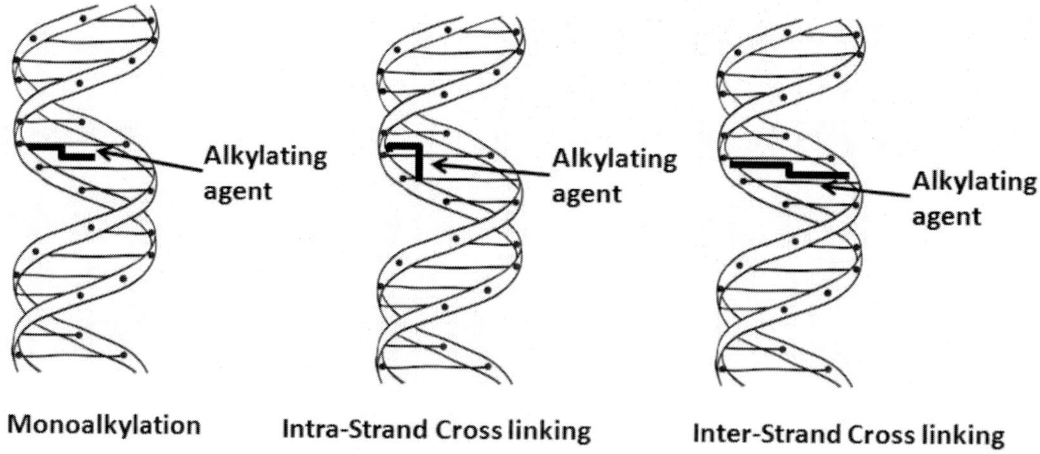

Figure 2. DNA cross linking using alkylating agents.

Cleavage

If we want to destroy the helix then chelating mechanism is used which breaks the DNA strand and cleave the backbone (Phosphate linkage). Normally the minor groove binder is used for cutting the DNA strands. The strand cutting agent should be hydrophobic in nature and should give rise to active species.

Example: Calicheamycin √$_1$ is used as antitumor drug. It binds to the minor groove of DNA and acts as a chain cutter (figure 3).

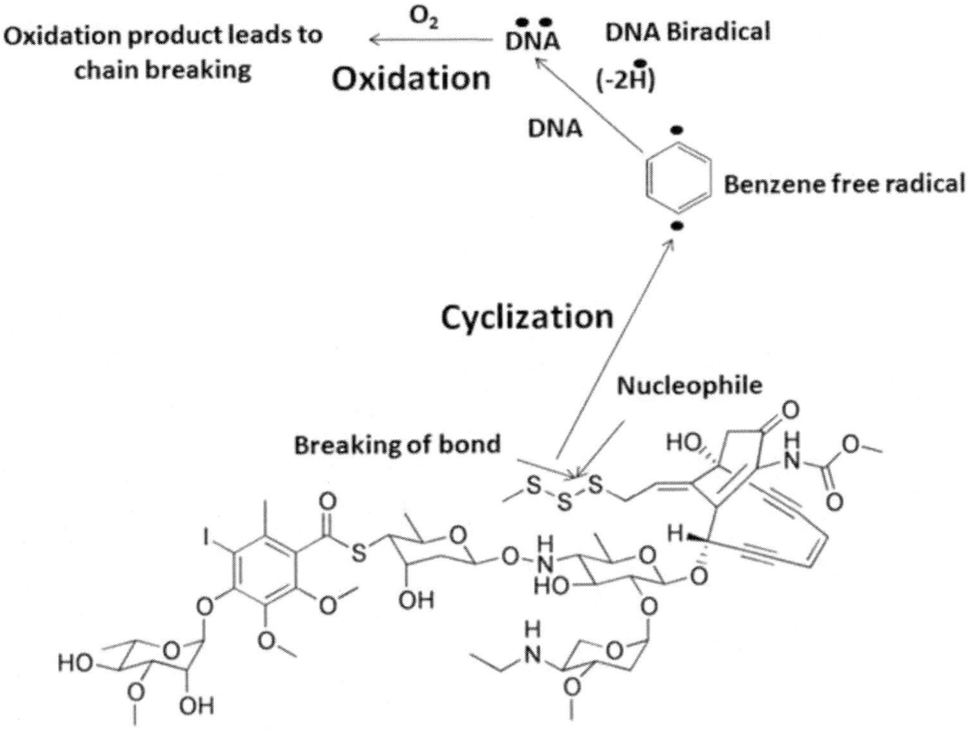

Figure 3. Mechanism of DNA cleavage by Calicheamycin √$_1$.

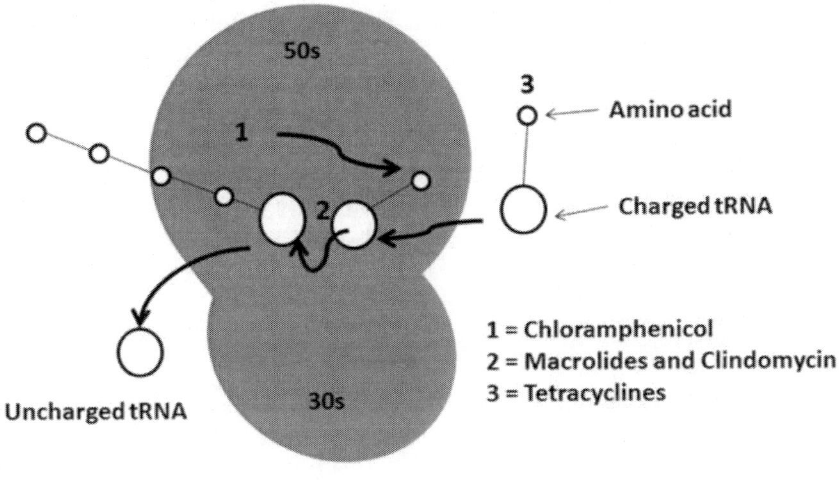

Figure 4. Illustration of mechanism of action of some antibiotics with reference of RNA as drug target

5. Ribonucleic Acids (RNAs)

RNA can be used as drug targets. Many antibiotic agents work by targeting RNA.
Example: Chloramphenicol, Tetracyclines, Erythromycin, Streptomycin etc.

Chloramphenicol, Macrolides and Clindamycin binding targets are close to each other on 50s ribosomal subunit of the bacterial ribosome (figure 4).

Chloramphenicol indirectly inhibits transpeptidation (catalysed by peptidyl transferase) by blocking the binding of aminoacyl moiety of the charged tRNA molecule to the acceptor site on the ribosome mRNA complex. Thus the peptide at the donor site cannot be transformed to the amino acid acceptor.

The peptidyl tRNA at the donor site donates the growing peptide chain to aminoacyl tRNA at the acceptor site in the reaction catalysed by peptidyl transferase.

6. Other Drug Targets

Cell membrane as drug target e.g., Polymixin B (Antifungal agent)
Lipid carriers as drug target e.g., Vancomycin (Used in place of penicillin)

Carbohydrates as drug target e.g., Glustat, Zavesca, Glyset, and Glucobay mimic the transition state of the hydrolytic reaction and are used for the treatment of diabetes [25].

Drug Target Identification

Drug target identification methods can be distinctly divided into three types [26]:

1. Direct biochemical methods
2. Genetic interaction methods
3. Computational inference methods

Direct methods involve labeling the protein or small molecule of interest, incubation of the two populations and direct detection of binding, usually following some type of wash procedure [27]. Genetic manipulation can also be used to identify protein targets by modulating presumed targets in cells, thereby changing small-molecule sensitivity [28]. In contrast, the target hypotheses can be produced by computational inference, using pattern recognition for comparative analysis of small-molecule effects to those of known reference molecules. A combination of these methods is used now a days. Where, scientists use both direct measurements and inferences to test highly specific target hypotheses.

Direct Biochemical Methods

Biochemical affinity purification gives a direct method to find target proteins that bind small molecules. As they are based on physical interactions mammalian or human proteins, these approaches can give information about the molecular mechanisms of efficiency or toxicity of relevant human disease. Biochemical approaches can complement the molecular optimization especially when the three-dimensional structure about the target is known.

Some basic steps to a direct biochemical method:

- Extraction of molecules from source
- Compound immobilized on a column
- Elution of affinity chromatographic fractions
- Monitoring chromatographic fractions for enzyme activity

Challenges with above approach are a requirement of the large amount of extracts, stringent wash conditions and pre-fractionation of extracts. Number of targets have been identified in natural and synthetic small molecules. Example: Mechanism of teratogenic side effect of Thalidomide.

Genetic Interaction Methods

Target identification based on genetic methods gives the relative ease of working with DNA and RNA to perform large-scale measurements and modifications. These methods are based on the principle of genetic interaction, relying on the scheme of genetic suppressors or enhancers to create target hypotheses. Gene knockout organisms, RNAi and small molecules with well-defined mechanisms can each be used to modify the functions of putative targets uncovering dependencies on activity. Example: A promising genetics-based technique for target identification involves combining results from small-molecule and RNAi perturbations. This approach enables parallel testing of small-molecule and RNAi libraries for induction of the same cellular phenotype, RNAi experiments can be performed on a genome-wide scale to find phenotypes similar to those induced by small molecules [29].

Computational Inference Methods

Computational methods are used to find out protein targets of small molecules. Moreover, they give analytical support for genetic and proteomic techniques. These methods are also used to discover novel targets for existing drugs, with the aim of putting a drug to new reposition or explaining off-target effects. Profiling methods depend on pattern recognition to combine results of parallel or multiplexed experiments [30]. Example: COMPARE algorithm, has allowed scientists to hypothesize new activities for small molecules.

Drug Target Validation

Drug target validation is first step for drug design and development. A novel target validation is the foundation of completely new drug exploration. New drug target validation may prove to be a substantial help to new drug research and development. In addition, it provides great insight into the pathogenesis of diseases that are target related.

Drug target validation can be divided into six different steps [31]:

1. Discovery of relevant bio-molecule.
2. Evaluation of its potential to be a drug target.
3. Measurement of biological activity (requires a design of bioassay).
4. Construction of a high-throughput screen.
5. Hit identification using screening process
6. Evaluation of the hits.

A target should be selected in such a way that upon pharmacological modulation, it provides meaningful efficacy and acceptable safety for specific human disease in long-term clinical usage. Basic knowledge of the disease and pathogenic pathway helps in a selecting a suitable biological molecule.

The next step is to get the readout of biological activity. Bioassay of biomolecule under investigation helps substantially.

Once an assay that measures the biological activity of the target, by some direct or indirect means, has been developed, then compounds can be tested in the bioassay to see if they inhibit, enhance, or do nothing to this activity [32].

After bioassay, the next key step is the beginning of a high-throughput screening (HTS) method.

HTS is a robust method to screen a large number of samples. Preliminary, screening gives 'hits', which can be rescreened to find out more positive results. These rescreened hits are then investigated in terms of their chemical characteristics, i.e., stability, toxicity (both *in-vivo* and *in-vitro*), and its pharmacological evaluation. Effects in cells and animal models are studied in particular.

If the hit obtained from HTS exhibits a pharmacological effect in animal models, then it may be promising. However, most of the times 'hit' displays no effect in an animal model and care should be taken while interpreting the results.

References

[1] Drews, J. & Ryser, S. (1997). The role of innovation in drug development. *Nature Biotechnol.* 15, 1318–1319.

[2] Drews, J. (2000). Drug discovery: a historical perspective. *Science*, 287(5460):1960-1964.

[3] Burgess, J. & Golden, J. (2002). Cracking the druggable genome. *Bio-IT World* [online], http://www.bio-itworld. com/archive/100902/firstbase.html.

[4] Hopkins, A. & Groom, C. (2002). The druggable genome. *Nature Rev. Drug Discov.* 1, 727–730.

[5] Gloriam, D.E., Fredriksson, R., Schioth, H.B. (2007). The G protein-coupled receptor subset of the rat genome. *BMC Genomics*. 8, 338.

[6] Lagerstrom, M.C., Schioth , H.B. (2008). Structural diversity of G protein-coupled receptors and significance for drug discovery. *Nat. Rev. Drug Discov.* 7, 339–357.

[7] Dunworth, W.P., Caron, K.M. (2009). G protein-coupled receptors as potential drug targets for lymphangiogenesis and lymphatic vascular diseases. *Arterioscler. Thromb. Vasc. Biol.* 29, 650–656.

[8] Hille, B. 2001. *Ion Channels of Excitable Membranes.* Third edition. Sinauer Associates, Inc., Sunderland, MA. 814.

[9] Ashcroft, F. 2000. *Ion Channels and Disease.* Academic Press, San Diego, CA. 481.

[10] Garcia, M.L., and Kaczorowski, G.J. (2005). Potassium channels as targets for therapeutic intervention. *Sci. STKE.* 302, 46.

[11] Gregory J. Kaczorowski, Owen B. McManus, Birgit T. Priest, Maria L. Garcia. (2008). Ion Channels as Drug Targets: The Next GPCRs. *J. Gen. Physiol.* 131(5), 399–405.

[12] Bennasroune, A., Gardin, A., Aunis, D., Crémel, G., Hubert, P. (2004). Tyrosine kinase receptors as attractive targets of cancer therapy. *Crit. Rev. Oncol. Hematol.* 50(1):23-38.

[13] Doan, T., Melvold, R., Viselli, S., Waltenbaugh, C. (2007). *Lippincott's Illustrated Reviews: Immunology,* edt. 1, 20p. Lippincott Williams & Wilkins, Philadelphia.

[14] Ottow, E. and Weinmann, H. (2008). *Nuclear Receptors as Drug Targets.* pp 1-24, WILEY-VCH Verlag GmbH & Co. KGaA, Weinheim.

[15] Sladek, F.M. (2003). Nuclear receptors as drug targets: new developments in coregulators, orphan receptors and major therapeutic areas. *Opin. Ther.* 7(5), 1-6.

[16] Robertson, J.G. (2005). Mechanistic basis of enzyme-targeted drugs. *Biochemistry*, 44 5561–5571.

[17] Koppitz, M., Eis, K. (2006). Automated medicinal chemistry. *Drug Discov. Today.* 11 (11): 561–68.

[18] Imming, P., Sinning, C., Meyer, A. (2006). Drugs, their targets and the nature and number of drug targets. *Nature Rev. Drug Discov.*5, 821–834.

[19] Saier, M.H., Jr. (2000) A functional-phylogenetic classification system for transmembrane solute transporters. *Microbiol. Mol. Biol. Rev.* 64, 354-411.

[20] Rothman, R.B., Silverthorn, M.L., Glowa, J.R., Matecka, D., Rice, K.C., Carroll, F.I., Partilla, J.S., Uhl, G.R., Vandenbergh, D.J., Dersch, C.M. (1998). Studies of the biogenic amine transporters. VII. Characterization of a novel cocaine binding site identified with [125I]RTI-55 in membranes prepared from human, monkey and guinea pig caudate. *Synapse.* 28(4):322-38.

[21] Yamashita, M., Fukushima, S., Shen, H.W., Hall, F.S., Uhl, G.R., Numachi, Y., Kobayashi, H., Sora, I. (2006). Norepinephrine transporter blockade can normalize the prepulse inhibition de"cits found in dopamine transporter knockout mice. *Neuropsychopharmacology* 31, 2132–2139.

[22] Race, J. E., Grassl, S. M., Williams, W. J., Holtzman, E. J. (1999). Molecular cloning and characterization of two novel human renal organic anion transporters (hOAT1 and hOAT3). *Biochem. Biophys. Res. Commun.* 255: 508-514.

[23] Masereel, B., Lohrmann, E., Schynts, M., Pirotte, B., Greger, R., Delarge, J. (1992). Design synthesis and biological activity of a series of torasemide derivatives, potent blockers of the Na+ 2 Cl− K+ cotransporter: in vitro study. *J. Pharm. Pharmacol.* 44, 589–93.

[24] Diogo, F. A., Santos, P.S., Duque, A.S., Cezário, R.C., Gontijo Filho, P.P. (2006) Experimental model in the qualitative and quantitative assessment of non-Helicobacter gastric microflora under proton pump inhibitors action. *Acta Cir. Bras.* 21, 279-284.

[25] http://www.cdriindia.org/Ihighlightconent/RND2010/R02-10.pdf [accessed on 12-05-2013].

[26] Schenone, M., Dančík, V., Wagner, B.K., Clemons, P.A. (2013). Target identification and mechanism of action in chemical biology and drug discovery. *Nature Chemical Biology*. 9, 232–240.

[27] Burdine, L., Kodadek, T. (2004). Target identification in chemical genetics: the (often) missing link. *Chem. Biol.* 11, 593–597.

[28] Zheng, X.S., Chan, T.F., Zhou, H.H. (2004). Genetic and genomic approaches to identify and study the targets of bioactive small molecules. *Chem. Biol.* 11, 609–618.

[29] Moffat, J. et al. (2006). A lentiviral RNAi library for human and mouse genes applied to an arrayed viral high-content screen. *Cell.* 124, 1283–1298.

[30] Feng, Y., Mitchison, T.J., Bender, A., Young, D.W. & Tallarico, J.A. (2009). Multi-parameter phenotypic profiling: using cellular effects to characterize small-molecule compounds. *Nat. Rev. Drug Discov.* 8, 567–578.

[31] Chen, X.P., Du, G.H. (2007). Target validation: A door to drug discovery. *Drug Discov. Ther.* 1(1), 23-29.

[32] John, G.H., Martyn, N.B., Bristol-Myers, S. (2002). High throughput screening for lead discovery. Burger's Medicinal Chemistry and Drug Discovery, sixth edition, Vol 2: *Drug Discovery and Drug Development*, Wiley Press, pp37-70.

In: Introduction to Drug Designing and Development
Editors: R. Kumar, A. Sharma and R. Kumar Tiwari
ISBN: 978-1-62948-556-0

Chapter 7

Screening of Drugs

Swati Srivastava*
Lovely Professional University- Phagwara, Punjab, India

Abstract

The screening of drugs is an important technique to access unique drug candidates during the drug discovery process. Various computational software or tools have been developed for easy and fast screening of drugs against a chemical library. To understand various aspects of the drug screening processes, one has to understand the fundamental concepts of the computational approaches which are running behind these techniques. This chapter deals with the comprehensive analysis of the drug screening processes and various available methods till date.

Advances in In-silico drug designing and Information technologies have significantly improved the drug design processes. The advance technology involves Combinatorial Chemistry, Cheminformatics, Genomics, Proteomics, automation, various screening process such as High-throughput screening and Virtual Screening has increased the lead generation process and further enhanced Drug development process.

Combinatorial Chemistry has emerged as an innovative technique for synthesizing multiple compounds at a single instance. It has reduced drug development cost and time as large populations of structurally different molecules called chemical libraries can be prepared at one instance [1]. These libraries need to be screened with the help of various In vitro and In vivo techniques.

Drug screening is a process which is used to identify a putative drug by screening of large chemical libraries on the basis of their ability to interact with the biological target. The experimental approaches for screening of billions of biological compounds are still arduous task, and therefore computational approaches emerge as important alternatives. Such as a

* Email: swati051@gmail.com.

High throughput screening, Virtual screening, Robotic techniques etc. to filter out lead molecule which has possibility from "Hit- to Lead". Pharmaceutical industries are adopting this technology for the faster and efficient discovery of new drugs. Drug screening is useful to predict putative binding affinity between the ligand and target. Drug Permeability, solubility and other key properties are always estimated prior drug administration especially for oral available compounds [2] these are screened by various computational and experimental methods before selecting candidate lead and moving to the next stage of Drug development. It has been proved that Absorption, Distribution, Metabolism, Excretion and Toxicity (ADMET) are the key properties which have to be primarily focused during the screening process.

ADME Property

Chris Lipinski and coworkers [3] analysed a subset of 2245 drugs from World Drug Index (WDI) to understand Common molecular features of orally available drug. They then concluded that better absorption of a drug molecule occurs when

- The Molecular Weight (MW) is less than 500 Dalton.
- The log P value is less than 5.
- HBD (Hydrogen Bond Donor) should be less than 5
- HBA (Hydrogen Bond Acceptor) should be less than 10.

As the above rule is formulated by Lipinski were in a multiple of five, therefore this rule is now known as "Lipinski Rule of Five". In addition to above rule other reactant based properties can be used to filter drug from whole library. such the presence of highly flexible unsubstituted , unbranched alkyl chains e.g., more than 8 CH2 groups, compounds which exceed maximum accepted numbers of rings or ionisable groups. Drugs which are reactive towards protein target should also be avoided, such as Michael acceptors, ketones, aldehydes and all types of suicidal inhibitors. [4]

Virtual Screening

Virtual Screening (VS) [5, 6] has emerged as an adaptive response to massive throughput synthesis and screening paradigm. This method is used for accurate prediction of Binding affinity, pharmacokinetic properties etc., to filter lead molecules. Massive compounds generated by Combinatorial chemistry are filtered or screened with the help of Virtual screening method (figure 1). Bioactive conformers are derived either by X-ray or by NMR techniques. We can compute or predict binding affinity of Ligand molecules with these conformers by various Ligand based Virtual Screening methods which are included in various sequential computational phases in order to rank ligand molecules by 3D similarity searching or Pharmacophore pattern matching [7]. Structure based drug screening methods are used to dock the known target molecules against unknown ligands. This leads to the analysis of electrostatic and steric properties. It can automatically analyse the large number of chemical compounds against protein-binding or active sites.

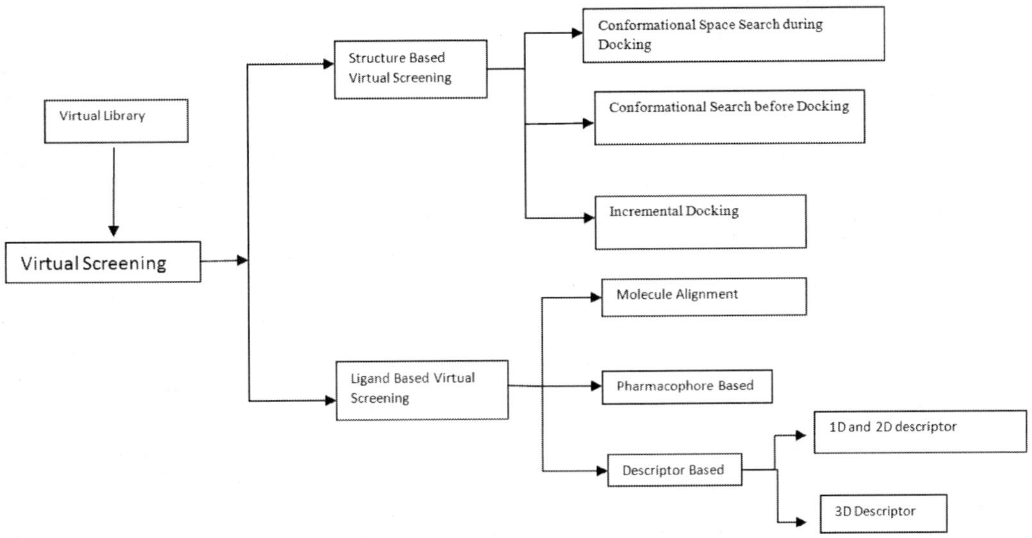

Figure1. Virtual Screening and its types.

Methods of Virtual Screening

1. Structure Based Virtual Screening

Structure based virtual screening can be done if target is known. If drug target is known then various docking algorithms can be used to dock ligand with the known target and then rank them based on interaction energy. This method involves various automated and fast docking algorithm simultaneously docking various chemical compounds. Target sites can be anything like various transporters, carriers, active sites in enzymes, an assembly site with another macromolecule are communication site, etc. Energy of target and chemical compounds are calculated based on the interaction which involves hydrophobic, hydrophilic, hydrogen bond, electrostatic and Van der Waal's forces (Non-interacting forces).

For Structural Based Virtual Screening mainly docking technique is used.

Docking

Docking is a technique by which one can predict the preferred orientation of the two molecules that makes complex by their interaction [8]. The docking methods involve two steps:

1. Searching Method: Which involves exploring various conformation space of Target site, analysing the binding site and its characteristics where the Ligand molecule will go and bind.

2. Scoring Function: After Docking has occurred the interaction of both Ligand and Target are ranked based on the interaction energies and Binding Affinity.

Both Searching and scoring methods are tightly coupled in Docking. Hence it is important to rank ligand based on highest ordered conformation with high Binding affinity and least energy with receptor to give them "Drug Likeness" property. Some of the docking tools are listed in table 1 for reference.

Searching Methods

Searching Method involved in docking technique is of three types:

a) *Conformational Space Search during Docking*: This method involves optimization of small molecule conformations and its orientation in the binding site. Binding energy, affinity etc. are calculated by placing the ligand in active site of receptor. Stochastic algorithms such as Monte Carlo Method, Simulated Annealing or Genetic algorithm is generally employed due to the complexity of this combined optimization technique [9].
b) *Conformational Search before Docking:* In this method, ligands are not placed in the binding site of receptor. GRID methodology is used to map the binding site. In GRID method, suitable probes are used to calculate various force fields and possible interactions. All low-energy rigid conformers are placed on the binding site and only six rotational and translational degrees of freedom are calculated. Programs like Slide and Fred involves this Docking method.
c) *Incremental Docking:* This method involves breaking of ligand molecules at various feasible rotating bonds and then docking these fragments at different favourable positions in binding starting from base fragment or the largest fragment. Possible orientation of ligand fragments with better docking ability are screened and then the chain is grown in various orientations and scored till the entire ligand is assembled back. Some of the program which uses this technique is FlexX, Hammerhead, HOOK.

Scoring Functions

Various scoring functions are used for docking. Firstly, it helps in calculating energy for different poses of the same ligand in receptor-binding site. Secondly, it helps in ranking diverse sets of compounds after docking based on their binding affinity in receptor-binding site. Ligand-binding to receptor are governed by kinetics and thermodynamics. The scoring function is calculated by various interaction energies such as hydrophobic effects, Van der Waal's and dispersion interactions, hydrogen bonding, steric, electrostatic interactions and solvation effects. [10, 11]

Various available scoring functions are categorized as:

a) *Force-field based-* force field describes the potential energy of a system in the form of mathematical functions. It sums up contribution of different Molecular Interaction Forces between ligands and target atom. Since these scoring functions are shaped in order to model enthalpic gas phase for energetic and structure, they do not have the ability to calculate entropy and solvation terms. [12].

b) *Empirical based-* Empirical functions are based on approximations similar to force fields. Various coefficients are calculated based on regression analysis using experimentally determined binding energies and potentially from X-ray structural information. These include non-enthalpic values also.
c) *Knowledge based-* this scoring function is based on ligand-target complexes, calculating simple atomic interactions-pairs interactions. Due to its computational simplicity it is efficient in screening large dataset of compounds.
d) *Consensus scoring-* Consensus Scoring method utilizes information from different scores to balance errors in single scores and enhances the probability of identifying 'true' ligands. X-CSCORE, which combines GOLD-like, DOCK-like, Chem-score, PMF and FlexXscore are some exclusive examples. They utilize consensus scoring function. [13, 14].

Table 1. Tools and Software currently used for Docking

S. No	Program	Methodology	Web site	References
1	DOCK	Determines the binding modes between target and ligand complex, can search the database of the ligands for compounds that can inhibit the enzymatic activity, bind the particular protein, bind nucleic acid target.	http://dock.compbio.ucsf.edu	15
2	AutoDock	Able to predict the binding ability of the lignad with known 3D target molecule. It uses Monte Carlo simulation annealing techniques, genetic and Lamarckian genetic algorithm.	http://autodock.scripps.edu	16-75
3	GOLD	Flexible docking between ligand and target, It uses genetic algorithm for conformational search, accuracy and reliability is very high.	http://www.ccdc.cam.ac.uk/ products/life_sciences/ gold	17-18
4	Darwin	To optimize the molecular confirmation it uses a combination of genetic algorithm and gradient minimization search strategy. CHARM is used for energy calculation.	http://citeseerx.ist.psu.edu	19
5	FlexX	Predicts the geometry of protein-ligand complex by using pose clustering algorithm,	http://www.biosolveit.de/FlexX	20,21
6	GLIDE	Grid Based Ligand Docking with Energetics, uses a series of hierarchical filters for searching conformational location.	http://web.chem.ucsb.edu/~kalju/chem162/public/docking_glide.html	22

2. Ligand Based Virtual Screening

Ligand Based Virtual Screening is also known as 'Neighborhood-behavior search'. It gives results based on closely related active molecules and poses same or common

Pharmacophore (substructure). The similarity searching method is adopted which is carried out based on descriptors. It has been observed that compounds with similar Pharmacophore produce similar effects. The Pharmacophore generated by similarity searching are ranked by various algorithms based on scores.

3. Pharmacophore Based Screening Method

Alignment is generally carried out for small molecules. Here small molecules are superimposed on each other and similarity is checked. Superimposed structure are ranked and screened. For superimposition generally reference molecule is taken as rigid or flexible molecule but the test molecule is generally preferred as flexible. Some of the tools which can be used for superimposition are Flexs algorithm [23] here reference molecule is considered as rigid. This algorithm is based on incremental construction procedure. In this method flexible ligand is broken down into small fragments and base fragment is identified first and then remaining are added based on stepwise manner.

4. Descriptor Based Screening Method

The molecular descriptor is the final result of a logic and mathematical procedure which transforms chemical information encoded within a symbolic representation of a molecule into a useful number or the result of some standardized experiment [24]. The descriptors are generated by statistical correlation techniques like Quantitative Structure Activity Relationship (QSAR). QSAR, Lipinski Rule of five and various ADMET are used for calculating descriptor which in turn provides a useful approach for drug designing. The descriptors are further grouped in three categories based on dimensions and information provided such as 1D, 2D and 3D. These may be further linear, scalar or nonlinear. Various programs are available which helps in calculating descriptor for a chemical molecule taking dataset input as ‘sdf’ or ‘mol’ format.

i) 1D and 2D descriptor

The chemical formula constitutes for 1D descriptor such as Molecular Weight, Molecular refractivity, Log P, atom number, atom type etc., where as Chemsketch draw or chemical structure represented in graphical form constitutes for 2D descriptor. In addition to the information provided by 1D descriptor it provides more information such number of Hydrogen bond donors., Hydrogen bond acceptors, number of rotatable bonds, number of rings etc.

ii) 3D descriptor

3D descriptors are calculated based on the spatial or conformational arrangement of molecules in space. It contains all conformation, topological and Microscopic information. Apart from the information provide above in 1D and 2D descriptor. It also provides information for Molecular Volume, surface area and Dipole Moment. Various can be used to generate the 3D structure such as 3D-FEATURE [25], CORINA [26].

5. Machine Learning Techniques for Screening

Machine learning is an artificial network approach, which is widely used in various fields of science and technology. Classification is an indispensable issue on machine learning. It involves the categorization of dataset relying on one or more characteristics. Learning algorithm constructs a classifier for a given data set to separate data into discrete classes based on the properties associated. The constructed classifier is then enforced on the unknown dataset to predict class labels. There are number of methods present for classification of a given data set. Apart from various statistical techniques and learning method there are various algorithms such as genetic algorithm which are used for virtual screening process. Other examples are an Artificial Neural Network (ANN) and Support Vector Machine (SVM).

Support Vector Machine

It is an efficient computational machine learning technique developed by Vladimir Vapnik. SVM is generally used for Binary classification as it gives best outcome; many endavours were made to use SVM for multiclass classification. SVM basically constructs a hyperplane in a boundless dimensional space; this hyperplane is favorable in classifying the data and for regression analysis. It follows a plan of separating data samples in different classes leading to maximization of margin to different classes (figure 2).

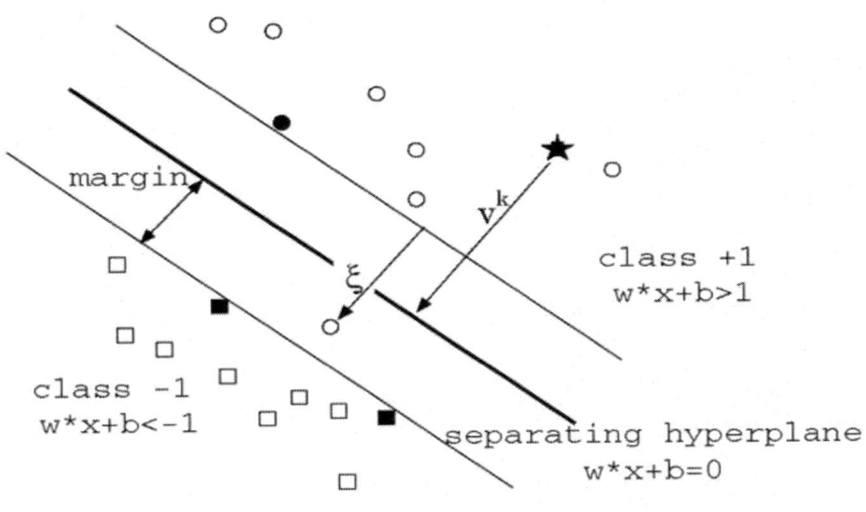

Figure 2. Binary Classification of linearly separable data by Support Vector Machine.

Let $\{x_i, y_i\}$ be training set for data x and class labels are y, $y_i \in \{-1, +1\}$. If there are linearly separable data then it is facile to separate these two data by a linear hyper plane with the help of SVM. With the help of linear hyper plane using maximum margin it will separate two classes of training set, for the point lying on a hyper plane it can be elucidated as (1)

$$W.X + b = 0 \quad (1)$$

where

'W' represents perpendicular to hyper plane

[|b| / |w|] represents normal to the distance of a hyper plane which is coming from an origin. If d_+ and d indicates the distances from the closest points to ahyper plane in classes +1 and -1. The points are contained by the support vectors and other training points are present to the side different from supportive vectors. The minimum distance between different classes was used to separate support vectors, i.e., separated distance is [2/ ||w||]. 'w' and 'b' can be extracted as a classification rule for SVM:

[XW + b >=1 (positive)]
[XW +b <= -1 (negative)]

If the training dataset points are nonlinear then result of both of the above given equations are not satisfactory at the synonymous time. Some slack variables are employed such as ξ_i's (non-negative) to solve this problem giving soft margin linear SVM. These slack variables are used in imparting flexibility in constraints for separating outliers which cannot be linearly separable during support vector design. A cost factor C is introduced which minimizes error while training and maximizes the margin. The cost factor C ranges from 2^{-5} to 2^{15}.

SVM apart from classification it provides an excellent generalization for different types of problems of time series calculation and regression.

SVM Kernels

SVM kernels are used to clarify the basic function. There are many kernels available in SVM some of this includes: Linear, Sigmoid, Polynomial kernel, RBF and Gaussian kernel.

Linear Kernel: This is most simple kernel available in SVM. It is used to classify linearly separable datasets using a single hyper plane. This kernel can be depicted as:

$$K(x, y) = < x, y >$$

Sigmoid Kernel: This kernel also performs well as above kernels. It can be depicted as follows:

$$K(x, y) = \tanh(gamma * < x, y > + coeff)$$

Polynomial Kernel: This kernel's performance depends upon the value of the degree. This kernel can be represented as:

$$K(x, y) = (gamma * < x, y > + coeff)\deg ree$$

Radial Basis Function (RBF): This is most commonly used Kernel for SVM classification. It maps high dimensional space, therefore data become linear separable. This kernel can be further represented as:

$$K(x, y) = \exp(-gamma * \|x - y\|^2)$$

Artificial Neural Network (ANN)

Artificial neural network is a computational model. It is derived from structural and functional specifications of biological neural networks. It comprises of interconnected processing elements called as "neurons". It comprises of different layers with first layer called input layer, sending data to model. Outer layer is known as the output layer showing or giving result. The central layer is the hidden layer; which is not visible to the user hiding all kinds of internal processing of the network and may comprise of any number, but generally 2 layers are good. In this output generated by one hidden layer is considered as input for another hidden layer. The output generated by the final hidden layer is considered as input for the output layer, which functions as finally emitting the prediction result. There is a multi-layer feed forward network which is having many number of hidden layers. As a biological neural network is interconnected via synapse, same here the neural network are interconnected by a synapses which stores units represented as "weights", applied in manipulating the data while calculation. The Network learns by a learning algorithm called as supervised learning algorithm. For obtaining an expected result of this algorithm synaptic weights are modified. Here each neuron as an input calculate the product of weight and inputs such as w_ix_i for i=1, 2, 3........... n. w_i represents weights and x_i represents inputs. This adduct is, used to estimate the activation function of ANN represented by the equation.

$X_i = w_ix_i$;
Whereas $Y = +1$ if $X >= \theta$.
-1 if $X <= \theta$.

The above equation is sign function, applied in various kinds of network model like: sigmoid, linear and step function. The merest form of feed forward ANN is: linear classifier (Perceptron) which is bi-classifier (figure 3). It maps its given input "x" vector to:

$f(x) = 1$ when $w_ix_i + b > 0$
$f(x) = 0$ else.
'b' is bias constant, independent of any input value.

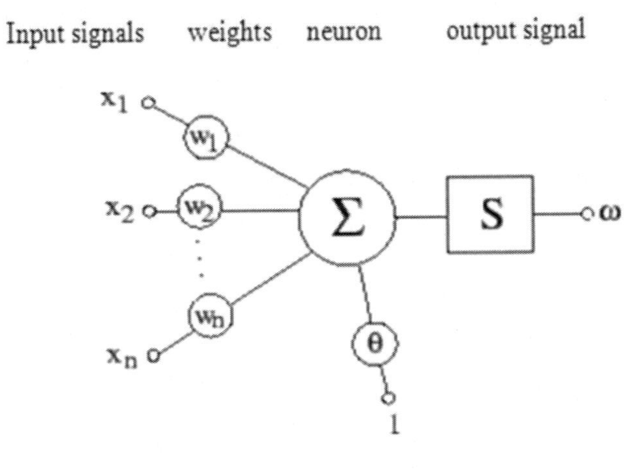

Figure 3. A simple neural network: Perceptron.

Classification by Back-propagation

A back-propagation NN is learning algorithm. During learning process the network adjusts its weights for anticipating correct class label for input data set. This learning algorithm has two phases: learning phase and back-propagation phase. Firstly, in training input data is subjected to network by input layer. It is then transferred layer to layer till the output is predicted via the output layer. Weights are assigned ranging from -0.5 to 0.5. Now each unit in network is associated with some bias. This association is again initialized randomly.

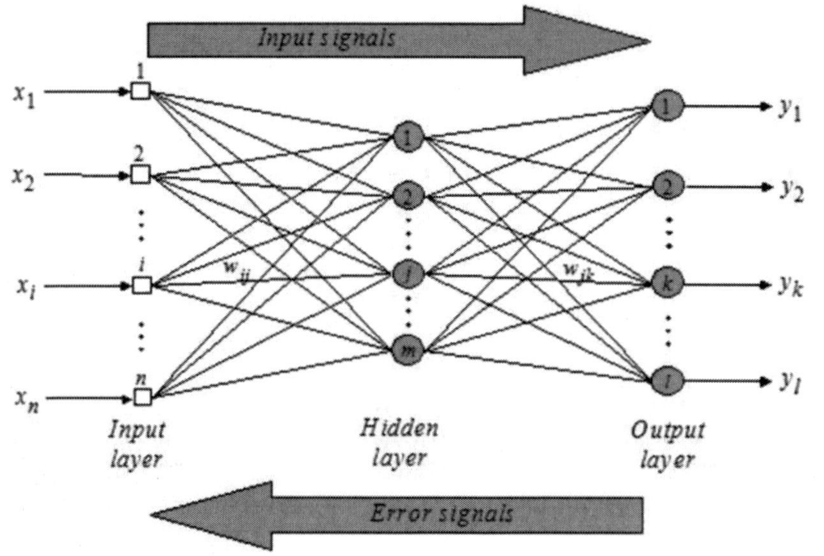

Figure 4. Error Back-propagation.

The input and output of neurons are determined by adduct of weighted signal and bias. In this method class labels are the target value of the dataset we are having. After input is subjected to the unchanged data, the values of the weights are reformed based on the variance between desired and actual output. Weights are modified to decrease the rms error calculated and then modified weights are propagated backwards through the network's output layer to the input layer, this phenomenon is called as the Back-propagation (figure 4).

The process continues till weights converge and wrongly classified data in previous process is lower than the threshold or till the number of epoch get over than prescribed. The training process stops and the time spend on training the network decides the back-propagation efficiency. Before training the network user should elucidate the topology of the network i.e., total no. of input, hidden and output layers. Normalizing the data feature is also urged, so as to maximize accuracy using network for a good classification and prediction.

Conclusion

Virtual screening has emerged as a potential technique for drug discovery process. Numbers of Bioinformatics methods have been discovered for fast screening of drugs to get putative hits. Various methods and software packages are available for the target and ligand based drug designing. However, lots of issues still have to be considered for effective use of the virtual screening in drug discovery process like pharmacokinetics, pharmacodynamics and toxicity etc. Machine learning approaches are effectively being used to accelerate the process of drug screening.

References

[1] Pandeya, S. N., Thakkar, D. (2005). Advances in Contemporary Research: Combinatorial chemistry: Anovel method in Drug discovery and its application. *Indian Journal of Chemistry* , 44B, 335-348.

[2] Anonymous. (2000). Waiver of in vivo bioavailability and bioequivalence studies for immediate-release solid oral dosage forms based on a biopharmaceutics classification system. URL: http://www.fda.gov/cder/OPS/BCS_guidance.htm.

[3] Lipinski, C. A.; Lombardo, F.; Dominy, B. W.; Feeney, P. J. (1997). Experimental and computational approaches to estimate solubility and permeability in drug discovery and development settings. *Adv. Drug Deliv. Rev.* 23, 3-25.

[4] Rishton, G. (2001). Personal communication.

[5] Walters, W. P.; Stahl, M. T.; Murcko, M. A., (1998). Virtual screening - an overview. *Drug DiscoveryToday,* 3, 160-178.

[6] Fox, S., Farr-Jones, S., Yund, M.A. (1999). High throughput screening for drug discovery: continually transitioning into new technology. *J. Biomol. Screening*, 4, 183-186.

[7] Kitchen, D. B., Decornez, H., Furr, J. R., Bajorath, J., (2004). Docking and scoring in virtual screening for drug discovery: methods and applications. *Nature,* 3, 935-948.

[8] Cohen; C.N. (1996). Guidebook on Molecular Modeling in Drug Design, edition 1, *Academic Press*, New York.

[9] Taylor, R.D., Jewsbury, P.J., Essex, J.W., (2002). A review of protein-small molecule docking methods. *J. Comput Aided Mol. Des. 16,* 151–166.

[10] Perez, C., Ortiz, A.R., (2001). Evaluation of docking functions for protein-ligand docking. *J. Med. Chem.* 44, 3768-3785.

[11] Helperin, I., Ma, B., Wolfson, H., Nussinov, R. (2002). Principles of docking: An overview of search algorithms and a guide to scoring functions. *Proteins Struct. Funct. Genet.* 47, 409-443.

[12] Halgren, T.A., (1996). Merck molecular force field. II. MMFF94 van der Waals and electrostatic parameters for intermolecular interactions. *J. Comput. Chem.* 17, 520-552.

[13] Charifson, P. S., Corkery, J. J., Murcko, M. A., Walters, W. P., (1999). Consensus scoring: a method for obtaining improved hit rates from docking databases of three-dimensional structures into proteins. *J. Med. Chem.* 42, 5100-5109.

[14] Clark, R. D., Strizhev, A., Leonard, J. M., Blake, J. F., Matthew, J.B. (2002). Consensus scoring for ligand/protein interactions. *J. Mol. Graph. Model.* 20, 281-295.

[15] Morris, G. M., Goodsell, D. S., Halliday, R. S., Huey, R., Hart, W. E., Belew, R. K., Olson, A. J. (1999). Advances and Challenges in Protein-Ligand Docking. *J. Mol. Biol.* 266, 424-440.

[16] Morris, G. M., Goodsell, D. S., Halliday, R.S., Huey, R., Hart, W. E., Belew, R. K. and Olson, A. J. (1998). Automated Docking Using a Lamarckian Genetic Algorithm and and Empirical Binding Free Energy Function. *J. Comput. Chem.* 19, 1639-1662.

[17] Jones, G., Willett, P., Glen, R. C., Leach, A. R., Taylor, R. (1997). Development and validation of a genetic algorithm for flexible docking. J. *Mol. Biol.* 267, 727-748.

[18] Aparna, V., Rambabu, G., Panigrahi, S. K., Sarma, J. A. R. P., Desiraju, G. R., (2005). Virtual screening of 4-anilinoquinazoline analogs as EGFR kinase inhibitors: importance of hydrogen bonds in the evaluation of poses and scoring functions. *J. Chem. Inf. Model.* 45, 725-738.

[19] Taylor, J. S., Burnett, R. M. (2000). DARWIN: a program for docking flexible molecules. *Proteins.* 41, 173–191.

[20] Rarey, M., Kramer, B., Lengauer, T., Klebe, G., (1996). Docking of hydrophobic ligands with interaction-based matching algorithm. *J. Mol. Biol.* 261, 470-489.

[21] Schellhammer, I., Rarey, M., (2004). FlexX-Scan: Fast Structure-Based Virtual Screening. *PROTEINS: Structure, Function, and Bioinformatics*. 57, 504-517.

[22] Kirkpatrick, P. (2004). Virtual screening: Gliding to success. *Nature Reviews Drug Discov.* 3, 299-299.

[23] Schnecke, V. Kuhn, L.A. (2000). Frontiers in *Drug Design* and *Discovery*. *Drug Des. Discov.* 20, 171–190.

[24] Putta, S., Lemmen, C., Beroza, P., Greene, J. (2002). A novel shape-feature based approach to virtual library screening. *J. Chem. Inf. Comput. Sci*. 42, 1230-1240.

[25] Todeschini, R., Consonni, V. (2008). Handbook of Molecular Descriptors. *Wiley Vch.* Germany.

[26] Brown, R.D., Martin,Y. C. (1996). Use of structure-activity data to compare structure-based clustering methods and descriptors for use in compound selection. *J. Chem. Inf. Comput. Sci.* 36,572-584.

In: Introduction to Drug Designing and Development
Editors: R. Kumar, A. Sharma and R. Kumar Tiwari
ISBN: 978-1-62948-556-0

Chapter 8

Structure-Based Drug Designing

Anju Sharma and Rajnish Kumar*
Amity Institute of Biotechnology, AMITY University-Uttar Pradesh,
Lucknow, Uttar Pradesh

Abstract

Drug design and development is a complex process. Selection of method for designing a drug molecule is highly dependent upon the available knowledge of protein/receptor and/or ligands. Availability of structural knowledge of protein/receptor is a suitable condition to adopt structure based drug design. De-novo drug design is structure based drug design and involves analysis of active site, molecular docking and use of various connection methods to generate a promising drug candidate. In this chapter we will study various approaches for analyzing active site of proteins, docking and connection methods.

Computational drug design can be broadly divided into two categories:

1. Indirect drug design or Ligand based drug design
2. Direct Drug Design or Structure based drug design

Indirect drug design is based on knowledge of ligand. This kind of drug designing can generate a model of biological target on the basis of knowledge of what is binding to it. Pharmacophore modeling comes under indirect drug designing where basic knowledge of ligands/drug candidates is available.

Direct drug designing is based on knowledge of protein or target. On the basis of structure of target, ligands/drug candidates are generated. As this type of drug designing is based on the structure of protein or target, it is also known as Structure based drug designing.

---

* Email address: 12.rajnish@gmail.com, rkumar2@lko.amity.edu.

De-novo ligand designing is example of structure based drug designing. De-novo ligand designing is carried out as an alternative to a screening experiment when lead structure is not available.

De-novo (Latin word) means 'from the beginning'. The most important challenge with this approach is to derive ligands which can easily be synthesized. Generally, fragment-based approach is used to design ligands that can be synthesized easily in laboratories. The central step in these approaches is to dock a library of small ligands or fragments into the active site of target receptor [1].

Classes of Ligand Design Methods

All De-novo design methods fall into one of three categories

1. Methods that analyze the active site
2. Methods that dock whole molecule
3. Methods that connect molecular fragments or atoms together to produce a ligand

Methods that Analyze the Active Site

These are used to determine which types of functional groups and atoms are best able to interact with the active site. This method does not construct ligands rather they analyze properties of the active site and determine favorable-binding locations for individual atoms or small fragments. The result of the analysis may be a set of preferred locations for simple fragments. Since fragment location techniques do not directly generate ligands, therefore this approach is not considered as true de novo design. It is an important perquisite for De-novo drug design.

Though these methods are conceptually very simple but they are quite useful for successful ligand design.

Now, let us understand what is active site of a protein or receptor?

The region of the enzyme containing the binding and catalytic sites is called the active site. It usually occurs near or on the surface of the protein as a cleft for the substrate to fit. In 85% of cases largest cavity or second largest cavity is considered as active site among all other cavities on protein surface.

Active site solely defines the probable function of protein. The active site is located in three dimensions, with amino acids or cofactors comprising binding and active sites. The active site depends on a variety of factors from the sequence of amino acids (primary structure) to arrangement of protein chain in space and time (secondary, tertiary and quaternary structures). The active site is dynamic with interactions at a variety of physical and chemical factors in the surroundings. Identification of binding and catalytic sites is a complex process, involving a variety of processes including the use of substrate analogues, modification of amino acid side chains of enzymes, generation of fusion protein and by site-directed mutagenesis etc.

Let's see that what are various approaches available for active site identification?

We need couple of assumptions while prediction of protein site:

I. Protein is already modeled.
II. Its 3D structure is known to us.

There are following approaches available to predict active site of protein/receptors:

1. Geometrical approach
2. Physicochemical approach
3. Machine –learning approach

Geometrical Approach

In this set of algorithm rely on the fact that if it is protein-ligand interaction then there should be cavity or convex area, and first or second largest cavity act as the active site. After finding the cavity find the volume information, which is calculated by filling the active site by spheres of particular size (size of water molecule).

Volume of active site = number of spheres in the cavity * volume of each sphere

It does not involve any Phylogenetic information.

Various geometrical methods to predict active site are as follows:

a) Probe and Ball Concept

Step 1. Protein 3D model is known.
Step 2. Start with a ball of size of water molecule (1.4 angstrom)
Step 3. Roll the ball over the surface
Step 4. The surface in contact with the sphere is called solvent accessible surface. It is a kind of expanded Van der Waals surface (figure 1).
Step 5. On increasing each atom's van der Waals radius by the probe radius, we get so-called expanded atom radii.

The union of the expanded atoms is what Tim Richmond (1984) calls the solvent-excluded volume. It is the region enclosed by the accessible surface. If groove size is more than water atom size then only probe can touch the surface. Few regions are there where probe cannot touch the surface, this region is called Re- Entrant surface. Molecular surface = Reentrant surface + accessible surface.

Challenges with this method is in 3D apart from moving the ball direction of movement is also crucial which is not considered in this method In another attempt by Jonathan Greer and Bruce Bush (1978) Probe spheres are rained down upon the atoms from above, stopping just before a collision (Van der Waals overlap) would occur. A finer set of lines is used for the next step. The lowest intersection point between each of these finer lines and the bottom of the lowest sphere defines a point of the molecular surface. In three dimensions this produces a grid. The method works well for fairly flat surfaces, but cannot handle irregular topographies with overhangs [2].

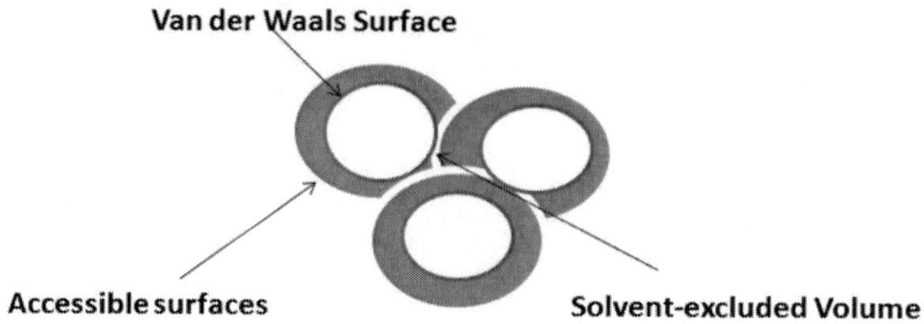

Figure 1. Elucidation of Van der Waal surfaces, Accessible surfaces and Solvent-excluded volume.

b) Arc Concept

In this instead of taking a ball, arc was used.

Step 1. Arc size should be twice the radius of circle
Step 2. Start with the center position of arc
Step 3. Give it some angle, whenever it touches the surface, its exposed area
Step 4. Move the arc center point to that point and again give some angle and so on.

Both the methods are highly used now days to determine the active site

Physicochemical Approach

It takes into consideration secondary structure composition, exposure, hydrophobicity, active residues, Phylogenetic analysis, homology patch etc.

a) Secondary Structure Composition

Raghav group IMTECH and Nussinov studied active site prediction on the basis secondary structure composition. Active site is part of protein surface. Most of the coiled region is present on the surface. Therefore active site is present in coiled region than helix.

It is just a statistical study; they took complex structures whose active site was known. Choose all the residues of the active site and checked whether they are part of helix or coil or sheet.

b) Exposure

One of the ways to predict active site is multiple alignments of related sequences.

The sequences of all organisms for a particular protein are gathered and a multiple sequence alignment is performed. Output of the MSA is fed as the input to the prediction algorithm in chunks of 60 amino acids for each of the organism.

c) Active Residues

It is found in most of the cases that Lysine, Arginine, Hystidene, Glutamine, Aspartic acid, Serine, Cystene have acid and basic moiety to mingle. They are largely present in the active site. Trypsin is also present as it alters hydrophobic value within pocket and is bulkier also.

d) Phylogenetic Analysis

In this method it seen that phylogenetically, how one function is similar to another. It is most widely used method. 5-6 residues of active site are known carry out multiple sequence alignment and quantify how their function is similar to each other. This approach is also called evolutionary trace method to find the active site.

Machine Learning Approach

Using Support Vector Machine (SVM) and Artificial Neural Network (ANN) active site of a protein can be predicted.

Prediction of active site using machine learning:

Step 1. Quantify the structure of protein. Take 3D model of protein. Sort it out on basis of Z axis. Divide it into slices (of some thickness), thickness cannot be less than 1.4 angstroms. Put all slices on surface, it will give two-dimensional map.

Step 2. Surface estimation: Now roll any probable probe and find residues on surface or take grid box concept.

Step 3. Cavity estimation (90% cases first or second largest cavity is active site)

Step 4. Feature selection: In general fifteen different properties are used to define each amino acid example helix, sheet, polar, non-polar etc.

Minimum three residues are required to find active site this is known as CATALYTIC TRIAD.

Step 5. Apply ANN and SVM to generate active site prediction model.

Methods that help in analyzing active site include GRID, HINT etc.

GRID: It computes the interaction of small organic fragments with an enzyme. Lattice is constructed, around the active site, which is further divided into equal grids. The method places probes at regularly spaced grid points and determines the regions with the most favorable scores by checking if there is any clashing of probe with protein or not (complete clash or partial clash). Each probe represents a functional group such as water or methyl etc. It is simple but inaccurate method.

HINT stand for hydrophobic interactions. It evaluates and visualizes the binding interactions between enzyme and ligand. It is a novel empirical molecular modeling system with new methods for *de novo* drug design and protein or nucleic acid structural analysis.

1. Estimates LogP for modeled molecules or data files.
2. Numerically and graphically evaluates binding of drugs or inhibitors into protein structures and scores *DOCK* orientations.
3. Constructs hydropathic (LOCK and KEY) complementarily maps that can be used to predict an ideal substrate from a known receptor or protein structure or to propose the hydropathic structure from known agonists or antagonists.
4. Evaluates/predicts effects of site-directed mutagenesis on protein structure and stability.

Methods That Dock Whole Molecule

Docking is a term used for computational schemes that attempt to find the "best" matching between two molecules: a receptor and a ligand. Molecular docking can be thought of as a problem of "lock-and-key", here, the protein can be thought of as the "lock" and the ligand can be thought of as a "key". Molecular docking may be defined as an optimization problem, which would describe the "best-fit" orientation of a ligand that binds to a particular protein of interest. Docking problem can be defined as follows:

Given the atomic coordinates of two molecules, predict their "correct" bound association [3]. The association of the molecules is based on the interactions like hydrogen bonds, salt bridges, electrostatic, Van der Waal etc. In its most general form, no additional data are provided. While it is assumed that the primary (known) site would be the one to participate in the bound conformation, there is no guarantee that this will be the case.

Docking problems can be best classified by the type of input molecules involved in docking. In *macromolecule docking*, two macromolecules like proteins and DNA are docked. The major characteristics of these problems are that the complex typically has large contact area and the molecules-although still flexible-have a fixed overall shape. Second class contains docking problems in which a small molecule is docked to a macromolecule. The macromolecule can be DNA fragment or a protein, in latter-case problem is called *protein-ligand docking*. Small molecule is an organic molecule. Small molecule docking differs substantially from macromolecular docking in the fact that the ligand is typically not fixed in its overall shape. The conformational flexibility of ligand is important and geometric properties alone are not sufficient to determine low-energy complexes. Protein-ligand docking problems can further be distinguished by the size of ligand molecule. Typical ligand molecule occurring in drug design docking has about 5-12 rotatable bonds, thus, the question of placing only a part of ligand in active site emerges [4].

1) Rigid Docking
2) Flexible docking

Different algorithms differ from each other on the basis of scoring function they use, searching function and how they change the orientation of the molecule.

Rigid-body Docking Algorithms

They constitute first approaches for screening sets of ligands according to their fit to a given target proteins. Main assumptions are:

- Protein is rigid
- Ligand is rigid

They are fixed in conformational space therefore no need to search for the lowest energy conformations of the two molecules. It is geometric base docking. Major component is steric clash between the two molecules.

A) Clique-search Based Approaches

Docking is method for matching characteristic features of the two molecules in three dimensional spaces. By match means assignment of ligand feature to a protein feature. Feature can be a volume of active site of protein or the ligand or an interaction between the molecules.

DOCK program is based on the idea of searching distance-compatible matches. It is most widely used software for molecular docking. Initially it is used for rigid body docking but now DOCK6 is used for carrying out flexible docking [5].

DOCK has two algorithms:

1) Algorithm 1: SPHGEN (Sphere Generation)

Starting with molecular surface of the protein, a set of spheres is created inside the active site till they touch any surface residues. Spheres represent the volume which could be occupied with by the ligand molecule. Cluster spheres and remove those which are highly similar or those with very large radius. Select clusters defining the active site.

2) Algorithm 2: MATCH

Create sub-graph and try to see that sub-graph is manifested in the known ligand or not. If not then rotate ligand's rotatble bonds and see whether matches the sub-graph or not, then add another point to the sub-graph. Calculate a matching between ligand atoms L and protein spheres K. To find compatible matches, following graph G is used. Vertices of graph G denote possible matches between protein and ligand. Edges connect pairs of vertices representing compatible matches. Compatibility is implemented as distance compatibility within a fixed tolerance ε i.e., the matches (l1, k1), (l2, k2) are distance compatible if $|d(p1,p2) - d(l1,l2)| < \varepsilon$ Search for sets with up to four compatible matches.

A search procedure maximizes the number of matches under the constraint that are compatible in 3D-space. Therefore an algorithm for enumerating cliques i.e., fully connected graph, can be applied to G. By superimposing the matched features of a clique one obtains an initial orientation of ligand molecule in active set of the protein. Position of the ligand is optimized and scored.

Several extensions were later introduced in DOCK.

Instead of using a single protein, an ensemble of protein structure is used for docking calculations. Initial DOCK algorithm uses volume as the feature to be matched, other use chemical interactions [6].

Another example of programs that uses distance-compatibility to screen fragment orientations are the well known de novo ligand design program LUDI and rigid body docking program CLIX.

CLIX is a rigid body docking program. It takes energetically favorable regions for functional groups of ligand as the underlying model. These regions are recalculated with GRID program. CLIX uses only two points for an initial matching. After fitting the two matched sites, the rotation about the common axis between the matched sites remains as an open degree of freedom. This rotation is then sampled in regular intervals.

B) Geometric Hashing

It originates from the area of computer vision and was first applied to molecular docking problems by Fischer et al. It consists of two phases;

1) Preprocessing Phase

A hash table is created from the set of models. For each model, each pair of points define so-called basis. For each basis every third point belonging to the model is expressed in coordinates relative to basis. A tuple is stored in a hash table addressed by the relative coordinates of the third point

2) Recognition Phase

Every pair is considered as a basis. Once basis are defined all other points are expressed by relative coordinates with respect to the basis resulting in a query for the hash table created before. Query votes for all matching tuples stored in hash table. Finally, models with many votes are extracted**.** Transformation is calculated from the matching points, and the match is verified [7]. Two aspects make Geometric hashing attractive for Docking:

- It is time-efficient.
- It deals with partial matching.

C) Pose Clustering

Pose clustering is a different approach from pattern recognition applied to the molecular docking problem. For applying pose clustering to docking the LUDI model of molecular interactions is used as the underlying representation. For each interaction group, interaction center and an interaction surface is defined. The interaction surfaces of the protein are approximated by discrete points.

The centers of ligand interactions are the object points which have to be matched to the scene.

Preprocessing: construct hash table for all interaction type pairs a, b:

Store all pairs of interaction-points p, q with address d (p, q). Chain lists twice, sorted by point id of p and q.

Search of initial ligand orientations:

Triplets (a, b, c) of ligand interaction centers:

Generate a list of all type- and distance-compatible pairs of interaction points for (a, b) and (a, c). Construct all distance-compatible triangles (p, q, r) by list merging. Triangles (p, q, r): Generate ligand transformation, overlap test. Cluster orientations by pair wise (Root Mean Square Distance) RMSD.

For remaining ligand orientations extend matching, overlap test and scoring [8].

D) Superposition of Point Sets

In rigid body docking, the superposition of point sets is a fundamental sub-problem.

It is defined as given two sets X, Y with n vectors.

Find a transformation $T = (\Omega, t)$ minimizing the RMSD between X and transformed vector Y

RMSD X, Y (T) = sqrt ((1/n) Σi (xi – Ω yi – t)2)
Ω describes a rotation around the centroid of Y.

Flexible Ligand Docking Algorithms

The major limitation of the rigid-body docking algorithms is that they do not consider conformational flexibility of the ligand molecules. Often small molecules have large conformational spaces with several low energy states. Even for small molecules with only few rotatable bonds significant differences between the bound conformation and the calculated low energy conformation can occur.

In flexible ligand docking, two heuristics are involved
Ligand is considered to be flexible i.e., it can rotate and take n number of orientations.
Proteins remain static.
Part of active site that is close to ligand is flexible.
Protein is taken as series of static structures. Different snapshots of protein structures at different time frames are taken and each snap shot is docked with the ligand molecule.

Flexible docking based on fragmentation. To handle conformational flexibility directly in a docking algorithm is by fragmentation. Ligand is divided into several fragments. Each fragment is either rigid or has small number of conformations which can be handled by conformation ensemble.

It differs from de novo design method in a way is that in this method fragment stems from a single molecule, in de novo fragment is picked from the database [9].

a) Place and Join Algorithms

In this multiple fragments are all docked independently. Then placements of adjacent fragments in which the connecting atoms overlap are identified and reconnected.

First ligand is manually divided into two fragments having one atom in common called hinge.

Then placements list are created for each fragment using DOCK. For each ligand atom triplet of a fragment, a hash table entry is created and addressed with the pair wise distance between the atoms.

The entry contains fragment identification as well as the location of the hinge. In matching phase, protein sphere triplets are used to extract ligand atom triplets with similar distance. Result of vote is counted for a hinge location for each match. Hinge locations with many votes are then selected. Finally fragments are reconnected, energy minimized and scored. It is advantageous if molecule consists of a small set of medium-sized rigid fragments. If fragments are too small, it is difficult to place them independently.

b) Incremental Construction Algorithms

In this method instead of placing all fragments of ligand independently, the algorithm begins with placing one fragment into the active site of the protein.

Then the algorithm adds the remaining parts of the ligand to the already placed fragment iteratively.

It has three phases:

- Selection of base fragments.
- Placement of base fragments.
- Incremental construction phase.

Search Strategies:

GREEDY: after adding a fragment, select the high scoring ones and reject the rest (GROW, FlexX, Hammerhead).Scales linear with the number of fragments. Optimal solution may be sub-optimal during buildup (the larger the considered set and the lower the number of fragments, the lower is the risk of missing the optimal placement).

BACKTRACKING: Performs a recursive (depth first). Search through the whole configuration tree (Leach). Scales exponentially with the number of fragments. No risk of losing the optimal solution due to tree pruning.

GOLD software uses genetic algorithm to provide docking of flexible ligand and a protein with flexible hydroxyl groups. This makes it a good choice when binding pocket contains amino acids that form hydrogen bonds with the ligand.

GOLD uses scoring function that is based on favorable conformations found in Cambridge Structural Database (CSD) and on empirical results on weak chemical interactions. The development of GOLD is currently focused on improving the computational algorithm and adding a support for parallel processing.

Other Docking Algorithms

1) Tabu Searches

These methods are based on stochastic processes, in which new states are randomly generated from an initial state (referred as current solution). These new solutions are then scored and ranked in ascending order. The best new solution is then chosen as the new current solution and the same process is then repeated again. To avoid loops and ensure diversity of the current solution a tabu list is used. This list acts as a memory. It contains information about previous current solutions and a new solution is rejected if it reminds a previous solution too much. An example of docking algorithm using tabu search is PRO_LEADS [10].

2) Docking by Genetic Algorithm

A genetic algorithm is a general purpose optimization scheme which mimics the process of evolution. The individuals are configurations in the search space. A so-called fitness function is used to decide which individuals survive and produce offspring.

First of all, a linear description of configurations is needed for describing all degrees of freedoms. It should be free of redundancy and models constraints of the configurations space directly such that configurations violating constraints are never generated during the optimization. Second, a fitness function is developed. It is closely related to scoring functions for molecular docking. The genetic algorithm is implemented in software tool GOLD.

A configuration is GOLD is represented by two strings.

The first string stores the conformations of the ligand and selected protein side chains by defining the torsion angles of each rotatable bond.

The second string stores a mapping between hydrogen bond partners in the protein and the ligand.

For fitness evaluation, a 3D structure is created from the chromosome representation by first generating the ligand conformations. According to mapping stored in second string, H-bond atoms are superimposed to H-bond site points in the active site.

Finally a scoring function evaluating hydrogen bonds, ligand internal energy as well as protein-ligand Van der Waals energy is applied as the fitness function and calculate docking score [11].

3) Docking by Simulation

Instead of trying to enumerate a discrete low-energy subspace of the problem, these approaches begin their calculation with a starting configuration and locally move to configuration with lower energy.

a) Simulated Annealing

SA is well-known simulation technique which is also frequently used for solving complex optimization problems.

Starts with configuration having energy or score value E(A).

Randomly move to new configuration B and energy E(B) is calculated.

The new configuration is accepted based on the Metropolis criterion, which means that it is accepted if E (B) ≤ E (A) or with probability.

$$P = e - (E(B) - E(A))/ kBT$$

Over the simulation the temperature T is reduced based on a so-called cooling schedule.

AUTODOCK program for protein-ligand docking is based on this strategy [12].

b) Hybrid Methods

It constitutes a multi-step approach based on rigid-body docking and Molecular Dynamics (MD). Fist a set of low-energy conformers is created. Each conformer is docked rigid into the active site using DOCK. The high scoring placements are then optimized using an MD-based simulated annealing optimization in combination with the AMBER force field.

4) Docking by Point Complimentary Methods

These methods are based on evaluating the shape and /or chemical complementarities between interacting molecules. The interacting molecules are usually modeled in an easy way, example using spheres or cubes as atoms. The ligand description is then rotated and translated to obtain maximum number of matches between ligand and protein surfaces, minus the number of volume overlaps. Additional constraints may be present, for example a demand for interacting surface normal to be approximately in opposite directions [13].

Some algorithms use a 3D grid, which is placed over the protein and over the ligand.

Each grid point is then labeled either open space or inside the ligand or protein. Then a correlation function is created and this function is optimized using rigid body translation and rotation. This often involves using traditional shape recognition algorithms like Fast Fourier Transforms (FFT) with Fourier correlation theory.

A high correlation score denotes good surface complementarities between the molecules. Examples: FTDOCK, SANDOCK, FLOG

5) Docking by Monte Carlo Methods

The Monte Carlo simulation method occupies a special place in the history of molecule docking. In molecular docking the expression Monte Carlo usually means importance sampling or Metropolis method, which generates random moves to the system and then accepts or rejects the move based on a Boltzmann probability. Monte Carlo methods play an important role in molecular docking [14]. Example AutoDock, ProDock, ICM, MCDOCK etc.

6) Distance Geometry Methods or Golden Search Method

Many types of structural information can be expressed as intra- or intermolecular distance. The distance geometry formalism allows these distances to be assembled and three-dimensional structures consistent with them to be calculated. The crucial feature is that it is not possible to arbitrarily assign values to the inter-atomic distances in a molecule and always obtain a low-energy conformation. Rather, the inter-atomic distances are closely interrelated and many combinations of distances are geometrically impossible. Example: DockIt.

Connection Methods

These methods are truly de novo design ligand design methods. These methods fall into a few categories depending upon the approach they use [15]:

a) Site-point Connection Methods

It determines desirable locations of individual atoms in the active site and then place suitable fragments at those locations.

First the site points for active points are generated. We get to know about the electrostatic mapping; within the active site try to find out where binding is maximum or where accumulation of positive or negative charges will be more. Then a similar prototype molecule is positioned in the active site so that it overlaps with several of site points. Finally additional building blocks are attached to make contact with other site points.

The site points may be generated with energy-based or rule based approaches. They can also be generated from the output of active site analysis programs.

Site-point connection methods include CLIX and LUDI

Advantages

1. Fast methods, only those site points that are near each other are compared, which limits the complexity of the 3D search process and fragments are selected rapidly.
2. They are versatile.

3. Ligands are constructed in a fragment-by-fragment fashion
4. Find reasonable bridging groups between two separate pieces
5. In this method user may select the number of site points that must be satisfied, allowing a more or less rigorous criterion for compound selection.

Disadvantages

1. They dependent on proper site-point placement. Ligands designed to superimpose on poorly selected site points are poor ligands
2. Slop factor: if site points need to be matched perfectly, most fragments will miss those site points and be rejected. On the other hand if large tolerances are allowed for matching the site points, the search may be slow and most compounds will not make optimal contacts with the receptor.
3. Lack of flexibility of the individual fragments.

CLIX is either a site-point or a whole-molecule-docking method. It uses the output from GRID calculations, carried out with a variety of probes, to characterize the receptor site in terms of an ensemble of favorable-binding positions for different groups of fragments. This information is then used to query a chemical database for candidate molecules having good coincidence for individual fragments with members of ensemble. The receptor is rigid throughout the process. Binding energy is estimated using the energy information in the GRID potential maps to suggest possible changes in the structures, to improve their binding.

LUDI is similar to CLIX. It is a method for fitting molecular fragments to site points within an active site in such a way that hydrogen bonds can be formed with the enzyme and hydrophobic pockets are filled with hydrophobic groups.

The program works in three steps. First it calculates interaction sites, which are discrete positions in space suitable to form hydrogen bonds or to fill a hydrophobic pocket. The interaction sites are derived from distributions of non-bonded contacts generated by a search through the Cambridge Structural Database. An alternative route to generate the interaction sites is the use of rules. The second step is the fit of molecular fragments onto the interaction sites. Currently they use a library of 600 fragments for the fitting. The final step in the present program is the connection of some or all of the fitted fragments to a single molecule. This is done by bridge fragments.

b) Fragment Connection Methods

Start with previously positioned fragments and find “linker” or “scaffolds” to connect those fragments without moving them i.e., isolated fragments that are selected in a variety of ways are connected. It relies on the concept that a small number of well-placed fragments, each making favorable interactions with the enzyme, is capable of providing a significant overall binding energy. A key feature of these methods is that although the linker contributes to binding but its contribution is not considered a critical part of compound evaluation. Linker is used to avoid bumping into the receptor and possess suitable geometry to ‘stitch together’ the isolated fragments. Fragment connection methods use a variety of database types.

Example: Methods in this category include: CAVEAT and HOOK, NEWLEAD, PROLIGAND

Advantages

1. Information about favorable fragment locations may be obtained from source.
2. If set of candidate fragments are already known then methods allows one to quickly stitch those binding elements.
3. Compounds suggested by this method can be quite rigid which lowers the overall entropy of the system.
4. Many choices of scaffolds are available.

Disadvantages

1. Slow in searching for those methods that perform flexible 3D searching or use large multi-conformational databases.
2. Any scaffold, no matter how good it may be may be rejected if some portion of it overlaps the receptor.
3. Molecules suggested by fragment connection methods are complicated and impractical to synthesize.

Example: CAVEAT is designed to identify scaffolds that can link together any number of isolated ligand fragments. Bonds are treated as vectors and the method works by comparing the relation between those vectors in the isolated ligand fragments with those of each molecule in the database. It allows any number of isolated ligands to be connected simultaneously with a single scaffold.

NEWLEAD automatically generates candidate structures by connecting two isolated ligand fragments with spacers assembled from small chemical entities. The building blocks for the connecting linker may be single atoms, library spacers or fused-ring spacers. It generates new structures that are chemically unrelated to the reference molecules, providing an unbiased starting point for the design of new generations of lead structures.

HOOK uses molecular skeletons from a database to connect multiple isolated functional groups. Each skeleton has two or more "hooks" which are specific bonds designated as connection points. Skeletons are treated as rigid, so if a skeleton is actually flexible, it is treated as set of distinct, rigid conformations.

c) Sequential Buildup Methods

It constructs a ligand atom-by-atom or fragment-by-fragment. Construction need not to be linear means each new piece may be added anywhere on the existing ligand. In this method we begin with a core fragment of ligand, place it at suitable position in the active site and in each subsequent step additional functional group is added until the entire ligand is assembled.

An important issue for sequential build up methods is referred as "speed versus coverage". If a program builds ligands quickly, it probably does so by sampling poorly or we can say it fails to consider all possibilities while constructing new molecule. On the other hand if exhaustive search is carried out then the method is fairly slow. This approach includes: GROW, GROWMOL etc.

Advantages

1. Ligands suggested by this method are smaller and more efficient than molecules derived from fragment connection methods.
2. Each piece is added sequentially therefore it is possible to perform more detailed conformational analyses, leading to fewer misses.

Disadvantages

1. Problem of crossing "dead zones"-open spaces of the active site where few enzyme contacts are possible.
2. Sequential build-up methods are more prone to "combinatorial explosion" i.e., there are huge number of ways to piece together atoms or small fragments in an active site.
3. Many ligands will be impossibly to generate because these methods use a finite set of building blocks.
4. Ligands suggested do not guarantee that the ligand will be easy to make, unless care is taken in developing suitable rules to guide the ligand construction process.

Example: GROW builds ligand in linear fashion. At each step the location, atom functional group etc. are randomly chosen. Scoring is based on "chemical complementarity" to the receptor. Following the generation a series of preprocessing steps takes place. First, ligands not making a sufficient number of hydrogen bonds and hydrophobic contacts with the enzyme are eliminated.

Next molecule is energy-minimized and strain energy of bound conformation is used to eliminate compounds that are binding in high-energy conformations. Next the potency of each remaining compound is estimated, using a regression equation derived from the experimental data available for that particular receptor. Finally, the remaining compounds are clustered into families.

d) Random Connection Methods

It is a special class which combines some of the features of site-point, fragment connection and sequential build-up methods along with bond-disconnection strategies and other methods to introduce randomness.

These methods begin with a "soup" of building blocks, either individual atoms or slightly larger fragments. These building blocks may be unconnected at the start of the run, or there may be connections between some or all fragments. Regardless of the choice of fundamental building blocks, these methods are all similar in that they slowly construct ligands by making and breaking the connections between building blocks. Although the building blocks can be held fixed, all known methods allow the molecules to move under a molecular dynamics or a Monte Carlo protocol. Decisions about whether to accept or reject any changes are not random, but are based on evaluation procedure.

Advantages

1. Randomness of these approaches is one of attractions, as random connection and disconnection approaches construct any molecule imaginable and do so in a bias free manner.
2. Have superior ability to explore "drug space" more broadly then other methods and generate more diverse compounds. This category includes: MCDNLG, CONCEPTS, CONCERTS, LigBuilder.

MCDNLG stands for Monte Carlo De Novo Ligand Generator and is relatively unbiased method. It has no fragment library or pre-stored information about the types of molecules desired. Rather the method starts with a random collection of atoms packed tightly into the active site of the receptor and slowly anneals it into a chemically stable molecule. Each atom is represented by its element type, hybridization, H-boding possibilities and so on. Changes to the ligands are made randomly from a list and include make-change-break a bond; delete-change-reappear-move a particle; rigidly translate-rotate the ligand and rotate a bond. Bonds are automatically assumed to exist between two atoms within 2.1 Angstroms. Scoring is based on a combination of intra- and intermolecular force-field terms. During the run, a standard metropolis-based Monte Carlo algorithm is used along with a simulated annealing protocol. Typically several hundred thousand Monte Carlo steps are taken. This procedure takes only a few minutes. LigBuilder does not have any database. It builds ligand atom-by-atom therefore ligands generated are sometimes not synthesized.

References

[1] Schneider, G., Fechner, U. (2005). Computer-based de novo design of drug-like molecules. *Nat. Rev. Drug Discov.* 4(8), 649-63.

[2] http://www.netsci.org/Science/Compchem/feature14e.html [Accessed on: 26-04-2013]

[3] Mihasan, M. (2012). What in silico molecular docking can do for the 'bench-working biologists'. *J. Biosci.* 37, 1089–1095.

[4] http://bioinfo3d.cs.tau.ac.il/Education/CS99b/class_notes/class6.html [Accessed on 28-04-2013]

[5] Halperin, I., Ma, B., Wolfson, H., Nussinov, R. (2002). Principles of Docking: An Overviewof Search Algorithms and a Guide to Scoring Functions. *Proteins: Structure, Function, and Genetics* 47:409–443.

[6] http://www.csb.yale.edu/people/core/pjf/mbgcourse/dock_demo.html [Accessed on 27-04-2013]

[7] Wolfson, H. J., Rigoutsos, I. (1997). Geometric Hashing: An Overview. *IEEE Computational Science and Engineering*, 4 (4), 10-21.

[8] Bouvier, G., Evrard-Todeschi, N., Girault, J. P., Bertho, G. (2010). Automatic clustering of docking poses in virtual screening process using self-organizing map. *Bioinformatics* 26 (1), 53-60.

[9] http://vred.bioinf.uni-sb.de/downloads/bioinfo_ws01/PL-Docking.pdf. [Accessed on 2-05-2013]

[10] Baxter, C. A., Murry, C. W., Clark, D. E, Westhead, D. R., Eldridge, M. D. (1998). Flexible docking using tabu search and an empirical estimate of binding affinity. *Proteins: Structure, Function, and Bioinformatics*. 33 (3), 367-382.

[11] Gardiner, E. J., Willett, P., Artymiuk, P.J. (2001). Protein docking using a genetic algorithm. *Proteins*. 44 (1), 44-56.

[12] http://edges-grid.eu/c/document_library/get_file?folderId=63854&name=DLFE-1629.pdf [Accessed on 14-05-2013]

[13] http://gcl.cis.udel.edu/courses/cisc849011_sp08/project_xiang.pdf. [Accessed on 14-05-2013]

[14] Lorenzen, S., Zhang, Y. (2007). Monte Carlo refinement of rigid-body protein docking structures with backbone displacement and side-chain optimization. *Protein Sci.* 16 (12), 2716–2725.

[15] Rotstein, S. H., Murcko, M. A. (1993). GroupBuild: A Fragment-Based Method for *De Novo* Drug Design. *J. Med. Chem.* 36, 1700-1710.

In: Introduction to Drug Designing and Development
Editors: R. Kumar, A. Sharma and R. Kumar Tiwari
ISBN: 978-1-62948-556-0

Chapter 9

Concepts of Combinatorial Library

*Anju Sharma**
Amity Institute of Biotechnology, AMITY University-Uttar Pradesh,
Lucknow, Uttar Pradesh, India

Abstract

Combinatorial chemistry is a high throughput technique which enables the rapid synthesis of thousands of compounds followed by screening these compounds for a particular activity. The basic principle is to synthesize a large number of compounds in a single experimental setup in contrast to the conventional one-at-time synthesis method. It was first applied for peptide and oligonucleotide synthesis and is now frequently used to synthesize library of proteins, chemical compounds, oligosaccharides, oligomers etc. The nature and diversity of the combinatorial library depends on synthetic strategy used to generate the library. Different strategies for generating combinatorial libraries, requirements and screening techniques are discussed in this chapter.

1. Introduction

Combinatorial chemistry (CombiChem) is an innovative and new technique to synthesize a large library of chemical compounds in a short time interval. The term 'combinatorial chemistry' is strictly used when a library of compounds is generated by treating different building blocks in one reaction vessel. These intentionally created libraries contain a population of structurally diverse compounds which are synthesized in a single vessel under the same experimental conditions. Combinatorial chemistry has accelerated the time-consuming and labor intensive traditional method of synthesizing compound. Earlier chemists were able to synthesize hardly 100-200 compounds in a year but with the emergence of combinatorial technique chemists can synthesize many hundreds or thousands of compounds

* Corresponding author: Email:anjusharma.online@gmail.com, asharma3@lko.amity.

in a single experiment. Combinatorial libraries are usually represented by one or more basic structure-having a small number of R-group positions where each R-position is substituted by lists of known alternative groups.

By definition combinatorial chemistry is defined as the systematic and repetitive, covalent connection of a set of different "building blocks" of varying structures to each other to yield a large array of diverse molecular entities [1, 2]. The essence of combinatorial chemistry is to generate large numbers of compounds very quickly. Large numbers of analogues are synthesized using the same reaction condition and same reaction vessel. Traditional or orthodox approach for synthesis is a stepwise process where one compound is synthesized at a time using fundamentals of basic chemistry. For example Compound X would be reacted with compound Y to yield compound XY (eq. 1). After completion of reaction newly synthesized compound XY would be isolated followed by a purification process via crystallization, chromatography or distillation.

$$X + Y = XY \tag{1}$$

On the other hand instead of an individual one to one reaction between parent compounds, large numbers of compounds are synthesized directly in parallel or in mixtures. (Figure 1) Every possible combination of compound from X_1 to X_n with Y_1 to Y_n is synthesized.

After the completion of the reaction, the structure of resultant compounds is not known with certainty. Compounds produced are not separated or purified rather the mixture is tested for desirable biological activity as a whole [3]. If desired activity is observed then the entire mixture is marked for further analysis i.e., mixture is analyzed to identify its active components. Synthesized molecules are tested using a variety of high-throughput techniques for their activity. On the other hand if no activity is observed then the mixture is discarded. Combinatorial chemistry is summarized in three steps:

a. Preparation of library,
b. Screening of library compounds
c. Determination of chemical structures of active compound

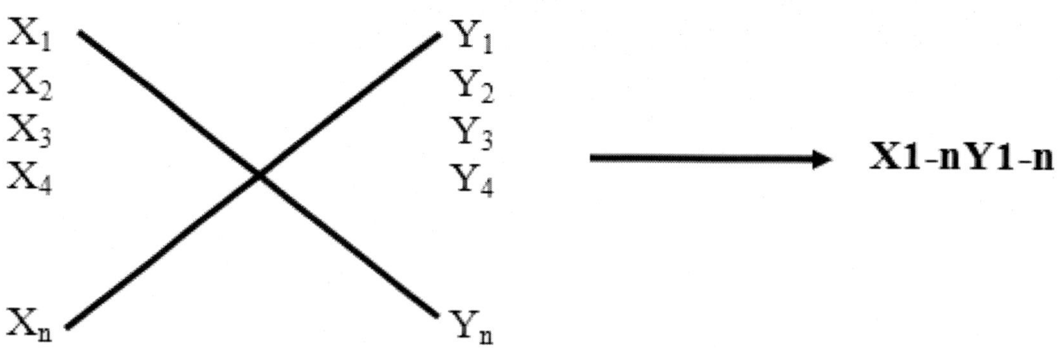

Figure 1. Schematic Illustration of Combinatorial Synthesis.

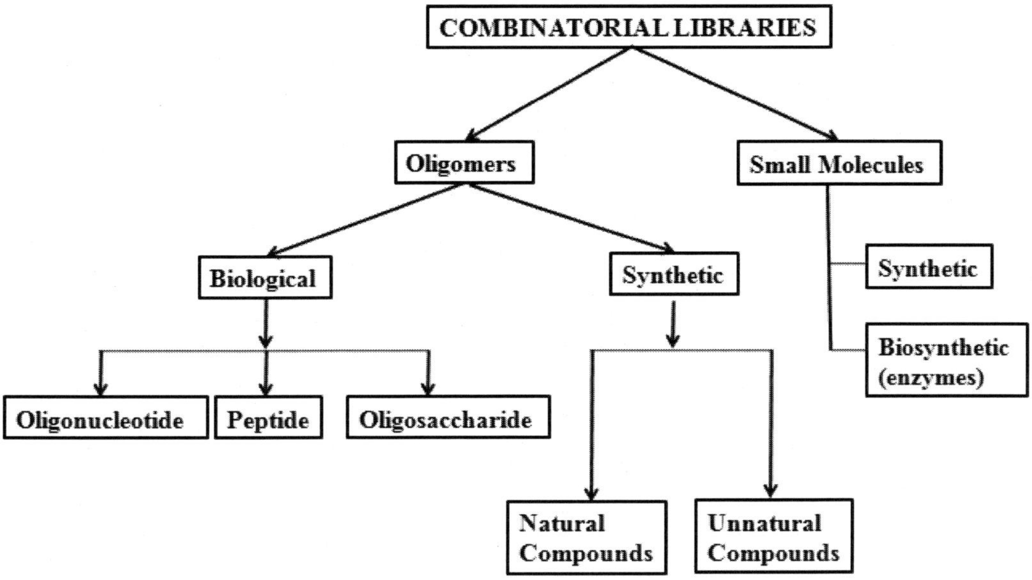

Figure 2. Types of Combinatorial Libraries.

Combinatorial chemistry offers various advantages over traditional approach:

- Synthesis is fast and efficient in combinatorial chemistry
- Cost of production is reduced
- Time efficient: Millions of compounds are produced in the same time as it takes to make one compound.
- It is a powerful method of generating diverse compounds.
- Provides a means to quickly and efficiently find a lead compound.
- Final product is easily cleaved out in the end and does not require any further purification.

Over the last few years combinatorial chemistry has evolved rapidly and has profound impact in different branches of science (chemistry, biology and other fields like semiconductors, superconductors, catalysts, polymers) but more specifically in pharmaceutical sciences. It has reduced the time and costs associated with producing effective and competitive drugs molecules. In a short time interval from its inception combinatorial chemistry has become the focus of scientific and research activities.

1.1. Brief History of Combinatorial Chemistry

The combinatorial library method was first applied to synthesize peptides and oligonucleotides. The history of combinatorial chemistry can be traced back to the year 1963 when a researcher in Rockefeller University, Bruce Merrifield, conducted solid-phase synthesis of peptides [4], which earned him a Nobel Prize. He marked the beginning of large scale synthesis of compounds and offered necessary tools to generate a library of small organic compounds (peptides). However it's only by early 1990's the concept resurfaced and got a jump start when H. Mario Geysen in 1984 developed a technique to simultaneously synthesize diversified peptides on pin-shaped solid supports. Since then combinatorial chemistry was used to generate libraries of peptides, organic and inorganic compounds, polymers and organo-metallic compounds (figure 2). During last decades a lot of research and development work in combinatorial chemistry is carried out in order to discover new compounds and improve high-throughput screening technologies.

2. Combinatorial Chemistry Approaches

Combinatorial libraries are constructed using two major approaches: a) Solid Phase Synthesis, b) Solution Phase synthesis. Both approaches will be explained one by one in this section.

2.1. Solid Phase Synthesis

The solid phase synthesis is an important approach in combinatorial chemistry as most of the combinatorial synthesis is done by this method. In this approach synthesis is carried out on a polymeric solid support attached with building blocks (resins, beads or linkers). Building blocks are masked by protecting groups thereby making initial experimental set up inert. The synthesis process begins by removing the protection of building block thereby making it active followed by addition of excess of reagents and monomers to force a reaction. After the initial coupling of unwanted materials or excess of reagents is removed by simple filtration and washing. Intermediates in a reaction sequence are attached to the beads and need not to be purified. Individual beads are separated at the end of reaction to get individual products. The solid support can be reused if the appropriate cleavage conditions and suitable anchor/ linker/ resins are used.

Solid phase synthesis is further divided into two categories:

a) Solid Phase Organic Synthesis
b) Mix and Split Synthesis

2.1.1. Solid Phase Organic Synthesis (SPOS)

Traditionally peptides are synthesized in solution from properly protected amino acids.

$$\text{Z-NH-}\underset{\displaystyle R_1}{\underset{|}{\text{CH}}}\text{-COOX} + \text{H}_2\text{N-}\underset{\displaystyle R_2}{\underset{|}{\text{CH}}}\text{-COOB} \rightarrow \text{Z-NH-}\underset{\displaystyle R_1}{\underset{|}{\text{CH}}}\text{-CO-NH-}\underset{\displaystyle R_2}{\underset{|}{\text{CH}}}\text{-COOB}$$

Figure 3. Traditional approach of synthesizing peptides.

The carboxyl group of one amino acid is protected (by protecting group **B**) while the amino group is free. The amino group of the other amino acid is protected (**Z**) and the carboxyl group is activated (**X**) in order to make it capable for forming a peptide bond with other amino acids (figure 3).

To grow peptide chain amino-protecting group of the di-peptide is removed and treated with another amino-protected and activated amino acid. After every step product is isolated from the solution and purified, thus makes it a tedious job [5].

Solid phase synthesis of peptides was first carried out by Merrifield in 1963. He developed reaction series for synthesizing proteins. The direction of synthesis is opposite to what is followed by the cell. In solid phase synthesis carboxyl terminal of first amino acid is anchored to a solid support.

Next desired amino acid is added to the first anchored amino acid followed by sequential attachment of rest of amino acids to obtain desired peptide or protein chain. It was made functional by adding chloromethyl groups which made it possible to attach the first amino acid to the resin.

Steps involved in solid state synthesis of dipeptide are as follows (figure 4):

1. Solid support used by Merrifield is made up of polystyrene-divinylbenzene co-polymer in the fine bead form.
2. Chloromethyl group was added to solid support to make it functional. It also aids the attachment of first amino acid to the support/ bead.
3. Solid support is exposed to first amino acid whose all groups are protected (Z) except the α-carboxyl group.
4. In step 1 of synthesis first amino acid attach to the resin.
5. Excess of amino acids and reagents are removed by washing/ filtration.
6. Now protecting group from the α-amino group of first amino acid is removed so that it can couple with the second amino acid.
7. The second amino acid which is fully protected except α-carboxyl group, properly activated by group X is added in excess along with reagents.
8. The coupling takes place between α-amino group of first amino acid and between α-carboxyl group of a second amino acid.
9. Again excess of amino acids and reagents are washed.
10. Sequentially repeat the process from step 5 forming a cycle until the desired chain is synthesized on the bead.
11. After the addition of the last amino acid, peptide or protein chain is cleaved from the resin.
12. Cleavage usually involves the breakage of the peptide from the resin and removal of the protecting groups.
13. The synthesized peptide is then recovered from the filtrate.

Advantages of solid phase synthesis

i. Polymeric support simplifies the problem of isolation of final products from the reaction mixture.
ii. The large number and variety of supports are there, on the basis of which one can design receptor binding assay for library evaluation.

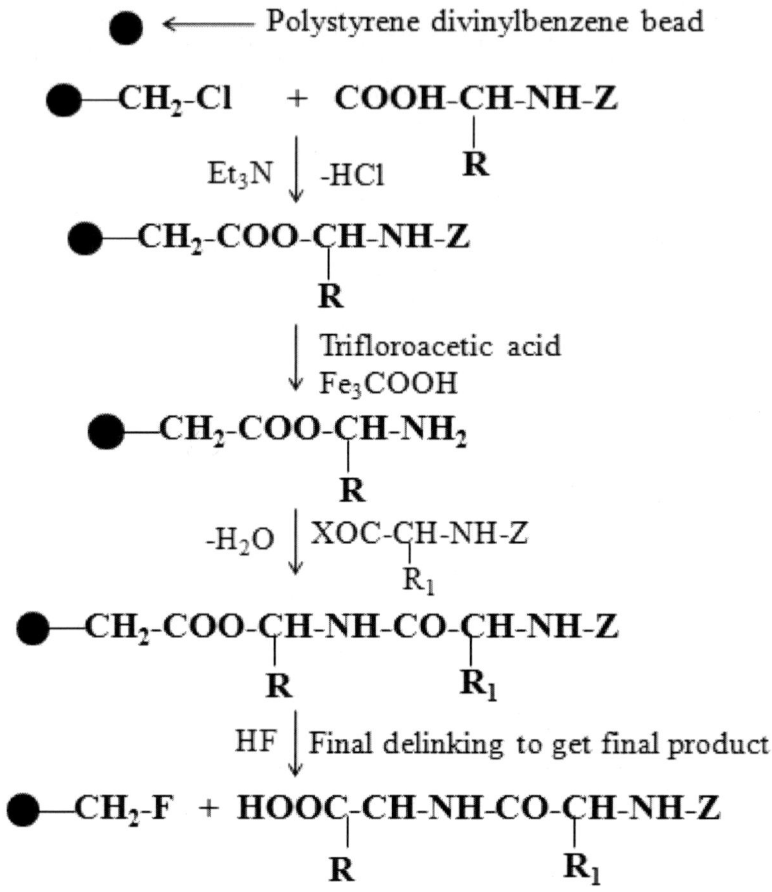

Figure 4. Merrifield solid phase synthesis of dipeptide.

2.1.2. Mix and Split Synthesis

Mix and split technique pioneered by Furka can generate a very large number of products. Like solid phase organic synthesis, mix and split method allows for sequential reaction of compounds attached to beads/ resins. Basic steps include:

1. Dividing the solid support into equal portions;
2. Couple each portion individually with different amino acids;
3. Mixing and homogenizing the portions.

The starting material i.e., sample of resin support material is divided into ‘n’ equal portions and each of the portions is then reacted with n different building blocks. After completion of the reactions, washing is carried out to remove excess of reagents and unbounded blocks. Individual portions are thoroughly mixed and again divided into ‘n’ equal portions. The process of addition of building blocks followed by reaction and removal of access of reagents and again mixing the portions is repeated till desired product is synthesized (figure 5). If the cycle is repeated for ‘x’ times, then x^n products are synthesized during the process.

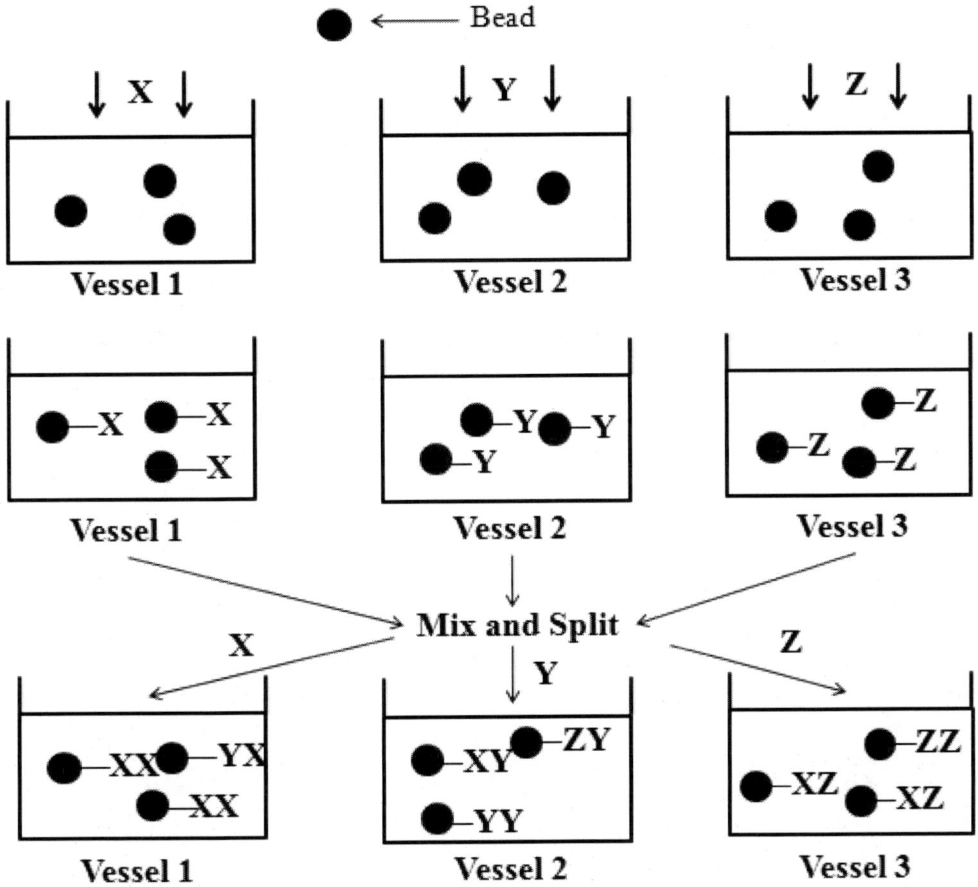

Figure 5. Mix and Split approach for solid phase synthesis.

The key features of the split-mix synthesis [5] are:

i. Number of peptides increase exponentially after each coupling step.
ii. All possible combinations of amino acid building blocks are represented in final peptides.
iii. It is applicable for the synthesis of different families of other kinds of organic compounds

Advantages

i. Large libraries are generated

Disadvantages [2]

i. Very complex mixtures are made.
ii. Tagging of molecules is required.
iii. Synergistic effect may be observed during screening, leading to false positives.

2.2. Solution Phase Synthesis

The solution phase synthesis approach is not widely used for synthesis, but in a few cases the libraries are successfully generated and screened by this method. In this method series of coupling reactions are realized in a different reaction vessel and all operations are carried out in parallel. In this number of operations practically remains the same. The advantage of this method is that it takes the same time to synthesize hundreds of compounds as required in preparing one compound. Compounds developed by this approach are called as compound libraries. This method is basically used for synthesis of nucleic acids with defined chemical structure. To obtain a specific oligonucleotide chain, building blocks are sequentially attached to the growing chain in the order required by a sequence of product (figure 6).

Advantages

i. It is used to identify active hit.
ii. End product is known beforehand.

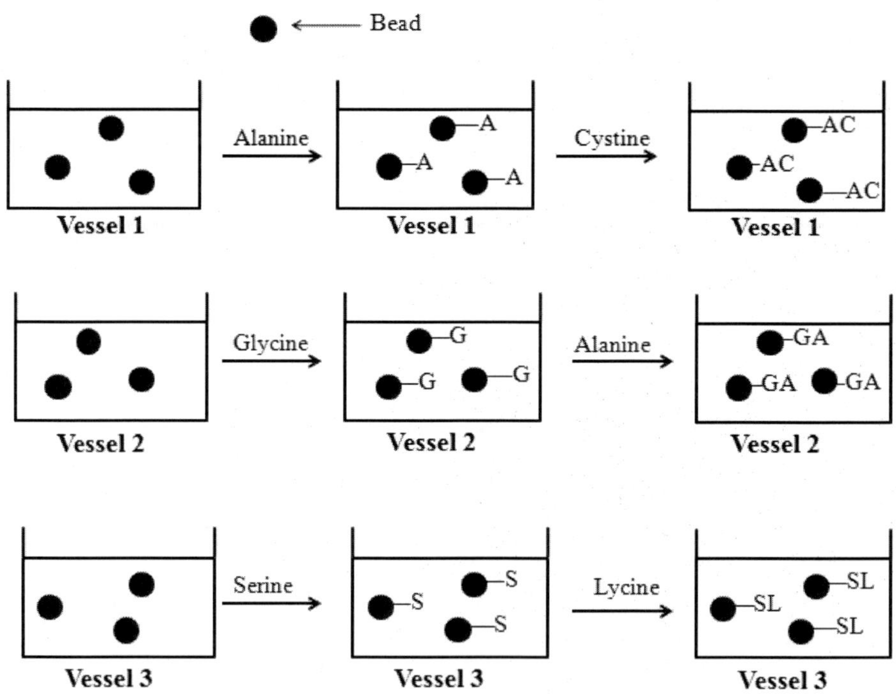

Figure 6. Parallel Synthesis Approach.

Disadvantages

i. It is useful for one or two step reactions.
ii. In multi-step reaction, products need to be isolated and purified thereby making it tedious and time consuming.
iii. There are chances of building up impurities in products.

2.2.1. Dendrimer supported synthesis [5, 6]

Dendrimers, branching oligomers, are used as support for synthesis. They are soluble and relatively large molecules as compared to the size of building blocks and reagents used in combinatorial syntheses. At the end of oligomer branches linkers are attached which serve as soluble supports for the synthesis (figure 7). After coupling step products are separated from the excess of reagents by size exclusion chromatography. This type of separation is comparatively faster than conventional separation and purification processes but is slower than simple filtration in the solid phase process.

3. Library Requirements

Synthesis of libraries both chemical as well as biological (proteins, peptides, poly-nucleotides) relies on three requirements:

a) **Polymeric solid support:** An inert cross-linked, insoluble, polymeric material for synthesis.
b) **Linker:** Linkers are means to link or bind substrate to solid phase that permits selective cleavage of some or all of the products from solid support during analysis and ultimately release the final product.
c) **Protecting groups:** A chemical protection strategy to allow selective protection and de-protection of reactive groups.

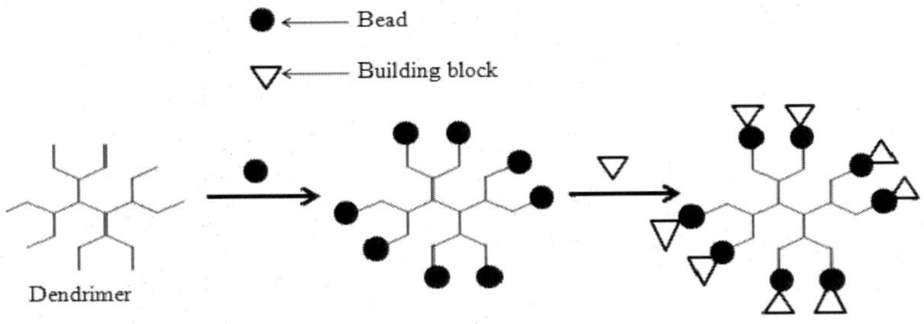

Figure 7. Dendrimer based synthesis.

3.1. Solid Support

Solid supports are used in solid phase synthesis to hold the first building block. Solid support has two parts: the core and the linker (figure 8). The core region ensures insolubility of support while the linker contains a functional group for the attachment of building blocks. A material must possess the basic characteristics in order to be used as solid support:

i. It should be insoluble in solvents used during synthesis.
ii. It should not react with the reagents used in synthesis.
iii. Linker should form a stable bond with building block under given reaction conditions of synthesis.

There are two types of supports. One in which reaction takes place only at the surface like polymer, glass beads etc. Second in which reaction takes place inside the body like resins that swell on the addition of solvents. Various types of solid supports are used now a day in solid phase synthesis [5], few of them are listed below:

3.1.1. Cross-linked polystyrene

Cross-linked polystyrene resins are the most commonly used supports in solid phase synthesis. They are synthesized as spherical beads of lightly cross-linked styrene and divinylbenzene. The ratio of styrene to divinylbenzene determines the density of cross links. If density is high the beads are mechanically stable. However if density is low then resin will swell on the addition of solvents during synthesis thereby increases the accessibility of functional groups buried inside the beads. Another important factor is size of beads. The reactions are faster when small beads are used, but small beads are difficult to filter out. If bead size is big in size then the reaction is slow. The bead size is characterized either by the diameter of the beads or by the inversely proportional mesh size.

3.1.2. Polyethylene glycol (PEG) grafted supports

PEG-grafted copolymers or Tentagel contains 1-2% crosslinked polystyrene core, covalently attached to polyethylene glycol chains through aromatic rings (figure 9). The substrate at the end of a flexible chain is more accessible to reagents. PEG-chains show hydrophilic characteristic, swells well in water and methanol but poorly in ether or ethanol [7]. PEG grafted polymers are unstable and have a tendency to become sticky hence becomes difficult to handle during synthesis.

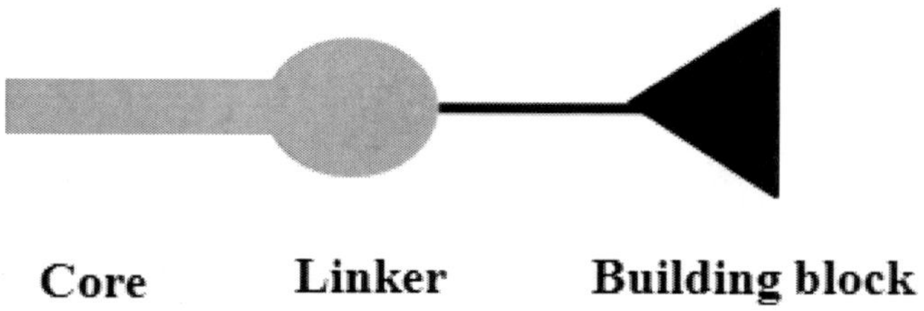

Figure 8. Structure of Solid support.

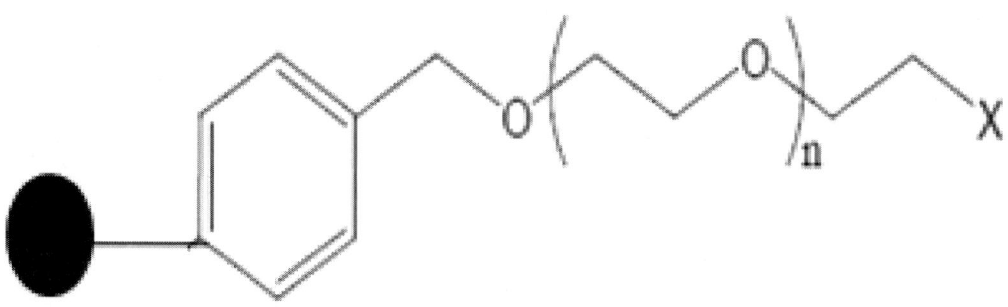

Figure 9. Structure of Polyethylene glycol grafted support. X is a functional group (Br, OH, SH or NH_2).

3.1.3. Inorganic supports

Functionalized glass beads with variable pore size and ceramics are used as inorganic support in solid phase synthesis. They do not swell in solvents but possess mechanical stability.

3.1.4. Non-bead form supports

Polymers are also used as supports in macroscopic state. To be used as a support, surface of polymers is attached to groups which serve as anchors to hold the substrate in a reasonable quantity. Non-bead supports are prepared by grafting polyolefin chains on the surface of objects with the help of radiations [8].

3.1.5. Polyamide Resins

Polyamide resins were designed by Sheppard. These resins mimic properties of peptide chains and possess good solvation properties. A mild protective or deprotective group (fluroenylmethoxycarbonyl (Fmoc)) is attached in polyamide resins which can be easily removed by base. Examples of polyamide resins are Dimethylformamide (DMF) or N-methyl pyrrolidinone (figure 10).

a) Dimethylformamide (DMF)   b)N-methyl pyrrolidinone

Figure 10. Structures of polyamide resins.

3.2. Linkers

Linker molecules are a link between first building block and solid support. Linker is a bi-functional molecule, on one side it forms an irreversible covalent bond with solid support and on the other side it is attached to the first building block via reversible covalent bond (figure 11). Linker molecule in a bounded state with solid support acts as anchor for synthesized compounds. Its role is to hold newly synthesized compounds attached to support till synthesis is carried out and in the end allows their smooth cleavage without destruction.

A large number of linker molecules attached to support or resins [5] are available commercially. Few linkers along with their structures (figure 12) are listed below:

i. **Merrifield resin** can attach to carboxylic acids. The final product is cleaved from the resin in carboxylic acid form using HF.

ii. **Hydroxymethyl resin** attaches to activated carboxylic acids and final product cleaved in a similar way as that of Merrifield resin.
iii. **Aminomethyl resin** forms amide bond with substrates which is resistant to cleavage. Therefore aminomethyl resin is used when the synthesized products are not cleaved but tested in bound form.
iv. **Trityl chloride resin** can attach to a variety of compounds like carboxylic acids, alcohols, phenols, amines, thiols. The final product is cleaved under mild conditions using a solution of trifluoroacetic acid (TFA) in different concentrations (2-50%).
v. **Wang resin** can also bind to carboxylic acids. During synthesis there is formation of stable ester linkages between resin and building blocks, but its cleavage conditions are milder than that of the Merrifield resin. Final products are cleaved using solution of trifluoroacetic acid (95% TFA).
vi. **Rink amide resin** contains protected amino group in the beginning. The first amino group is deprotected followed by attachment to carboxylic acids. The final product is cleaved using diluted (~1%) TFA in carboxamide form.
vii. **Photolabile anchors** are those in which final product is cleaved with the help of irradiation rather than chemicals. Anchors usually contain nitro groups which absorb UV light and cleave the bond between solid support and newly synthesized compound.
viii. **Safety catch linkers** are linkers which are cleaved by performing two different reactions instead of the single reaction. These linkers are usually unreactive to the conditions of the library synthesis but are activated by a simple chemical transformation to permit cleavage of final products.

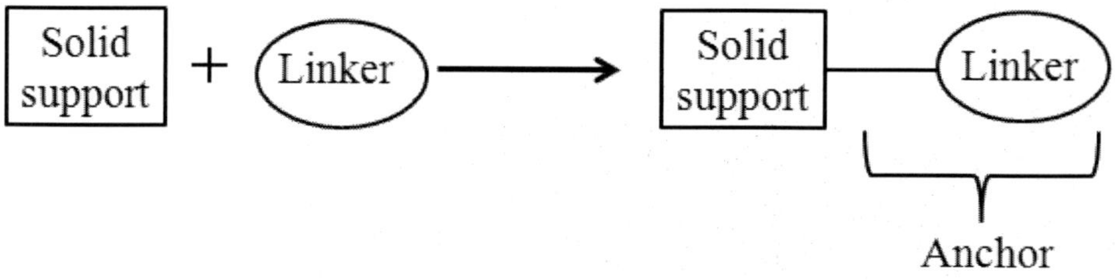

Figure 11. Linker molecule.

3.3. Protecting Groups

Protecting groups are used to block one or more functional groups of building blocks. They are reversibly attached to the functional group and make them less reactive or inactive. When the protection is no longer required, the protecting groups are cleaved and original functionality of functional groups is restored. Major requirement of protecting groups is to be stable under reaction conditions and should be easily cleaved as and when required during synthesis. A large number of protecting groups are available (figure 13). *t*-butoxycarbonyl (Boc) group protects amino group during peptide synthesis and can be removed using mild TFA at room temperature. 9-fluorenylmethoxycarbonyl (Fmoc) also protects the amino group and is removed under basic conditions. Usually 20% piperidine dissolved in DMF is used as reagent. Carboxyl groups are protected by converting them either to benzyl esters or *t*-butyl esters. The benzyl esters are cleaved by saponification, HF or catalytic hydrogenation. While *t*-butyl esters are cleaved by TFA. The t-butyl esters and Boc groups possess similar properties but are less sensitive to acidolysis. Thiol groups are protected by benzyl ether formation or by tritylation. The alcoholic and phenolic hydroxyl groups are protected by converting them to benzyl ether or t-butyl ether. The amide groups (present in asparagine and glutamine) is protected by tritylation. The -NH group of the imidazole ring present in histidine is protected in conjunction with the Fmoc strategy by tritylation. The indole ring of tryptophane is protected by Boc group.

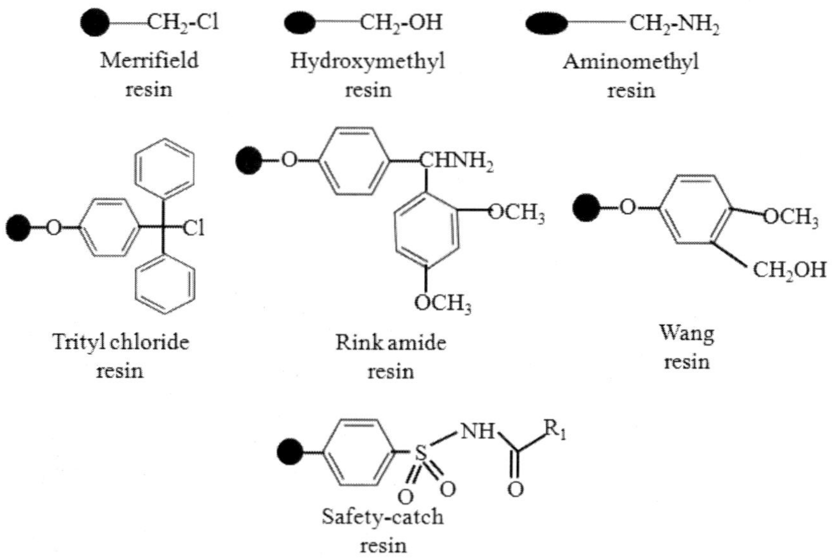

Figure 12. Example of linkers.

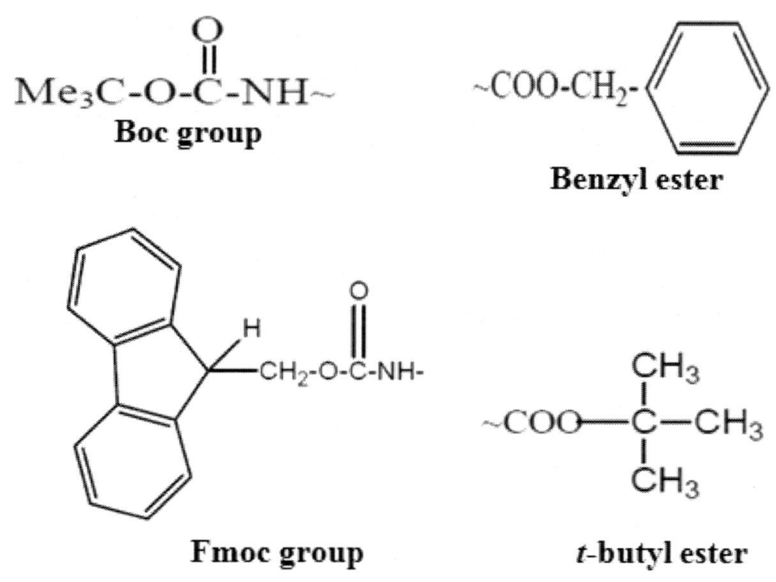

Figure 13. Example of protecting groups.

4. Experimental Techniques in Combinatorial Chemistry

Combinatorial libraries are generated by two fundamental techniques [1, 2]:

a) Biological Library Approach
b) Spatially addressable parallel solid phase library approach

4.1. Biological Library Approach

This approach is limited to peptide libraries with eukaryotic amino acids only. The biological system used to generate diverse peptide mimics evolutionary system of generating proteins. It takes advantage of protein folds by grafting random oligopeptides on tertiary folds. In this approach diversity is maintained by the structures of oligonucleotides/ oligopeptides. Different oligonucleotides are synthesized, cloned and expressed as peptides. Three approaches are used to build biological library:

i. Filamentous phage approach
ii. Plasmid approach
iii. Polysome approach

The filamentous phage approach is given by Parmley and Smith in 1988 [1, 2, 9] to develop small, random peptide library. With the help of ECoRI they inserted a stretch of random deoxynucleotide into P III gene of filamentous phage. P III gene mediates absorption to host cell as an interface to the entry of phage into bacterial cells. Random deoxynucleotide sequences were expressed and displayed as peptides on the surface of the bacteriophage particle, which were detected by anti-ECoRI antibodies. Later approach was implemented to synthesize millions of random peptide library from which specific ligand against monoclonal antibodies were isolated [10]. This method was also used as a tool for generating cDNA expression library cloning. On parallel line library of random peptides were expressed in plasmid and polysomes [11, 12]. There are two major limitations of the biological library approach:

i. It is limited to 20 eukaryotic amino acid.
ii. Unnatural amino acid or any other organic moiety cannot be incorporated into the library.

4.2. Spatially Addressable Parallel Solid Phase Library Approach

Spatially addressable synthesis is the one in which the identity of a compound can be determined by its location of the synthesis substrate. In this approach a solid support, attached with resins or linker molecules, is used for parallel synthesis of peptides. One end of resins or linkers is attached to solid support and the other end is open for peptide synthesis. This approach is applicable to peptides, non-peptides, oligomers, chemical compounds etc. Various methods are used to generate spatially addressable libraries:

i. Multi-pin methodology
ii. Tea bag methodology
iii. SPOTS membrane method
iv. Light directed peptide synthesis on resin support.

4.2.1. Multi-pin apparatus

A multi-pin method was developed by Geysen and his colleagues [8] for synthesizing a series of peptide epitopes. The apparatus consists of polyethylene pins, of size 4 * 40 mm, arranged on Microtiter plate consisting of 96 wells (figure 14). The wells were characterized by the coordinates: rows and columns. At the tip of the pin a spacer molecule (for example: NB-Frmoc-β-alanyl-1, 6-diaminohexane or polyacrilic acid) was attached whose other end act as starting point of peptide synthesis. The wells were filled with activated amino acid and coupling reagents. Pins were immersed into the wells and kept immersed till the coupling occurs. Washing is performed to remove excess of reagents and unwanted components. Newly synthesized peptides remain attached to the pins. Peptides were then screened after de-protection, without cleaving from the pins. Antibodies are used to screen out peptides, using an enzyme linked immunosorbent assay (ELISA) method, on the basis of their binding capabilities [8, 13]. Sequence of peptide attached to pin depends on the order in which amino acids are added into the particular well. Therefore by recording the order of adding amino acid in each well and position of well, the sequence of peptide can be determined.

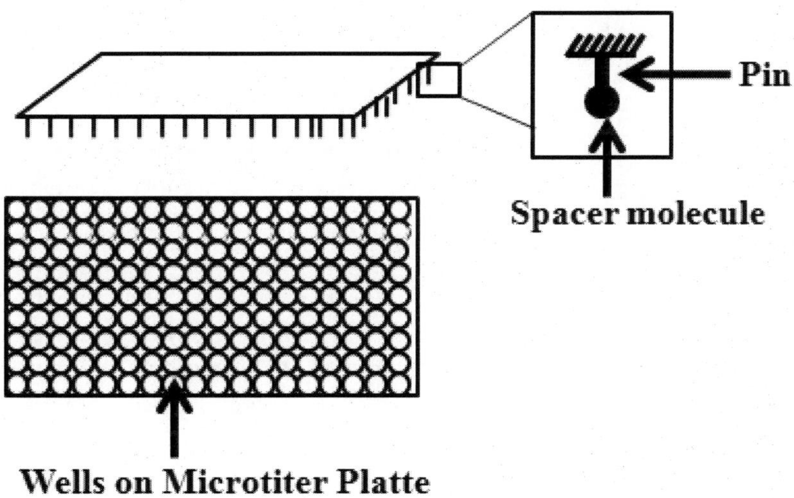

Figure 14. Multi-pin technology apparatus.

4.2.2. Tea bag method

A tea bag method was developed by Houghten for multiple peptide synthesis [14]. This method was used to synthesize a series of polypeptides on bead form polymer support. A porous polypropylene bag containing polymer beads is placed in solution of activated amino acids. Coupling reaction between resins and amino acids take place which is followed by washing. The deprotection of the amino group of newly added amino acid was performed on the solid support enclosed in the same bags. The process is repeated and in the end each bag contains a single peptide chain (figure 15). This approach has two advantages [5]:

- Less number of operations are needed than in a normal parallel synthesis.
- Number of reaction vessel is less than the number of the synthesized compounds.

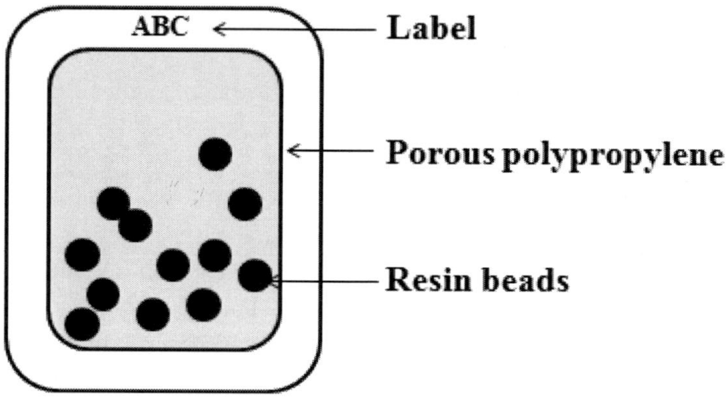

Figure 15. Tea bag approach.

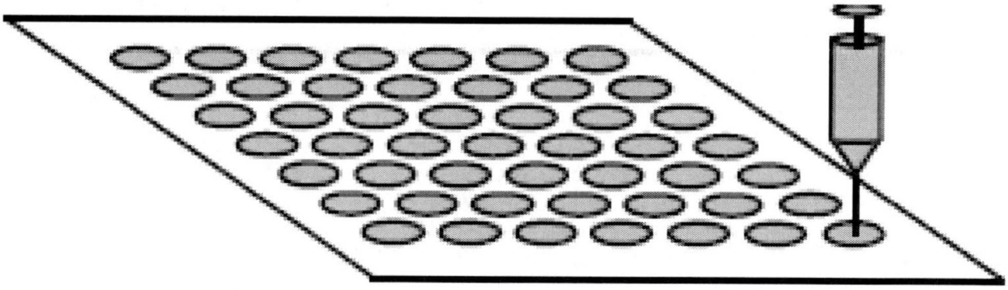

Figure 16. Spot synthesis method [5].

4.2.3. SPOTS membrane method

This approach was developed by Frank and his colleagues [15, 16]. Its mechanism is same as that of multi-pin method but differs in the type of solid support used for peptide synthesis. In SPOTS membrane method instead of polyethylene pins, cellulose membrane or paper was used as solid support for peptide synthesis. Amino acid and coupling reagents are dissolved in low volatility solvents. The small amount of solution is pipette onto predefined positions of membrane (figure 16). Spots generated due to pipetting act as reaction wells on which peptide synthesis takes place. The peptides can be screened on the paper after removing the protecting groups.

4.2.4. Light directed peptide synthesis on resin support

This approach is a combination of two key technologies: a) Solid phase synthesis b) Photolithography. A solid support is covalently attached to the amino linker. An amino linker is protected by photo labile nitroveratryloxycarbonyl (NVOC); this is known as first masking. Light is used to activate specific region on the solid support for synthesis of peptide. Solid support is exposed to light which removes photo labile protecting group resulting in de-protection and activation of specific regions of solid support. Now activated (specific regions) solid support is exposed to first set of amino acids, where the amino group of each amino acid is attached with the photo labile protecting group. On exposure, coupling takes place between the carboxyl group of protected amino acids and selectively activated regions of solid support. Excess of amino acids is removed, thereby left with masked amino acid coupled with solid support. Now substrate is again illuminated by light through a second mask, such that second protected building block (amino group of attached amino acid) is activated. Again support is exposed to second set of protected amino acids followed by coupling reaction. The process of illumination, thereby activation of the masked group followed by addition of amino group protected amino acids continues (figure 17). The order in which masks and sequence of amino acids are added defines the product and its location. Position of desired end product is known therefore it is easily identified, isolated and interaction with other molecules can be inferred directly. The only limitation is due to photolithography technique used to activate sites for synthesis. Specific resolution and sites are required to activate sites but there are a limited number of known sites that can be activated by appropriate resolution.

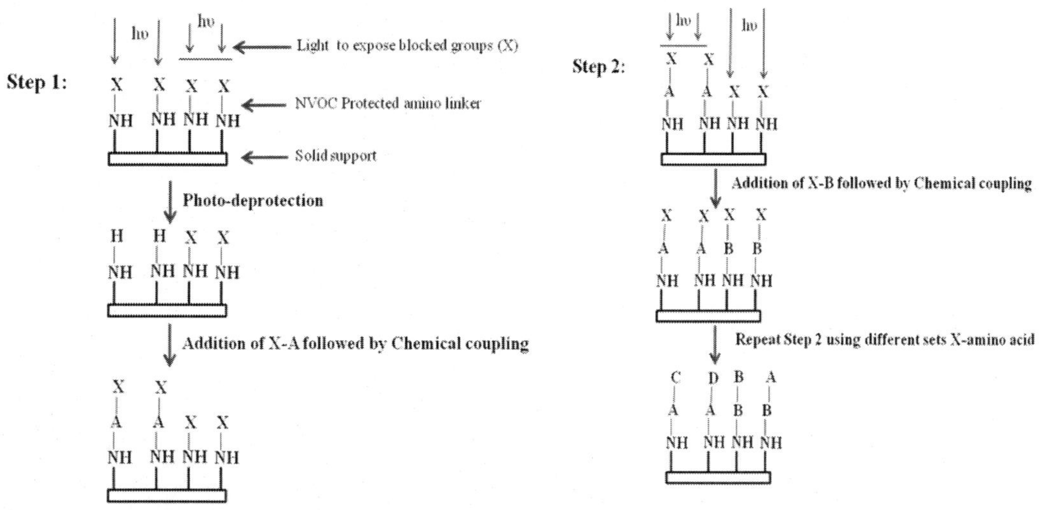

Figure 17. Light directed peptide synthesis.

5. Screening of Combinatorial Libraries

Combinatorial libraries containing thousands of compounds are searched for compounds having pre-determined properties. This process is called screening. Screening of combinatorial libraries is carried out with the help of assays that unambiguously show the presence or absence of components having the desired property. The results of the assays often appear as changes in color, fluorescence, radioactivity, conductivity etc. [5]. There are many approaches for screening of libraries. The classical method of screening of compounds for desired biological activity involves testing all compounds one at a time in a competition-binding assay or in cell-based assay. Compounds attached to the beads are released locally on a pool of confluent mammalian cells. This leads to activation of cells in the area surrounding the bead.

Bead responsible for cell activation is isolated and detected. The problem with this method is that activation of cells is basically a cumulative effect of all compounds, in which some compounds may have high affinity for the cells or some may have low affinity. As a result it becomes difficult to separate out compounds on the basis of simple activation of cells [2].

In one approach, the target molecule is covalently attached to an insoluble matrix. A chromatography column is filled with the matrix and dissolved library is passed through the column. The active components bind to the target and are retained in the column while the inactive components are eluted out. Similar to other affinity approaches, after washing the column the active molecules are eluted which are then sent for structure prediction.

In another approach both, the target protein molecule and the components of the library are dissolved in the same medium. The active molecules bind to the target protein on the basis of their binding affinity. The mixture is submitted to size exclusion chromatography. The protein molecule holding attached active molecule readily separates from the inactive small molecule library components. Applying appropriate conditions the ligand dissociates from the receptor and its structure can be determined [5].

5.1. High-Throughput Screening (HTS)

High throughput screening is a method for scientific experimentation which allows researchers to effectively conduct millions of biochemical, genetic or pharmacological tests in a short period of time. Through this process one can rapidly identify active compounds, which modulate a particular activity or property. HTS uses a brute-force approach to collect a large amount of experimental data -- usually observations about how some biological entity reacts to exposure to various chemical compounds -- in a relatively short time.

HTS equipment is a small container, usually made of plastic that features a grid of small, open divots called wells. Most of the wells contain experimentally useful matter, often a solution of dimethyl sulfoxide (DMSO) and some other chemical compounds synthesized by combinatorial synthesis.

Each well contains different compound. To prepare for an assay, the researcher fills each well of the plate with some biological entity and keep it for incubation. It allows the biological matter to bind or react with the compounds in the wells; measurements are taken across all the plate's wells, either manually or by a machine. The machine outputs the result of each experiment as a grid of numeric values, with each number mapping to the value obtained from a single well.

References

[1] Gallop, M. A., Barrett, R. W., Dower, W. J., Fodor, S. P. A. & Gordon, E. M. (1994). Application of combinatorial technologies to drug discovery.1. Background and peptide combinatorial libraries. *J Med Chem*, *37*(9), 1233-1251.

[2] Pandeya, S. N. & Thakkar, D. (2005). Combinatorial chemistry: A novel method in drug discovery and its application. *Indian Journal of Chemistry, 44B*, 335-348.

[3] Houghton, R. A., Pinnila, L., Blondelle, S. E., Appel, J. R., Doolley, C. T. & Cuervo, J. H. (1991). Generation and use of synthetic peptide combinatorial libraries for basic research and drug discovery. *Nature, 354*, 84-86.

[4] Merrifield, R. B. (1963). Solid Phase Peptide Synthesis. I. The Synthesis of a Tetrapeptide. *J. Am. Chem. Soc., 85*, 2149-2154.

[5] Furka, A. (2007). Combinatorial Chemistry: Principles and Techniques. Arpad Furka in electronic form, Budapest.

[6] Terrett, N. K. (1998). Combinatorial Chemistry, Oxford University Press. ISBN-13, 978-0198502197.

[7] Rapp, W. (1996). Combinatorial Peptide and Non-peptide Libraries. A Handbook (ed. G. Jung), Wiley-VCH VErlag GmbH Weinheim. 425-464.

[8] Geysen, H. M., Meloen, R. H. & Barteling, S. J. (1984). Use of peptide synthesis to probe viral antigens for epitopes to a resolution of a single amino acid. *Proc Natl Acad Sci.*, USA, *81*(13), 3998-4002.

[9] Lam, K. S. (1997). Application of combinatorial library methods in cancer research and drug discovery. *Anti-Cancer Drug Design, 12*, 145-167.

[10] Cwirla, S. E., Peters, E. A., Barrett, R. W. & Dower, W. J. (1990). Peptides on phage, a vast library of peptides for identifying ligands. *Proc Natl Acad Sci.*, USA., *87*, 6378-6382.

[11] Scott, J. K., Loganathan, D., Easley, R. B., Gang, X. & Goldstein, I. J. (1992). A family of concanavalin A-binding peptides from a hexapeptide epitope library. *Proc Natl Acad Sci.*, USA., *89*(12), 5398-5402.

[12] Cull, M. G., Miller, J. F. & Schatz, P. J. (1992). Screening for receptor ligands using large libraries of peptides linked to the C terminus of the *lac* repressor. *Proc Natl Acad Sci.*, USA. *89*, 1865-1869.

[13] Gordon, E. M., Barrete, R. W., Dower, W. J., Fodor, S. P. A. & Gallop, M. A. (1994). Applications of combinatorial technologies to drug discovery.2. Combinatorial organic synthesis, library screening strategies and future directions. *J Med Chem.*, 37, 1385-1401.

[14] Houghton, R. A. (1985). General method for the rapid solid-phase synthesis of large numbers of peptides: specificity of antigen-antibody interaction at the level of individual amino acids. *Proc Natl Acad Sci.*, USA. 82, 5131-5135.

[15] Frank, R., Güler, S., Krause, S. & Lindenmayer, W. (1991). Facile and rapid "spot synthesis" of large numbers of peptides on membrane sheets. In: Peptides 1990. *Proceedings of the 21st European Peptide Symposium*, eds. E. Giralt, D. Andreu, Leiden, ESCOM. 151-152.

[16] Frank, R. (1992). Spot-synthesis: An easy technique for the positionaly addressable parallel chemical synthesis on a membrane support. *Tetrahedron, 48*, 9217-9232.

In: Introduction to Drug Designing and Development
Editors: R. Kumar, A. Sharma and R. Kumar Tiwari
ISBN: 978-1-62948-556-0

Chapter 10

Quantitative Structure Activity Relationship

Anju Sharma
Amity Institute of Biotechnology,
AMITY University-Uttar Pradesh,
Lucknow, Uttar Pradesh, India

Abstract

The drug exerts its biological effect by binding to its respective receptors. This phenomenon is governed by the structure of drug molecule as well as the structure of the receptor.

Quantitative Structure Activity Relationship (QSAR) is based on the hypothesis that the structure of the molecule contains features responsible for its physical, chemical and biological properties. These features are termed as descriptors, which are used to formulate mathematical equations. After validation QSAR equations are used to predict the activity of newly synthesized molecules.

Traditional QSAR describes structure-activity relationship on the basis of physicochemical, steric, electronic properties (Hammet equation and Hansch analysis) or making use of some structural features (Free Wilson Analysis) and Multiple Linear Regression (MLR) to build a model. Developing a QSAR model is a multi-step process. Traditional QSAR models are simple to calculate and allow for relatively fast analysis, but they often fail to take into account the 3D structures of chemical structure. Three dimensional (3D) QSAR is another method based on the statistical correlation analysis enabling the comparison of 3D molecular forces produced in the vicinity of different compounds to determine correlation between biological activities and folds. QSPR (Quantitative Structure Property Relationship) is an extension of QSAR which tries to establish relationship between structure and molecular properties like solubility, cell permeability.

Theory and methodology of traditional and 3D QSAR are described in this chapter together with validation approaches. The overall goals of QSAR models remain focused on its prediction ability and its receptiveness to mechanistic interpretation.

1. Introduction

A *similarity principle* states that a set of molecules will typically display an understandable structure-activity relationship. In other words, *compounds with similar chemical and physical properties have similar biological properties.* This principle laid the foundation or forms the basis of QSAR, an acronym of Quantitative Structure Activity Relationship.

The relationship between the chemical structure and activity is quantified by QSAR. Activity here may correspond to any physical property like boiling point, solubility, water-ocatnol partition coefficient etc. In terms of toxicology and pharmacology activity corresponds to biological activity like antiviral, antibacterial activity. QSAR applies the similarity principle within a co- generic series of compounds or structural class to:

(a) Correlate affinities of ligands to their specific binding sites, rate constants, inhibition constants and other biological activities either with certain structural features or with atomic, group or molecular properties such as lipophilicity, polarizability, electronic and steric properties.
(b) Establish a link between the ability of certain molecules to perform its desired functions and properties of that molecule. This represented an effort to quantitatively relate the structure of a compound to its activity and resulting equations were aptly named QSAR.

2. Molecular Structure and Molecular Properties

It is often observed that all molecular properties are coded by and consequently result from molecular structure. The relationship between lipophilicity and unspecific biological properties, such as narcotic, bactericidal, fungicidal, hemolytic and toxic properties, has been known since the beginning of the century. In 1964 independent publications of the Free Wilson method [1] and of Hansch analysis [2], marked a milestone in the development of QSAR. QSAR basically correlates , within congeneric series of compounds, affinities of ligands to their binding sites, inhibition constants, rate constants and other biological activities , either with certain structural features (Free Wilson analysis) or with atomic, group or molecular properties, such as lipophilicity, polarizability, electronic and steric properties (Hansch analysis) [3-16] (figure 1).

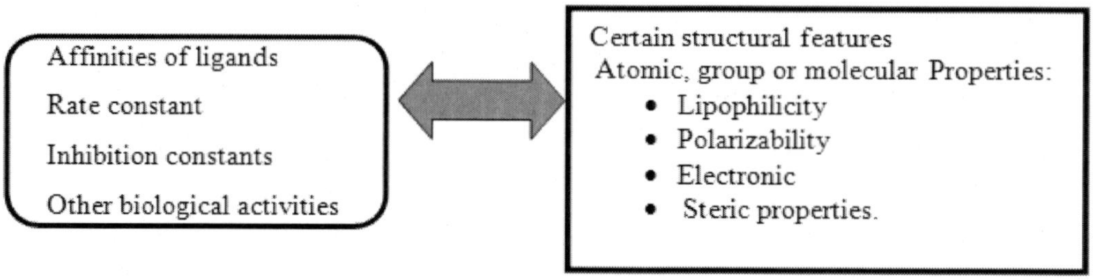

Figure 1. Illustration of correlation between activity and properties.

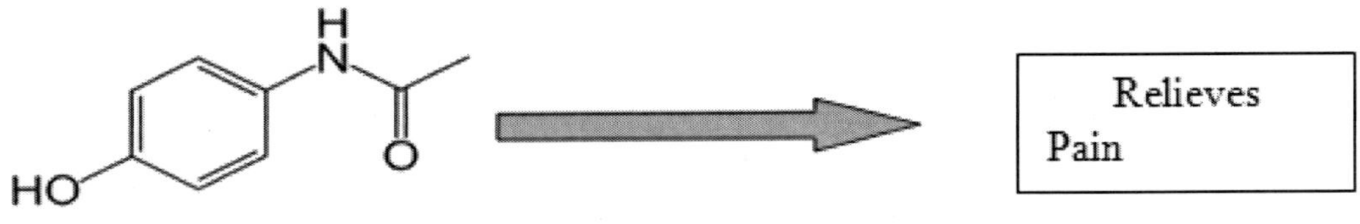

Figure 2. Illustration of relation between structure of paracetamol and its activity.

One example for understanding structure property relationship is of drug Paracetamol. Paracetamol selectively inhibits cyclo-oxygenase enzyme COX-3 found in the brain and spinal cord, thereby relieves pain and reduces fever.

Cyanide which is toxic in nature exerts its toxicity because of its structure. Cyanide inhibits terminal enzyme of the respiratory chain, cytochrome-c oxidase enzyme. This inhibition leads to insufficient utilization of oxygen and suffocation and thereby causing drastic effects on health. Inhibition of cytochrome-c oxidase occurs through binding to ferric ion of cytochrome.

The overall goal of QSAR is to retain their original essence and remain focused on the predictive power of the approach and its receptiveness to mechanistic interpretation. QSAR represents an effort to quantitatively relate the chemical structure (physicochemical properties) to the activity of the compound. Physicochemical properties are broadly classified into three general types: Electronic, Steric, Hydrophobic. A statistical analysis for a set of properties (descriptors) for a series of biologically active compounds is carried out to develop the equations.

The statistical equations thus developed are aptly known as QSAR equations (example equation 1) and are used to predict the activity of additional compound or compound not yet synthesized.

$$\textbf{Biological activity} = f\ \textbf{(Molecular structure)} \qquad (1)$$

3. QSAR Equations

All QSAR equations have molecular property expressed as a function of molecular descriptors. Equations differ from each other in the molecular property they are trying to correlate, descriptors they are using and the mathematical expression they use. Example:

Oral bioavailability = f (descriptor set 1)

Carcinogenicity = f (descriptor set 2)

The most common parameters that are correlated to molecular activity are electronic and lipophilicity i.e., "σ" is electronic parameter given by Hammett, "π" is lipophilicity parameter developed specifically for QSAR by Hansch. It's not that only these two parameters are tested various others are also tested but none finds wide acceptance as σ and π.

A typical QSAR equation is:

$$\log\left(\frac{1}{C}\right) = -K_1(\log P)^2 + K_2\log P + K_3\Pi + K_4MR + K_5E_s + K_6 \qquad (2)$$

Where, C is the concentration needed to carry out the desired effect, logP and $(\log P)^2$ terms are used to show the parabolic relationship of lipophilicty and activity, K_1, K_2, K_3, K_4, K_5, K_6 are all regression coefficients.

4. Molecular Descriptors

Molecular descriptors are the basic tool for any QSAR modeler. The descriptors are simply numbers which are derived from the specific molecular representations and encode structural chemical information. They are the outcomes of the logical mathematical procedure that transforms chemical information encoded within a symbolic representation of a molecule in a utilitarian manner. The descriptors are generally encoded by algorithmic techniques. Usually more than one descriptor is used to discriminate between compounds.

Molecular descriptors not only co-relate molecular structure (Figure 3) to properties but also describe different aspects of molecules, compare different molecular structure and different conformations of the same molecule, also used as database storage.

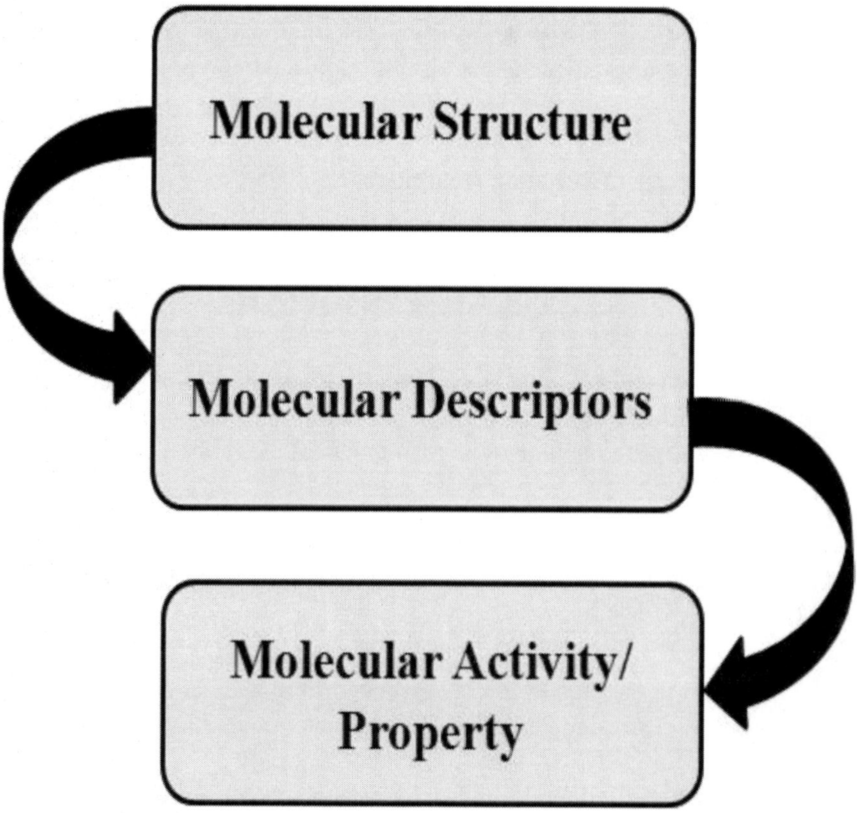

Figure 3. Relation between structure and property.

Three categories of descriptors are there:

1. Descriptors having an experimental counterpart (LogP)
2. Descriptors which represent properties of whole molecules (MR, viscosity) and that can be calculated (from 2D graphs, topological indices 2D-fingerprints etc.)
3. Descriptors which can be encoded by pharmacophores (3D representation)

Different type of properties have been used in developing QSAR models, this includes physicochemical, molecular, quantum chemical and binding properties. Example of physiochemical properties is hydrophobicity, electronic parameters, steric parameters, ionization constants and solubility etc. Molecular properties include geometry, shape, electron distribution, conformation etc. Quantum chemical properties include charges and energy values. Binding properties involve binding interaction between macromolecules which play important role in receptor-mediated responses. Physicochemical properties are of vital importance in understanding how drug-receptor interactions take place. Initially three broad parameters were suggested which still bore a huge impact namely Electronic, Steric, Hydrophobic [17].

4.1. Electronic Descriptors

Electronic properties are intimately related to chemical reaction and biological activities of compounds. Small electronic perturbation may bring about change in mechanism of reaction. Different substituent groups alter the reaction rates thus help in delineating the overall reaction mechanism. Electronic role of substituent's on rate constants was first studied by Burckhardt. However the role of electronic parameters and effect of substituent was firmly established by Hammett. He studied the dissociation constant of substituted benzoic acid and phenyl acetic acid. A dissociation of organic acids (HA) is a process which involves removal of protons from a neutral compounds leaving behind a negatively charged species (eq 3). The extent of reaction is measured by the dissociation constant (K).

$$HA \leftrightarrow H^+ + A^- \tag{3}$$

$$K = \frac{[H^+][A^-]}{[HA]} \tag{4}$$

Dissociation of bases (B) involves the addition of a proton liberating a water molecule as shown in equation 5.

$$B + H_3O^+ \leftrightarrow BH^+ + H_2O \tag{5}$$

Louis Hammett observed that dissociation constants of benzoic and phenyl acetic acid (Figures 4 and 5) are influenced by electronic properties of the substituent of the phenyl ring.

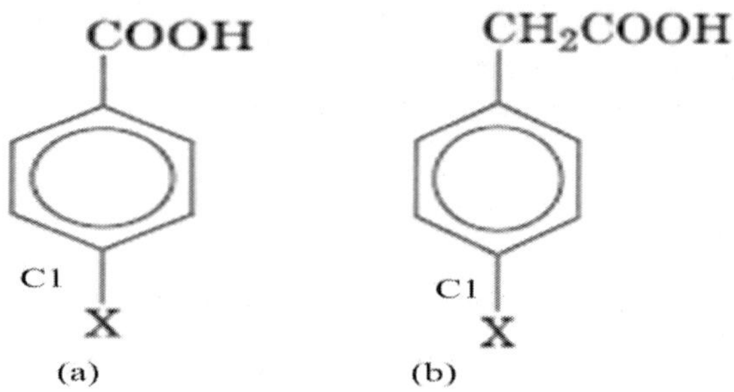

Figure 4. Structure of (a) Benzoic acid (b) Phenyacetic acid. Where X = H, CH3, NO2.

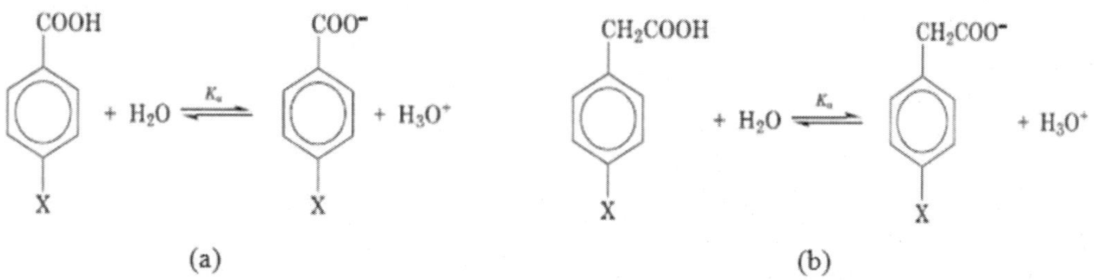

Figure 5. Dissociation reaction of (a) Benzoic acid, (b) Phenylacetic acid.

The electron withdrawing groups increase dissociation while electron donating groups decrease the same (Table 1). This led to an operational definition of first electronic descriptor "σ".

4.1.1. Sigma (σ) Descriptor

It describes the effect of the substituent on the dissociation reaction. Sigma measures the size of the electronic effect for given substituent and represents a measure of electronic charge distribution in benzene nucleus.

Substituent at phenyl ring can increase or decrease the equilibrium constant by stabilizing or destabilizing the anionic form via formation of positive (+) or negative (–) partial charge at C1 (Figure 4). Electron donating substituent's have negative "σ" values because hydrogen (H) will be more tightly held by the molecule and it becomes difficult to dissociate H from the carboxyl (-COOH) group. Electron withdrawing substituents have positive "σ" values, as it will be easy to take out H from structure. σ is calculated using equation 6.

$$\sigma_X = \log K_X - \log K_0 \tag{6}$$

Or

$$\log\left(\frac{K_X}{K_0}\right) = -pK_X + pK_0$$

where K_X and K_0 refers to substituted and un-substituted compounds respectively.

Table 1. Dissociation constants of Benzoic acid and Phenylacetic acid (where K and K_0 refers to substituted and unsubstituted compounds respectively)

Benzoic Acid			Phenylacetic Acid		
R	K	Log (K/K_0)	R	K	Log (K/K_0)
NO_2	$37.05 * 10^{-5}$	0.776	NO_2	$14.1 * 10^{-5}$	0.43
Et	$4.4 * 10^{-5}$	-0.15	Et	$4.2 * 10^{-5}$	-0.09
H	$6.2 * 10^{-5}$ (K_0)	0	H	$5.2 * 10^{-5}$ (K_0)	0

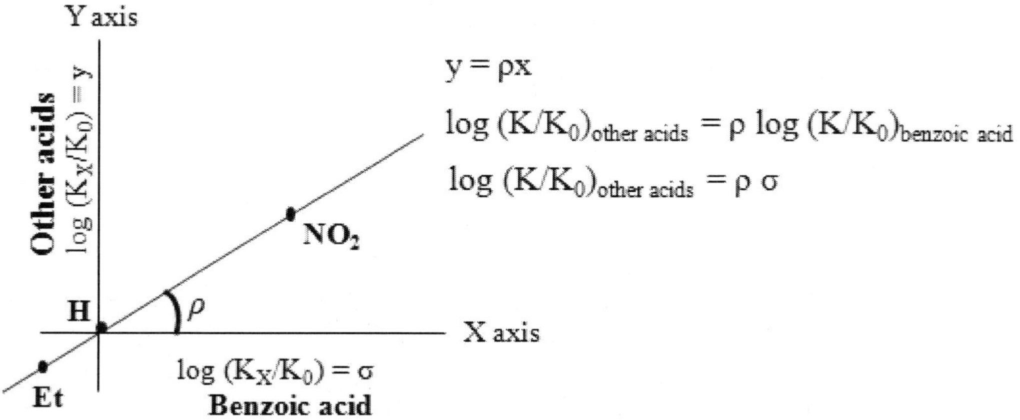

Figure 6. Plot between log (K_X/K_0) of substituted benzoic acids and phenylacetic acid; where ρ is related to the given scaffold (other acids), σ is descriptor of substituent and describes its influence on the dissociation constant.

During bond formation between atoms, free energy decreases i.e., ΔG becomes negative. While in bond breaking, free energy increases thereby ΔG becomes positive. Small changes in ΔG have profound effect on equilibrium constants. The change in free energy is related to equilibrium constant K, this phenomenon is known as linear free energy relationship.

$$\Delta G = -RT \log(K) \tag{7}$$

On plotting quantity log (K_X/K_0) for benzoic acids on the X axis and log (K_X/K_0) for phenylacetic acid on Y axis, Hammett obtained a straight line (figure 6).

Hammett also drew attention to the fact that a plot of log (KX/K0) for benzoic acids versus log (KX/K0) for ester hydrolysis for a series of molecules is linear, which suggests that substituent exert similar effects in dissimilar reactions. Owing to the association of dissociation constant to free energy (equation 7), this correlation was meaningful. It suggests that changes in structure produce proportional changes in activation energy of reactions. This finding is universally known as linear free energy relationship (LFER): Hammett equation (equation 8).

$$\log\left(\frac{K}{K_0}\right)_{otheracids} = \rho \log\left(\frac{K}{K_0}\right)_{Benzoicacids} \tag{8}$$

Table 2. Diagrammatic illustration of substitutions at mata, para and ortho positions

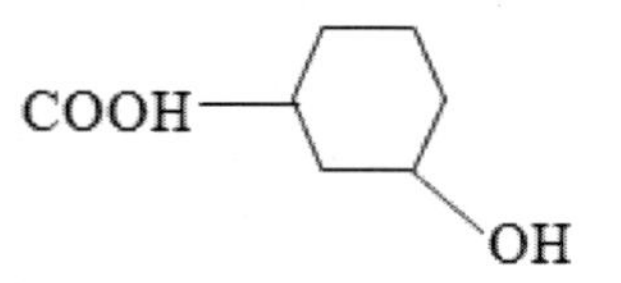	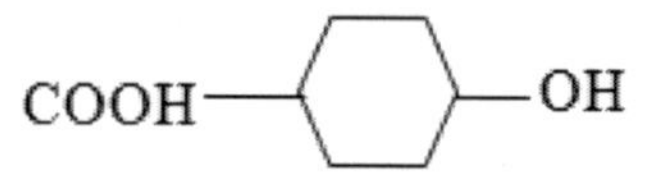	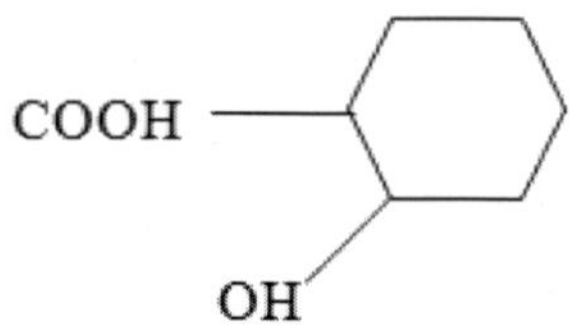
Meta substituted	Para substituted	Ortho substituted

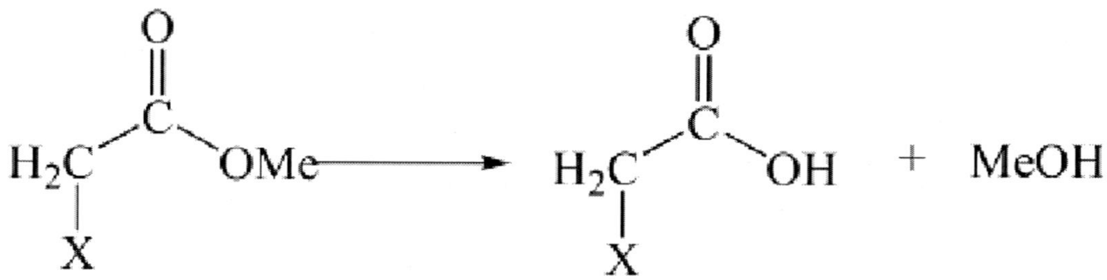

Figure 7. Hydrolysis of aliphatic compounds.

Or

$$\log\left(\frac{K}{K_0}\right)_{otheracids} = \rho\sigma$$

The σ values differ depending on whether the substitute is at meta/ortho/para positions in case of aromatic compounds. Substitution at para, meta and ortho position is shown in table 2.

At meta position: Oxygen is electronegative, can pull electrons due to inductive effect. σ_{meta} for phenol is 0.12 (due to inductive effect).

At para position: Oxygen at para position has electron donating effect because of resonance. Inductive effect is absent due to large distance. σ_{para} for phenol is -0.37.

At ortho position: Ortho-substituted molecules do not always follow Hammet equation and are subject to different parameterizations.

In case of aliphatic compound nature of substituent (X) affects the rate of hydrolysis (Figure 7).

Carbonyl C has a partial positive charge. In order to attach with OH^- it has to have more positive. If X is electron drawing, there will be a more positive charge on carbonyl C leading to more hydrolysis. If X is electron donating, it dilutes the positive charge on carbonyl C as a result hydrolysis is reduced. If substituent X is a bulky group it will hinder carbonyl C and may change the rate of reaction. Steric factors are difficult to measure experimentally.

Hammett equation was further expanded by Charton [18] and Fujita and Nishioka [19] by including the effect of substituent placed at ortho position. Charton divided the ortho electronic effect into its resonance (β), inductive (α) and steric (X) contributions.

$$\log K = \alpha\sigma_1 + \beta\sigma_R + Xr_v + h \tag{9}$$

Fujita and Nishioka modified equation by integrating new descriptors Taft's constant (E_s), Swain-Lupton field constants (F_{ortho}) and para sigma values (σρ) for ortho substituents (equation 10). Ortho-substituted aromatic molecules are processed differently. Reason being that changes in the rate or ionization constants mediated by meta or para substituent changes enthalpy (ΔH) not entropy (ΔS) of reaction while ortho substituents affect both entropy and enthalpy. Entropy is highly sensitive to even a small change in size of reagents, susbstiuents and degree of solvation.

$$\log K = \sigma\rho + \delta E_s^{ortho} + fF_{ortho} + C \qquad (10)$$

In a different study carried out by Bolton et al. (20) ionization of substituted benzoic acids was examined. He measured accurate values of change in free energy, enthalpy, entropy and established different scenarios under which LFER works:

1. The change in enthalpy is constant and change in entropy varies for a series.
2. The change in enthalpy varies while the change in entropy is constant.
3. Both change in entropy and enthalpy vary and are proven to be linearly related.
4. Precise experimentation and measurement suggested that category 3 was most prevalent in benzoic acids.

Limitation of Hammett equation:

1. Primary σ values are reliable and easy usable. They are obtained from thermodynamic ionization of benzoic acids at 25°C. However secondary values are unreliable as they are obtained experimentally rather by comparing with another series of compounds. Thus the chances of error are there because the comparison is dependent on the accuracy of measured series and regression analysis.
2. Discontinuities are observed in Hammett plots due to changes in the mechanisms and transition states. Those reactions which proceed by two concurrent pathways showed non-linear plots [21, 22].
3. Reaction mechanism differs if the solvent is changed. Therefore it is important to extrapolate σ values to include polar solvents and non-polar solvents as well.
4. Resonance or direct conjugation also breaks down the Hammett equation. In general when a bond is formed between a substituent and reaction centre through the pi-electron system, reactivity is increased, diminished or mitigated by separation. However in study of *X-cumyl chlorides* strong conjugate interaction between lone-pair para substituents and vacant p-orbital in a transition state, led to deviations in Hammet plot. [23].

4.1.2. ρ (rho)

It is defined as proportionality or reaction constant. It describes the magnitude of the effect exerted by substituent on the dissociation reaction of a given scaffold. As the distance between the substituent and the dissociated proton increases its influence on the dissociation reaction decreases and so does the value of ρ. If a reaction is aided by electron withdrawal from the reaction site then the value of rho is positive however if the reaction is assisted by an electron donation from the reaction site then the value of rho is negative.

4.1.3. pKa (Ionization Constant) Values

The relationship between ionization and biological activity was first established by Albert [24]. Ionization is based on electronic structure of molecules. pK_a values are now often used to describe physical organic reactions and biological systems. It is a composite of electronic components that are used directly in QSAR equation therefore caution should be made while interpreting the relationship between biological activities and pK_a.

4.1.4. Quantum Chemical Descriptors

Quantum mechanical descriptors are electronic descriptors that give information about the nature of intermolecular forces involved in the biological response. They are directly derived from the molecular wave functions due to the application of quantum chemical methodology. Most popular methods for calculating quantum chemical descriptor are Hartree-Fock (*ab initio*) and semi-empirical methods. There is no statistical error in quantum mechanical calculation. Examples of quantum chemical descriptors are net atomic changes, highest occupied molecular orbital/ lowest unoccupied molecular orbital (HOMO-LUMO) energies, super-delocalizabilties and frontier orbital electron densities.

4.2. Hydrophobicity / Lipophilicity Descriptors

Hydrophobic interactions are of vital importance in biological process as well as in chemistry. Molecular recognitions strongly depend on hydrophobic interaction between ligands and receptors. Term “hydrophobic” means “water fearing”. Hydrophobicity of solutes is determined by measuring partition coefficients (P). Partition coefficient basically deals with neutral species, whereas the distribution ratio includes concentration of charged and/ or polymeric species.

Lipophilicity is another term coined to describe hydrophobicity. Molecular lipophilicity is related to the presence of hydrophobic groups (aromatic rings) and with absence of polar groups. Lipophilicity increases with the addition of aromatic groups and decreases with the addition of polar groups (figure 8). Hydrophobicity/ Lipophilicity is defined as a tendency of a compound to prefer an organic phase rather than an aqueous phase usually *1-octanol* (equation 11).

$$P = \frac{[concentration]_{octanol}}{[conscentration]_{aqueous}} \tag{11}$$

Octanol is chosen as solvent for determining partition coefficient due to many reasons. It mimics bio-membrane because it shares the traits of amphiphilicty and hydrogen-binding capability of phospholipids and proteins found in biological membranes. Octanol is cheap, relatively non-toxic and chemically inert. Hydroxyl group present in the octanol act as both hydrogen bond donor and hydrogen bond acceptor as a result it is capable of interacting with a variety of polar groups.

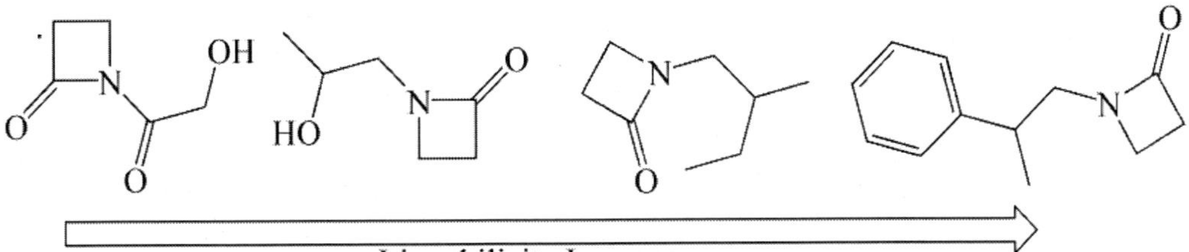

Figure 8. Diagrammatic illustration of increase in lipophilicity due to addition of aromatic groups.

It can dissolve many organic compounds as compared to alkanes, aromatic hydrocarbons and cycloalkanes. It is UV transparent over a large range and has a vapor pressure, low enough for reproducing the measurements.

To exert its biological effect, a drug must reach its site of action. On its way the compound encounters various biological barriers. The movement of drug from its site of application to its site of action depends on lipophilicity/ hydrophobicity of drug. Thus lipophilicity determines in part the concentration of drug that reaches the target site. Once a drug is at the site of action then binding affinity for its biological part be it enzyme or receptor depends on lipophilicity, the electronic properties and other linear free energy related properties.

The importance of lipophilicity was first recognized by Meyer and Overton. In their study they found a correlation between oil/ water partition coefficient and narcotic potencies of small organic molecules [25, 26]. Hansch and his colleagues demonstrated the importance of lipophilicity and laid the foundation for the development of QSAR approach. They gave multiparameter approach which included both electronic and hydrophobic terms to establish a QSAR for a series of plant growth regulators [27]. They gave two descriptors namely a) LogP, b) π. Lipophilicity based descriptors have generated huge impact, interest in the development of QSAR equations.

4.2.1. LogP

LogP describes the lipophilicty of a compound. It is the measure of partitioning of compound between a lipidic phase (normally 1-octanol) and an aqueous phase. It is represented by P or its log value (equation 12).

Compounds with $P > 1$ ($\log P > 0$) are lipophilic (12)

or

Compounds with $P < 1$ ($\log P < 0$) are hydrophilic

where $\log P = \frac{[drug]_{organic}}{[drug]_{aqueous}}$

In 1964 Hansch et al. published their study of structure activity relationships of plant growth regulators and their dependency on Hammett constants and hydrophobicity. They introduced linear free-energy-related Hansch model (also called the 'extra-thermodynamic approach') (equation 13).

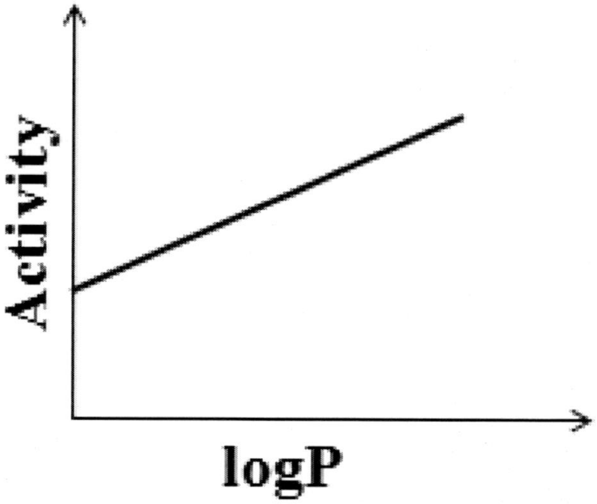

Figure 9. Linear Hansch model.

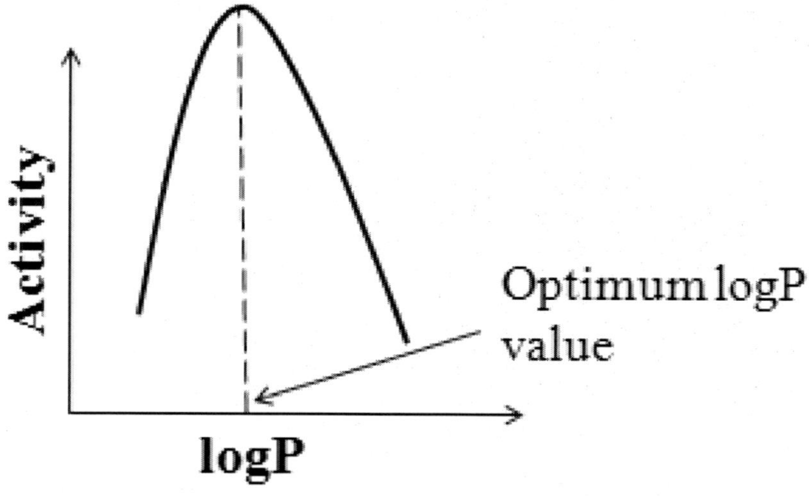

Figure 10. Parabolic nature of lipophilicity as observed by Hansch for large molecules.

Initially Hansch took small set of compounds and observed that biological activities correlated well with logP. Resulting QSAR expression turned out to be quite simple: a linear equation (figure 9).

$$Activity = 0.91 \log P + 0.14 \tag{13}$$

Linear free energy based Hansch model was applicable to a small number of compounds, as the number of compounds increases graph changes from straight line to parabolic curve. Also equation (13) worked well when the two solvents are both alkanols. However, when two solvent systems have different hydrogen bond donor and acceptor capabilities, the linear relationship fails [28, 29] and plot was parabolic in nature (figure 10).

In order to ameliorate his initial idea (only one descriptor) Hansch further refined his QSAR model and introduced other descriptors into model (equation 14) such as electronic (σ), Es (Taft), π (liphophilicty of substituent), MR (Molar refractivity) etc. that represent attributes which may influence drug action. QSAR equation became:

$$\log\left(\frac{1}{C}\right) = -K_1(\log P)^2 + K_2 \log P + K_3\Pi + K_4 MR + K_5 E_s + K_6 \tag{14}$$

Where C is the concentration needed to carry out the desired effect, logP and $(\log P)^2$ terms are used to show the parabolic relationship of lipophilicty and activity, K_1, K_2, K_3, K_4, K_5, K_6 are all regression coefficients.

Hydrophobicity is directly proportional to logP. Hydrophobicity of whole molecule can be computed by the above equation. For individual substituents that deliver a very low logP value which is usually absent in vivo, a new descriptor was introduced π.

4.2.1.1. Different Methods of Encoding LogP

1. *Simple Count:*

LogP is encoded by estimating the number of hydrogen bond acceptor/donor, rings, molecular weight etc. and frequency of their occurrence, which is often calculated from 2D connection tables. Limitation of simple count method is that it is applicable for congeneric molecules only (i.e., molecules having same nucleus) and not for different type of molecules.

2. *By Breaking Molecule Into Fragments:*

The molecule is broken into fragments first and then for each fragment descriptor value is calculated and summed up (eq 15).

Ex: Partition Coefficient = Sum of fragment values + series of correction features

Correction features are included to account for the internal fragment interactions.

$$\log P = \sum_{i=1}^{n} a_i f + \sum_{j=1}^{M} b_j f_j \tag{15}$$

where i represents type of molecule, a_i represent fragment of type i with f_i as correction factor, b_j represents occurrence of correction factor with F_j as correction factor.

ClogP is a automated system for calculation of logP, reported by Leo and Hansch in 1993. It is widely used for calculating logP values. It uses automatic fragmentation scheme to fragment a molecule:

a) By identifying the isolating carbons
b) Atom-based methods

By Identifying The Isolating Carbons/ Fragment:

Isolating carbons are those carbons which are not attached to any heteroatom (any atom other than C & H) by either a double bond or triple bond. The idea is that such carbons are attached only to hydrogen and are hydrophobic.

Example:

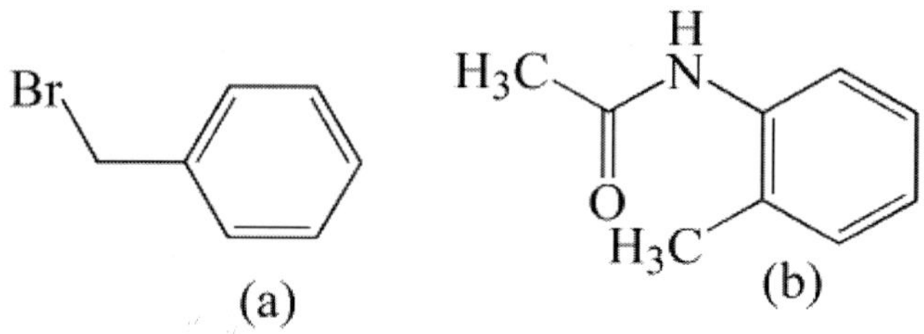

Figure 11. Structures to calculate logP values.

For each fragment of molecule of (figure 11a), experimental value of logP is calculated as follows:

Bromide fragment = 0.48
1 aliphatic isolating carbon = 0.195
6 aromatic isolating carbon = 0.78
7 H on isolating carbon = 1.589
1 chain bond = -0.12
Total = 2.924

For molecule 11(b) experimental value is calculated as follows:

-NH (amide fragment) = 1.510
6 aromatic isolating C = 0.78
1 chain bond = -0.120
1 ortho substitute = -0.76
2 aliphatic isolating C = 0.39
10 H isolating C = 2.270
1 benzyl bond = -0.15
Total = 0.90

The advantage of fragment method is that all electronic interactions are accounted for.

Disadvantage: Values for descriptors are determined experimentally, if due to any reason we cannot calculate values for fragments then this method is not applicable.

Leo and Halkman improved this method in 2000 and gave a recent version of ClogP which can give logP values of missing fragments.

Atom Based Method:

Atom based method calculates contribution of each atom to logP using formula given in equation 16

$$\log P = \sum n_i a_i \quad (16)$$

where n_i represents number of atoms of atom type i, a_i represents atomic contribution (this is calculated from regression analysis when training set of compounds are used in which all experimental values are known).

Gosh and Krippen had classified C, H, O, N, S and halogens into 110 atom types depending upon type of hybridization (sp^2, sp^3, sp) and nature of neighboring atoms. The problem with this method is that only electronic interaction with adjacent atom is considered, long range interactions were not considered.

4.2.2. Π Descriptor

In addition to the parabolic term for the nonlinear characteristics of lipophilicity, combination of different physiochemical properties was introduced in linear free energy related Hansch model.

Hansch and Fujita introduced lipophilicity parameters "**π**" of substituent X in the same way as Hammett had defined electronic parameter σ. **π** characterizes the lipophilicty of a substituent. It is defined as the difference between the logP value of the substituted and the unsubstituted compounds (equation 17).

$$\Pi = \log P_X - \log P_H \tag{17}$$

Substituent's that are more hydrophobic than H have positive π values. While substituent's less hydrophobic than H have negative π values.

Example: For para-bromo-amisol (figure 12), value of π descriptor is calculated as follows:

π of benzene ring is 2.13
π of bromine attached to benzene ring is 0.86
π of methoxy group is -0.02
Total = 2.97 Experimental = 2.97

Advancements are still being made in methodologies and programs for calculating partition coefficients till date. Many more descriptors were introduced to calculate hydrophobicity of a molecule. In a recent attempt to calculate logP led to development of solvatochromic parameters [30, 31]. This approach was proposed by Kamlet et al. and focused on molecular properties of molecule. In its simplest form it is expressed as equation 18.

$$\log P_{octanol} = aV + b\Pi^* + c\beta_H + d\alpha_H + e \tag{18}$$

Where V is a solute volume, π* represents solute ploarizability, β_H and α_H measures hydrogen bond acceptor and hydrogen bond donor strength, e is the intercept.

This model was again modified by Abraham et al. which was extensively used by researchers to characterize hydrophobicity scales [32-34].

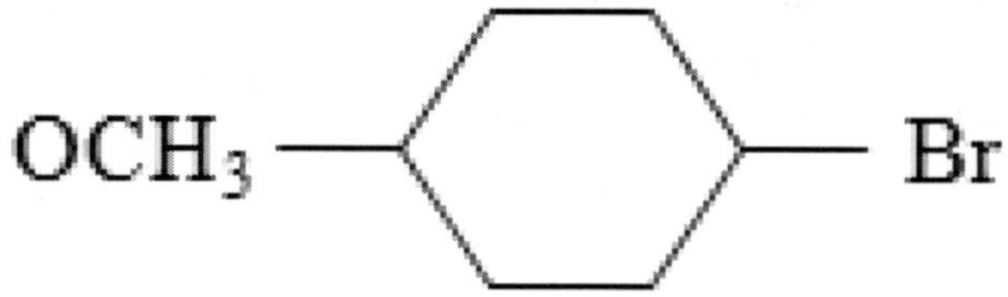

Figure 12. Structure of para-bromo-amisol.

4.3. Steric Descriptors

It is difficult to quantize steric effects at the molecular level. The difficulty level is increased when attempts are made to describe the shape and size of molecule. Inspite of all problems associated with steric factors and their calculations they have the overwhelming importance in both biological interactions as well as in transportation in cellular systems. The first steric parameter that was quantified and used in developing QSAR models was Taft's E_s constant. Later, many more were introduced like Molar refraction (MR) descriptor, Molecular weight (MW) etc.

4.3.1. Taft's E_S Constant

The Taft steric constant E_s is derived experimentally. It is based on the rate constants for a given model reaction. Taft constant is a measure of the steric effect exerted by a substituent (equation 19) on the equilibrium [35].

$$E_s = \log K_X - \log K_H \tag{19}$$

Where K_x and K_H are rate constants of acid hydrolysis of substituted and unsubstituted ester compounds (XCH_2COOR and CH_3COOR respectively). The Bulkier the substituent, the more negative is Es.

Hancock introduced small corrections on Es in order to correct hyperconjugation in α-hydrogens of acetate moiety. Corrections in Taft constant E_s^c is given in equation 20 where n represents number of α-hydrogens and 0.36 is a constant derived from molecular orbital calculations.

$$E_S^C = E_S + 0.306(n-3) \tag{20}$$

Another parameter upsilon υ_X (equation 21) for steric effect was developed by Charton who proved strong correlation between Es and van der Waals radii [36].

$$v_X = r_X - r_H = r_X - 1.20 \tag{21}$$

where r_X and r_H are the minimum van der Waals radii of the substituent and hydrogen respectively.

4.3.2. Molar Refraction (MR) Descriptor

It is described as "chameleon" parameter by Tute [37]. It is a crude measure of the overall mass of molecule still it includes polarizability component which describe cohesion and is related to London dispersion force as described in equation 22:

$$MR = \frac{4\Pi N\alpha}{3} \tag{22}$$

Where N is Avogadro's number and α is the polarizability of the molecule. It does not contain any information about the shape.

MR is also defined by the Lorentz-Lorenz equation (equation 23). According to which it contains information about the compound's volume corrected by the refractive index (the ratio of the velocity of light in vacuum to the velocity of light in the substance of interest).

$$MR = \frac{(n^2 - 1)MW}{(n^2 + 2)d} \tag{23}$$

Where d stands for density, n represents refractive index, MW/d equals to Molar volume.

Values of refractive indices are very low or there is hardly any difference among them, as a result nothing much can be inferred. Therefore molar MR values are considered instead of refractive indices. Molar volume is important because if we mix two compounds say protein and ligand; both have certain molecular weight and density individually. On mixing whether they are binding or not can be accessed by measuring Molar Volume as the total molar volume does not remain same as earlier. If there are more interactions between protein and ligand, their combined molar volume will be less, however if there is less interaction or no interaction between the two, molar volume will increase. Therefore by computing the total molar volume we can define the interaction. That is the reason why molecular volume is included in the Molar refraction calculation.

MR is scaled by 0.1 and used in QSAR models. Positive value of MR indicates that there are either dipolar interactions in the vicinity or a ligand is anchored in an opportune position for interaction. Negative Value of MR indicates steric hindrance at binding site or interaction site.

4.3.3. STERIMOL Parameters

Problem with MR was that it does not distinguish shape; as a result MR value for amyl (-$CH_2CH_2CH_2CH_2CH_3$) is same as that of (-C (Et) $(CH_3)_2$) i.e., 2.42. It fails to adequately address the three-dimensional shape of the molecule. As a result Verloop's STERIMOL parameters were developed which define steric constraints of a given substituent along different axes [38]. They measure standard bond angles, bond distances, van der Waal radii and possible conformations of the substituents.

Five sterimol parameters are required to define shape. They are L, B1, B2, B3 and B4 (figure 13).

- L represents the length of substituent along the axis of bond between the parent molecule and the substituent;
- B1 to B4 represents four different width parameters.

These five parameters were not utilized as efficiently as other parameters due to a high of co-linearity between B1, B2 and B3. Also large training data were needed to statistically validate sterimol parameters. Thus Verloop introduced a slight modification of existing five parameters and gave three parameters for QSAR analysis [39] which enhanced the prediction of correlation with biological properties. Newly defined parameters include:

- Modified length L,
- Minimum width B1
- Maximum width B5 orthogonal to L

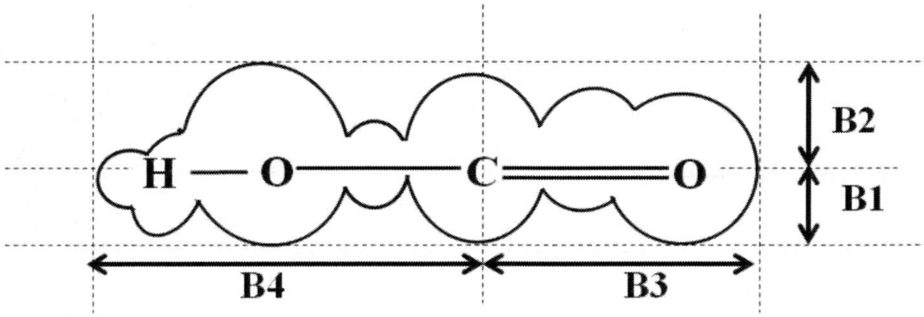

Figure 13. Diagrammatic illustration of Sterimol descriptors.

Sterimol is software that can calculate steric parameters known as Verloop steric parameters. Program CMR given by Leo and Weininger 1995 is also widely used to calculate steric parameters.

4.3.4. Molecular Weight (MW)

Molecular weight is the sum of weights of atoms of which molecule is comprised of. Molecular weight is also used as descriptor in QSAR analysis particularly in distribution/ transportation problems where diffusion is the mechanism or in cellular systems.

4.4. Topological Index

Topological index is also known as connecting index. It is determined on the basis of chemical graphs of a compound. Topological indices are numerical parameters derived from graphs (hydrogen-suppressed molecular graphs) in which the atoms are represented by vertices and the bonds by edges. The connections between the atoms are described by various types of topological matrices (e.g., distance or adjacency matrices). These connections are then mathematically manipulated to derive a single number i.e., graph-theoretical index or topological index [40, 41]. Topological descriptors are usually graph invariant i.e., they do not depend on the way the graph is depicted or labeled and no need of energy minimization of the chemical compound. Simple topological descriptors do not recognize double bonds and atom types like C, N, S etc. They ignore hydrogen bonds and are basically generated for undirected molecular graphs [42]. However sophisticated descriptors consider the hybridization state of every atom present in the molecule. Many indices were given by researchers but the first topological index was proposed by Hosoya et al. followed by Wiener index, Randic's molecular connectivity index, TAU descriptors, Balban's index, Bonchey and Polansky index etc.

Topological descriptors are divided into two categories:

- Global indices
  Indices, which describe entire molecule example: Hosoya and Wiener indices.
- Local / Differential indices
  Indices which describe every atom in a molecule example: Bonchev and Polansky index, Modified Hosoya Index.

4.4.1. HOSOYA Index

Hosoya indices were introduced by Haruo Hosoya in 1971 [43]. He gave the Z index which shows good coorelation between the boiling points of alkane isomers. The Z index for alkanes was calculated using a path graph which is described in terms of vertex and edges. A path graph or linear graph is basically an unbranched tree having two or more vertices, that is, it contains only vertices of degree 2 and 1. In particular, it has two terminal vertices (vertices that have degree 1), while all others (if any) have degree 2.

- Linear alkane is represented by a path graph without branching.
- Methane molecule is represented by a path graph with one vertex and no edges. It has one (empty) matching so its Hosoya index is one.
- Ethane molecule is represented by a path with one edge and two matching's (one with zero edge and one with one edge) therefore its Hosoya index is two.
- Propane has three matchings.

In general matching in path having k edges can form matching in the first k-1 or in k-2 edges together with the final edge of the path. Thus Hosoya indices obey Fibonacci series in case of linear alkanes.

4.4.2. WEINER Index

Weiner index was given by Harry Weiner in 1947. The Weiner index for any molecule is defined as the total length of shortest path between all pairs of vertices in a chemical graph [44]. Hydrogen atoms were ignored by Weiner.

WI = count number of bonds between each pair of atoms and summing the distance i.e., take a pair of atoms, measure distance between them and finally sum up the distances.

For example: Butane (C_4H_{10}) exists in two forms: n-butane and branched structure (figure 14).

The chemical graph of *n*-butane is a four-vertex path graph. The graph has three pairs of vertices at distance one from each other, two pairs at a distance two, and one pair at distance three, so its Wiener index is calculated as: 3 * 1 + 2 * 2 + 1 * 3 = 10. The chemical graph of isobutane is a tree with one central vertex connected to three leaves therefore it has three pairs of vertices at distances one from each other (the three leaf-center pairs), and three pairs at distance two (the leaf-leaf pairs).

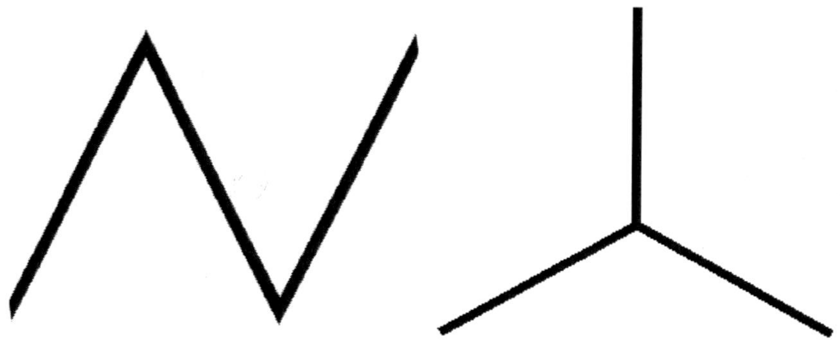

(a) n-butane (b) Isobutane

Figure 14. Isomers of butane.

The Weiner index for isobutene is 3 * 1 + 3 * 2 = 9. In general Weiner index of the molecule having a structure similar to n-butane i.e., having n-vertex is calculated by the formula $(n^3 - n) / 6$. For molecule having n-vertex star graph similar to isobutene, weiner index is calculated by the formula $(n - 1)^3$.

4.5. Two Dimensional Fingerprints

Two methods are there for encoding 2D-fingerprint

- Fragment dictionary
- Hashed method

4.5.1. Fragment Dictionary

Fragment dictionary contains a list of structural keys. In this we look for substructure in chemical data set this is exactly similar to looking for a bit in a string. Each fragment is checked in a new molecule to be added in the database and structural keys are assigned (shown in figure 15). In chemical abstract service twelve different types of screens are there according to which fragments are determined;

a. *Augmented atoms:* central atoms, neighboring atoms and bonds.
b. *Atom-sequence:* linear sequence of connected atoms with or without bond differentiation.
c. *Bond-sequence:* atom sequences with bond differentiation but not atoms.
d. *Ring-systems:* number of rings in a molecule or ring types.

Different Structural keys are as follows:

- as = acyclic single bond
- cs = cyclic single bond
- a = acyclic bond
- c = cyclic bond
- ad = acyclic double bond
- D = non-fused ring atoms
- T = fused or bridged ring atom
- *= any atom

MACCS and **ISIS** from **MDL** information system is widely used for this purpose. Also BCI fingerprints from Bernard Chemical Information are widely used to describe chemical compound.

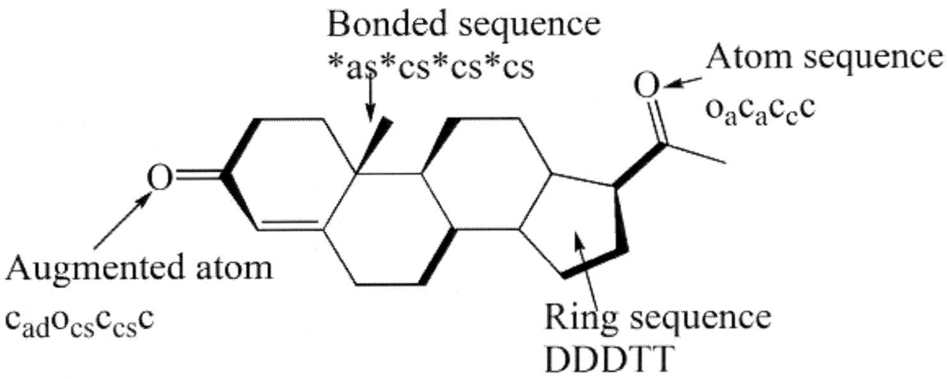

Figure 15. Schematic representation of structural keys.

4.5.2. Hashed Fingerprints

The chemical hashed fingerprint of a molecule is a bit string (a sequence of "0" and "1" digits) that contains information on the structure. It differs from fragment dictionary ways.

a) It does not require any dictionary.
b) Applicable to any type of molecular structure.
c) It is produced by generating all possible linear paths of connected atom between 1 and 7 path length range.
d) For zero path length means atoms are aromatic, aliphatic like c, C, O.
e) For path length one, atoms are cc, CC, C=O, CO, cO.
f) Each and every path is considered and all leads to another program.

4.6. Molecular Structure Descriptors

Molecular structure descriptors are derived from a two-dimensional representation of a chemical structure. Most widely used structure descriptors were given by Randic [45] and extensively developed by Kier and Hall [46]. No experimental data are required to determine molecular structure descriptors rather they are embedded in the hydrogen suppressed framework of the molecule.

4.6.1. Branching Index

This is calculated from hydrogen suppressed graph of any molecule based on δ_i of each atom type 'i' where δ_i calculates number of adjacent non-hydrogen atoms.

4.6.2. Bond Connecting Value

Bond Connecting Value or connectivity index is calculated for each bond as the reciprocal of the square root of product of degree of two atoms and is represented by C_k. For each bond C_k value is calculated using equation 24.

Finally all C_k values are summed up to get the X value which is known as a molecular connectivity index (equation 25).

$$C_k = \frac{1}{\sqrt{\delta_i \delta_j}} = (\delta_i \delta_j)^{-0.5} \tag{24}$$

$$^{1}X = \sum C_k = \sum (\delta_i \delta_j)^{-0.5} \tag{25}$$

^{1}X considers individual bond therefore it is first bond order and one bond path. ^{2}X and ^{3}X denote second and third bond order respectively. Similarly higher molecular connectivity indices represent more complex structures and longer paths.

4.6.3. Molecular Connectivity Indices

Molecular Connectivity Indices are closely related to many physio-chemical parameters.

They are introduced as an improvement of Kier and Hall proposed δ. δ_i as earlier it was dependent only on adjacent atom i.e., intrinsic nature was not taken into account, which is important. So δ_i is redefined in terms of sigma electron and the number of H-atoms associated with it and this is known as Valence δ_i value. In this all electrons present in σ electron, π electron and lone pairs all are encoded. Simple δ_i for atom i can be written as shown in equation 26. Modified δ_i i.e., valence δ_i is calculated using equation 27.

$$\delta_i = \sigma_i - h_i \tag{26}$$

where h_i represents the number of H-atoms bonded to atom I and σ_i represents the number of sigma electrons.

$$\delta_i^v = z_i^v - h_i^v \tag{27}$$

where z_i^V value is the total number of valence electrons including σ, π and lone pairs for atom i.

Therefore by using δ_i^V we can discriminate between CH3 =CH2 and –NH2 which is not possible with δ_i. In the periodic table for any element beyond fluorine, expression of delta is modified according to equation 28.

$$\delta_i^v = \frac{z_i^v - h_i}{z_i - z_i^v - 1} \tag{28}$$

Table 3. Comparison of δ_i and δ_i^2

	$-CH_3$	$-CH_2-$	$=CH_2$	-NH
δ_i	1	2	1	1
δ_i^V	1	2	2	3

4.6.4. Kappa Shape Indices

This descriptor is also given by Kier and Hall in 1991 and entirely depends on molecular shape. Molecules can have different shapes especially when the molecule contains flexible bonds. Shape indices depend on how the molecule is characterized by comparing with molecules of extreme shapes. Shape indices are of different orders depending upon whether counting is done over single bond fragment or from different paths/ graphs (Figure 16). First order (^1K) and second order (^2K) Kappa index are calculated by the formula given in equation (29 and 30).

$$^1K = \frac{2P_{max}^1 P_{min}^1}{\left(P^1\right)^2} \tag{29}$$

where P_{max}^1 is the number of edge and P_{min}^1 is a number of bonds in linear molecule or in one bond path, P^1 is the number of bonds in the molecule for which shape index is calculated.

$$^2K = \frac{2P_{max}^2 P_{min}^2}{\left(P^2\right)^2} \tag{30}$$

where P_{max}^2 is the number of edge and P_{min}^2 is a number of bonds in linear molecule or in two bond path, P^2 is the number of bonds in the molecule for which shape index is calculated.

Example: If the molecule contains A number of atoms then

$P^1_{\min} = (A-1)$ And $P^1_{\max} = \frac{A(A-1)}{2}$ therefore first order Kappa indices are $^1K = \frac{A(A-1)^2}{(P^1)^2}$.

Also $P^2_{\max} = \frac{(A-1)(A-2)}{2}$ and $P^2_{\min} = A-2$ as a result second order Kappa indices are calculated as $^2K = \frac{(A-1)(A-2)^2}{(P^2)^2}$.

The problem with Kappa indices is that they do not include any information about the identity of atoms as only shape and connectivity is considered while calculating the values. Therefore modifications were carried out to study the type of atoms. New α value for atom i is introduced which is a measure of size of molecule relative to standard molecule (sp^3 hybridized carbon). α is sum of α_i's in a structure where α_i is calculated using equation (31). Atom count 'A' is adjusted for each atom present in molecular structure and then it is compared with sp^3 hybridized carbon to check whether the volume is more or less. After modification new first ($^1K_\alpha$) and second order ($^2K_\alpha$) Kappa indices are computed by equations (32) and (33).

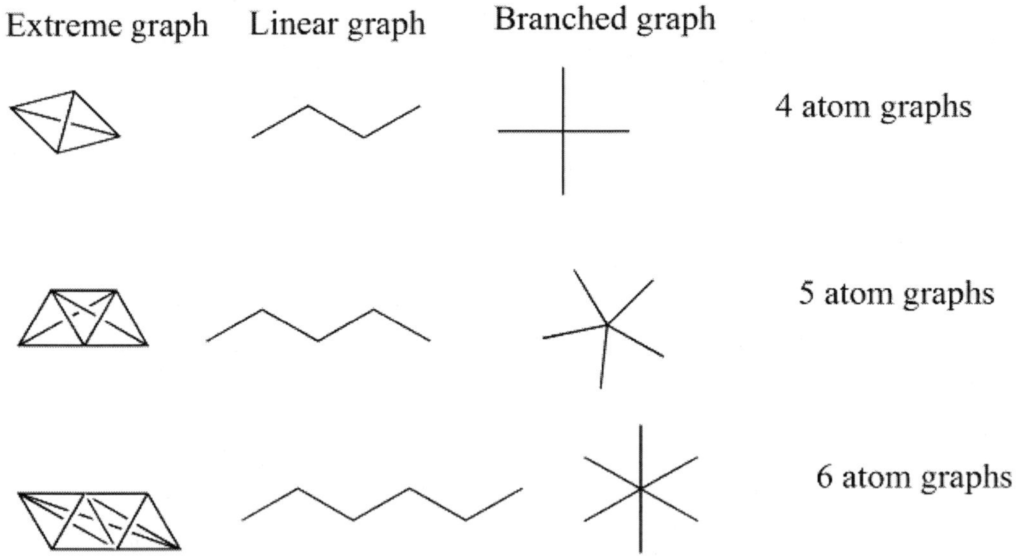

Figure 16. Illustration of different type of graphs present in molecular structures.

$$\alpha_i = \frac{r_i}{r_{c_{sp^3}}} - 1 \tag{31}$$

$$^1K_\alpha = \frac{(A+\alpha)(A+\alpha-1)^2}{(P^1+\alpha)^2} \tag{32}$$

$$^{2}K_{\alpha} = \frac{(A+\alpha-1)(A+\alpha-2)}{(P^2+\alpha)^2} \qquad (33)$$

5. Free Wilson Analysis

In 1964 Free and Wilson derived a mathematical model based on the hypothesis that overall biological activity is the essence of all elementary contribution of the substituent. This approach assumes that substituent effects are additive therefore presence and absence of certain structural features i.e., substituent's were represented by the values 1 and 0. If substituent is present it is assigned value 1 otherwise 0. Free-Wilson approach addresses structure-activity studies in a congeneric series in simplified manner (equation 34) for chemical structure (Figure 17).

$$\log(1/C) = R_1 \text{ contribution} + R_2 \text{ contribution} + R_3 \text{ contribution} \qquad (34)$$

or

$$\log(1/C) = \sum_{i=1}^{N} a_i x_i + \mu$$

Where x_i is indicator variable which describe the presence or the absence of substituents at each substituent position, a_i represents coefficients and μ is the overall average activity.

Free-Wilson QSAR model is built on the basis of the structural matrix filled with x_i indicator values. For example if R3 substituent is fixed with Bromine (Br), while R1 and R2 can have substituents from Fluorine (F), Hydrogen (H), Chlorine (Cl), Methyl (CH_3) substituent. Table 4 shows resulting structural matrix for different substituent at para and meta positions.

Equation 35 describes antiadrenergic activities for 22 different meta- and para- and meta,para-disubstituted analogs of N,N-dimethyl-α-bromophenethylamine, where C is the concentration that causes a 50% reduction of the adrenergic effect of a certain epinephrine dose [4-6].

$$\log\left(\frac{1}{C}\right) = -0.301[m-F] + 0.207[m-Cl] + 0.434[m-Br] + 0.579[m-I] + 0.45[m-Me] + 0.340[p-F] + 0.768[p-Cl] + 1.020[p-Br] + 1.429[p-I] + 1.256[p-Me] + 7.821 \qquad (35)$$

where "r" represents the correlation coefficient which is a measure for the relative quality of the model, "s" stands for standard deviation which is a measure for the absolute quality of a model and "F" represents Fisher value which measures statistical significance.

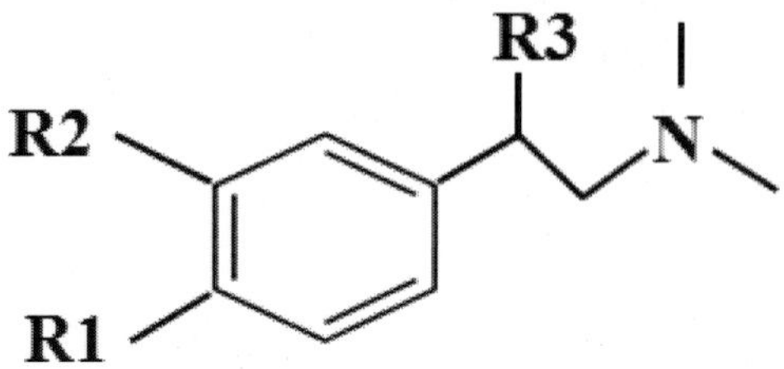

Figure 17. Schematic presentation of a molecule for Free Wilson analysis.

Table 4. Free Wilson relation between (a) experimental data and (b) structure matrix

Sr. No	Para position (R1)	Meta position (R2)	log(1/C) observed
1	H	F	7.52
2	F	H	8.16
3	F	Cl	8.19
4	Me	Me	9.3

(a)

Sr. No	Para position (R1)			Meta position (R2)			log(1/C) observed
	F	Cl	Me	F	Cl	Me	
1	0	0	0	1	0	0	7.52
2	1	0	0	0	0	0	8.16
3	1	0	0	0	1	0	8.19
4	0	0	1	0	0	1	9.3

(b)

The Free Wilson analysis gives a glance which physiochemical property is important for the biological activity and which is not. In above dataset following conclusion [47] was made on the basis of equation 35:

- Biological activities increase with increase in lipophillicity of substituent (F to Cl to Br and then I)
- Biological activities increase with electron donor properties of substituent
- *Meta*-substituent have lower group contributions than *para*-substituent.

The main advantage of Free Wilson approach is that it is necessary to know chemical structures of compounds as well their biological activity values. On the other hand it has certain limitations [47]:

- Minimum two different positions of substitutions must be chemically modified.
- Predictions cannot be made for the substituent which is not included in the analysis.
- Predictions can be formed from different combinations of substituent only if substituent is included in the analysis.
- A single occurrence of a structural feature in whole data set makes the vague statistical model.
- Every substituent is described by many degrees of freedom which may not exist.

6. QSAR Modeling

QSAR model development involves chemistry, biological, statistical and toxicological studies. It is an iterative process (Figure 18).

First a QSAR equation is derived from an initial set of descriptors. Attempts are then made to improve this model by adding or removing descriptors and refining the mathematical equation in an iterative fashion. There are three basic requirements of QSAR model:

- A data set with experimental values for a particular biological activity.
- Structure of molecules present in data set or descriptor values.
- Statistical methods to establish relationship between structure and experimental values.

6.1. Construction of Traditional QSAR

1. A set of compounds is taken that have similar structure i.e., the molecular skeleton is same, only the substituent's are changed or those that assure structural diversity even within a chemical class. If biological activity is not known then all compounds are synthesized and their biological activity is determined.
2. Calculate descriptor values for each compound.
3. Divide the dataset into two sets: One for training and one for testing.
4. Start with two or three descriptors which are likely to be related to the biological activity of interest.
5. Build a model: Formulate mathematical equation that reflects the relationship between the biological activity and the chosen descriptors.
6. Gradually improve the equation by adding more descriptors.
7. Validate the model using a test set using a variety of validation techniques like cross-validation, F-test, Student's T-test etc.
8. Since all compounds have the same structure but different substituent's therefore conclusion can be applied to new molecules with different substituent's but same structures.
9. The equation may does not work for some structures. These are known as OUTLIERS. It does not mean to omit the outriders. They might have some properties that is important for activity and must be included in equation.
10. Evolve equation by adding such properties and work on the betterment of the equation.

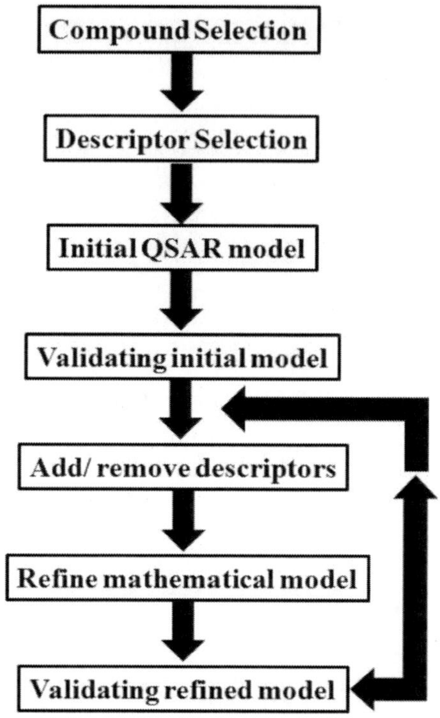

Figure 18. Flowchart of traditional QSAR.

6.2. Compound Selection

This is a first step in building the QSAR model. It consists of collecting sufficiently large and diverse set of compounds with their known biological activities. There are two limiting factor in developing a QSAR model:

- Availability of experimental data
- Accuracy and precision of the data
- Homogeneity of compounds

Therefore in order to develop a meaningful model, selection of the dataset must be done with great care. One should look for the following parameters while selecting compounds.

- Compounds may belong to congeneric series of chemicals or assure structural diversity even within a chemical class.
- Compounds in the dataset should have the same mode of action.
- Compounds should bind to the same receptor.
- Initially outliers should not be included in the dataset. (Compounds which give incorrect information).
- Compounds should cover a wide range of values for descriptors which are relevant to biological activity (initially based on intuition or research papers).

This increases the probability that future compounds will have descriptors in the range and prediction will be interpolative rather than extrapolate. As a rule, interpolative predictions are more accurate than extrapolative predictions (figure 19). Data is basically collected from either literature or is generated specifically for QSAR analyses. More diverse is the data more generalized and robust will be the resulting QSAR model. One drawback of QSAR model is that its applicability is highly dependent and limited by the type and quality of data from which it has been brought forth.

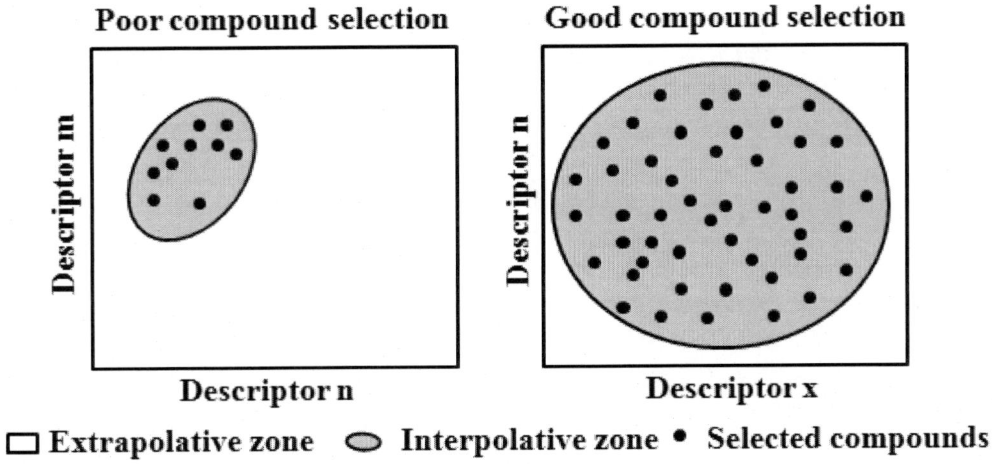

Figure 19. Illustration of interpolative and extrapolative selection of compounds.

It should be applied only within the model's applicability domain i.e., to compounds which are similar to the data set compounds.

6.3. Descriptor Calculation

Descriptors are different ways to represent a molecule. They encapsulate all features of chemical compound; one-dimensional descriptors like molecular weight, counting number of atoms and groups; two-dimensional descriptors like H-acceptors, H-donors, number of rings, topological graphs etc.; three-dimensional descriptors like overall volume, surface area, dipole moment etc. Once the dataset is ready with their experimental biological activity values then next step is to determine structural data i.e., descriptor or variables. Important issue with descriptors is their reproducibility especially when they are experimentally derived. Experimental values vary even when same compound is under experimentation [48]. Therefore approaches were developed to theoretically calculate descriptor values instead of performing experiments. More than 3000 molecular descriptors are now available and are summarized and explained [49-51]. There are many advantages of calculating theoretical descriptors:

- They eliminate the need of experimentation.
- Different kinds of descriptors which capture all structural aspects of molecules are calculated in one go.

- They are homogeneously calculated by tools for complete dataset.
- Values can be calculated for hypothetical structures i.e., compounds need not to be synthesized.
- They are reproducible.

Though descriptors calculated from theoretical approaches do have discrepancy of several orders of magnitude but is less as compared to experimentally derive value. Complete dataset is fed to a variety of feature/ descriptor calculating tools, to generate as many as possible theoretical descriptors for each and every compound in the data set. Various software are known which calculates a wide range of theoretical descriptors like DRAGON [52], CODESSA [53], OASIS [54] etc.

6.4. Division of Data into Training and Test Set

Randomly compounds are divided into training and test set. If the data set is large then division is done by 75:25 rule (i.e., If total100 compounds are in the data set, out of these 100, 75 random compounds will be in the training set and rest 25 molecules in the test set). If the data set is small then division is done on 50:50 basis (i.e., Half randomly selected compounds will constitute amtraining set and rest half will make up test set).

One care should be taken while division i.e., training set data should be diverse enough to remove the error of extrapolation and outliers. It is the training set that will give rule set/ model while test set will validate or gives an efficiency of QSAR model.

6.5. Scaling of Descriptors

Once a dataset is divided into training and test set, next step is to normalize descriptor values of training as well as test set. This is required because the descriptor represents a broad range of physio-chemical properties. If the values of all descriptors do not lie within a particular range, then there is a possibility that descriptor having large range of values dominates the descriptor selection as well as modeling process, thereby generating a model which will be biased to a particular property. To obviate this problem descriptors values need to be calibrated and brought into the same range (Figure 20). Normalization provides a good balance of descriptor respective influence when they are combined. Scaling treatment consists of a mathematical operation called "normalization" which defines limits for the variation of each descriptor. Different types of normalization techniques are:

- *Maximum Normalization*: Identifying the maximum value and divide each descriptor value by maximum value
- *Minimum Normalization*: Identifying the minimum values and divide each descriptor value by minimum value.
- *Standard deviation*: Calculate standard deviation and mean for each and every descriptor. The descriptors are scaled using following formula given in equation 36:

$$x_i' = \frac{x_i - mean(x)}{standard\_deviation(x)} \qquad (36)$$

Where x_i' represents normalized descriptor value, x_i represents the original value of descriptors and i varies from 1 to N.

- Another way is based on new maximum (say 1) and new minimum (-1 or 1) values as described in equation 37.

$$x' = (x - minA)(new\_maxA - new\_minA)/(maxA - minA) + new\_minA \qquad (37)$$

Where x' is the normalized descriptor value, x is the original descriptor value, maxA and minA represent original maxima and minima of concerned descriptor. New_maxA and new_minA represent maxima and minima defined for normalized descriptor value [55].

6.6. Descriptor Selection

Theoretical methods generates large amounts of descriptors which may influence the biological activity or may not be. A good QSAR model is developed from only those descriptors which are related to biological activity under consideration. Therefore small optimal descriptor set is chosen carefully.

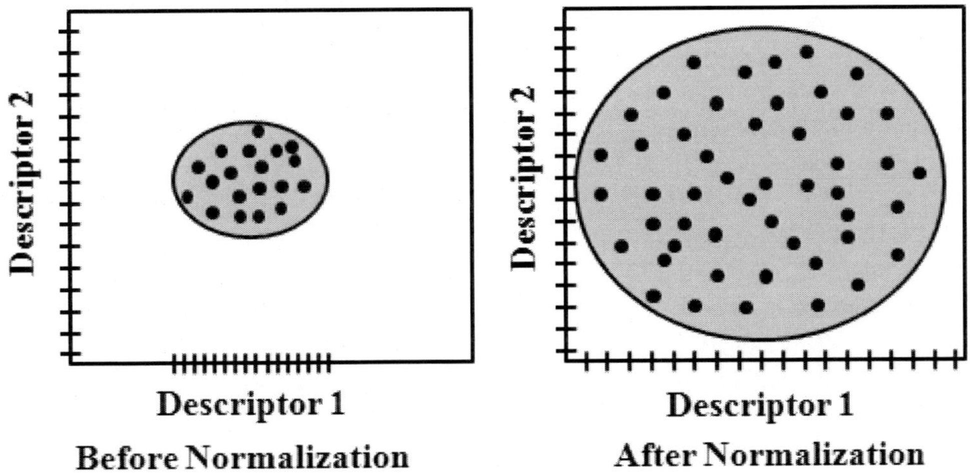

Figure 20. Illustration of effect Normalization on descriptors values.

The important point to mention here is that descriptor selection is carried out only on the training set compounds not on the entire data set. There are two methods to select optimal descriptors:

a. Manual Selection
b. Automated Selection

6.6.1. Manual Selection

Descriptor selection is tedious and time consuming process. According to Hansch, this process is influenced by the modeler's conviction to have a priori knowledge of mechanism of activity and presumption to assign mechanistic meaning to selected descriptor, which is normally well known and used repeatedly [56]. In the short thorough understanding of the structure-activity relationship is required which is exploited to generate analyses i.e., domain knowledge.

Example: If preliminary analyses indicate that steric or hydrophobic substituents may increase activity, then descriptors such as molar refractivity (MR) and hydrophobic substituent constants may be selected at first place. HOMO/ LUMO are always selected while modeling chemical reactivity.

6.6.2. Automated Selection

Automated descriptor selection is carried out by applying mathematical approaches with an aim to maximize the predictive power of QSAR model. The descriptors are selected in an automated manner using programs that score and rank them. In principle the identification of better descriptors is accomplished by a systematic evaluation of all possible combinations of descriptors. For each combination, QSAR equation is derived and ranked. The highest ranked equation reveals the best subset of descriptors.

However this systematic approach is not always feasible. If there are "n" numbers of the descriptor, it will generate $2^n - 1$ combination for evaluation, which is computationally NP hard problem. Various methods are suggested for selection of a subset of descriptors from a large descriptor pool.

a) Forward Selection
b) Backward elimination
c) Stepwise Regression

6.6.2.1. Forward Selection

It starts with the single descriptor which best correlates with the dependant parameter (which is evident from activity vs descriptor graph). At each subsequent step, method adds the next most contributing descriptor. The problem stops when the addition of a descriptor does not improve the model's performance as assessed by appropriate statistical indices.

6.6.2.2. Backward Selection

It starts with a model that includes all the descriptors in the beginning. At each step, it gets rid of those descriptors that degrade the model's performance. The process is stopped when performance begins to decline as assessed by relevant indices.

6.6.2.3. Stepwise Regression

It starts (like forward selection) with the single descriptor that best correlate with dependent parameter. At each subsequent step the method adds the next most contributing descriptor and can potentially remove non-contributing descriptors. The process is stopped when the addition of descriptor does not improve the model or when removing of descriptors causes the model's performance to decline, as assessed by appropriate statistical indices.

Once the optimal set is determined, it is cross-checked to remove correlated descriptors if any. Therefore efforts are made to identify and remove descriptors that convey the same information, about a series of molecules. For those among the selected descriptors, plot descriptor X versus descriptor Y and identify correlated descriptors. The descriptor that has the highest correlation with other is discarded. While discarding descriptors two criteria's are looked into:

- A descriptor that carries strong structural information is preferred and less intuitive one is removed.
- Among highly correlated descriptors, descriptor which is highly correlated to activity is retained and others are removed. This can be inferred by plotting descriptor X vs Activity. If there is observable trend then keep the descriptor otherwise discard the same.

The general consensus for establishing a meaningful SAR equation is that the number of molecules in training set should exceed the number of descriptor by a factor of 3 to 5 (equation 38).

$$p > 3n \tag{38}$$

where p measures number of molecules, n measures number of descriptors.

6.7. Model Generation / Qsar Equation Generation

The starting point for deriving the equation is the study table (Table 5). It consists of a spreadsheet with the molecules across the molecular characteristics (Biological activity, descriptor values) down the column. Typically first column indicates the molecular identification (ex: compound name, 2D structure), second column is activity value and subsequent columns contain corresponding descriptors.

Study table leads to graphical analysis. This step is of paramount importance and leaves room for "hunches" and preliminary interpretations. The trends in system are identified and correlation process begins. The initial analysis helps us to guide the selection of right mathematical equation – that contain information about the behavior of system and allows interpretation of the system. The next hurdle is the development of mathematical equations. The complexity of model depends on both: type of the mathematical equation and number of descriptors considered. More descriptors used for study more complex an equation will be and vice versa. Depending on the number of descriptors and complexity of data different types of models/ equations (linear or nonlinear) are developed based on complex statistical approaches like single linear regression, multiple linear regression (MLR) etc. QSAR models are broadly divided into two categories: linear models or non-linear models.

6.7.1. Linear Models

6.7.1.1. Single Linear Regression

The simplest QSAR equation is a linear equation (equation 39) having one descriptor and one compound. It is represented by a straight line (Figure 21) of the form:

$$y = mx + c \tag{39}$$

or

$$activity = m(descriptors) + c$$

where y represents activity, c is intercept on y axis, x is descriptor value and m represents slope.

Table 5. Illustration of study table

	Property of interest	Descriptors					
Compound	Activity	logP	MR	MW	..	..	Density
1	84	-2.55	80.43	300.8	-9.5	25.6	1.25
2	20	-8.25	57.08	489.65	-4.29	91.32	1.23
3	..	..	..	..	..	..	..
4	..	..	..	..	..	..	..
N	59	-6.87	10.95	387.43	-3.87	57.82	1.42

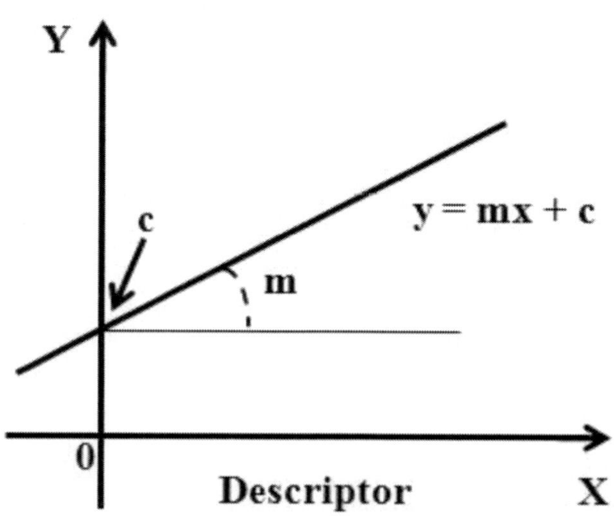

Figure 21. Simplest QSAR equation.

Since the model is not originated from just one compound, a series of compounds are used with their corresponding biological activity therefore previous model needs small modifications (equation 40 represents new model). Development process considers all compounds of the training set. As a result origin of the plot is moved to a point of average (X, Y). The regression equation becomes:

$$Y = mX + c \tag{40}$$

And regression coefficient

$$m = \frac{\sum XY}{\sum X^2} \tag{41}$$

Where $Y = (y - \bar{y})$ and $X = (x - \bar{x})$, $\bar{y}, \bar{x}$ means average of y and x respectively.

6.7.1.2. Multiple Linear Regression

It is not always possible to correlate biological activities with single descriptors. If biological activity is dependent on more than one descriptor than QSAR equation is extended to incorporate all descriptors. Indeed, the observation that several parameters used simultaneously can lead to better model prompted the development of a method commonly known as "Multiple linear regression (MLR)". Resulting model maintained linearity for each descriptor. In MLR activity is expressed as a linear combination of descriptors as shown in equation 42 and 43.

$$Activity = c + m_1x_1 + m_2x_2 + m_3x_3 + \ldots\ldots\ldots\ldots + m_nx_n + c \tag{42}$$

Or

$$y = c + m_1x_1 + m_2x_2 + m_3x_3 + \ldots\ldots\ldots\ldots + m_nx_n + c$$

where c, m_1, m_2, m_3, m_4,..., m_m are coefficients and x_1, x_2, x_3, x_4,........x_n are descriptor values and n is the number of molecules.

$$y = \sum_{i=1}^{n} m_i x_i + c \tag{43}$$

Where y is scalar and represent activity, x_i is the value of descriptor i and m_i is its associated coefficient, c is the intercept or error.

In matrix notation $y = x^T m + c$ (44)

Where x^T is a row vector of descriptors and "m" is a column vector of their associated coefficients.

Mathematics of Multiple linear regressions:

For multiple compounds activity values are put together into a vector y of length n, where n is number of compounds. The descriptors are collected into a matrix of order $n * m$, where n is again number of compounds and m is the number of descriptors. Coefficients are collected into a vector of length m and errors are collected into another vector of length n (Figure 22).

To get coefficients in MLR, we use matrix inversion:

$$y = xm + e \tag{45}$$

$$m = \left(x^T x\right)^{-1} yx^T \tag{46}$$

Where, m represents vectors of coefficients, x represents an original descriptor matrix, x^T is transpose of original descriptor matrix and y is vector of activities.

6.7.2. Non-linear models

Hansch's first model to correlate lipophilicity with biological activity was linear, but as he extended his study by including more compounds he observed that the relation is no more linear it became parabolic.

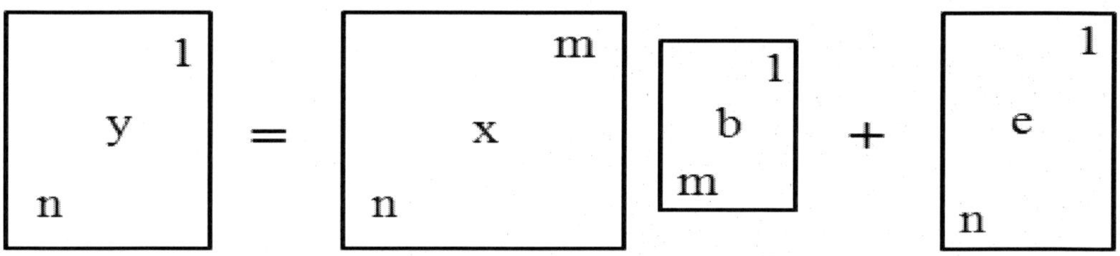

Figure 22. Matrix notation of MLR equation.

This is because an optimum value of logP is required to pass through the cell membrane and exert an effect, compound having logP value more than optimum value will not be able to cross the cell membrane and hence no biological activity will be observed. Similarly there are many more reasons for developing non-linear models like kinetics of drug transport, equilibrium control of its distribution, metabolism, solubility, pharmacokinetics etc. Following are the examples of non-linear models that are valid for special and complex biological system:

- Parabolic model (Hansch) : $$\log\left(\frac{1}{C}\right) = a(\log P)^2 + b\log P + c \tag{47}$$
- Probability Model : $$\log\left(\frac{1}{C}\right) = aloP - 2a\log(P+1) + c \tag{48}$$
- Equilibrium model: $$\log\left(\frac{1}{C}\right) = a\log P - \log(aP+1) + c \tag{49}$$

- Bilinear model: $\log\left(\frac{1}{C}\right) = a\log P - b\log(\beta P + 1) + c$ (50)

6.8. Choice of Model

There may be cases that more than one equation fits the data of a training set, and out of them few produces meaningless information if applied to molecules other than those present in the training set. This error is known as data-overfitting. A complex model with improved success rate can be generated by using curved lines across the space. Such model has distorted shape and will correctly classify the outlier thereby reflecting the scattering of the training set – it is therefore an overfitted data.

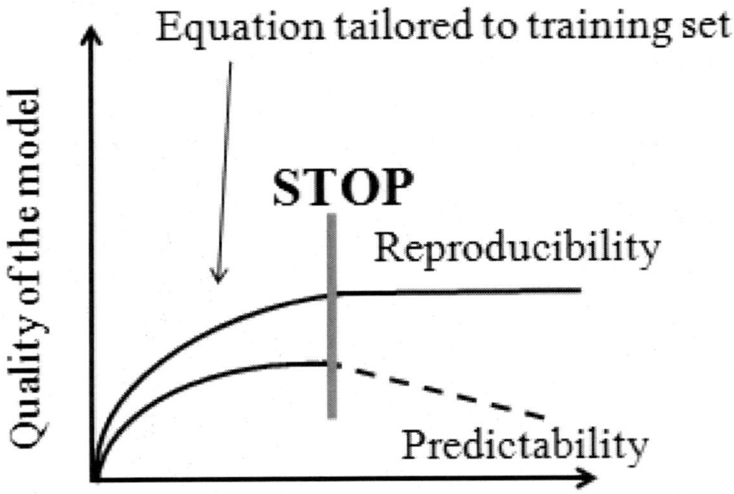

Figure 23. Diagrammatic illustration of balance between reproducibility and predictability of QSAR model.

Golden rule for selecting a model is if the number of classifier for two class problem is more than the risk of getting trapped into less predictability is more. Our aim is to find which classifier/model gives better predictability and less number of rules (not less that we lose reproducibility) (Figure 23).

Reproducibility means to get the same results with same training set, how good our training data is predicted.

Predictability means getting the correct result with test data.

An equation that fits the data of a training set precisely can yield an equation that is perfectly mathematical but meaningless for molecules in the test set. On the other hand equation that gives good predictability will definitely yield better reproducibility. Refinement of QSAR equation must be terminated early enough so that the predictive capabilities of the model are not lost.

6.9. Validation Methods

The first objective of any modeler should be validation for the predictive application of the QSAR model. Validation methods are used to check:

a) How well QSAR equation can reproduce the training set data?
b) How far it can be generalized to test set molecule or new molecule?
c) Difference between predicted activity and observed activity i.e., how good or bad it is?

Any line fitting the algorithm's effectiveness depends on R_{emp} and R^* or R (equation 51). Where R_{emp} is an empirical risk of prediction i.e., how much training data has been predicted correctly and R is risk data, how much new data is predicted correctly if given descriptor are chosen. Therefore the empirical risk should be less than risk of training set plus constant which depend on the type of algorithm multiplied by the square root of dimension of a training algorithm divided by the number of data.

$$R_{emp} \le R + C\frac{\sqrt{D}}{N} \tag{51}$$

where C is a constant which depends on type of algorithm, D is dimension of training algorithm/ classifier and N is the number of data used.

The aim is to minimize:

- R i.e., to make $R = R_{emp}$ if not high i.e., predictability = reproducibility
- To make $R_{emp} = R$, value of N should be large and value of D should be small. D is dimension of classifier. If number of classifiers is less $R_{emp} = R$.

A reliable QSAR model must have following information:

- Defined endpoint
- Unambiguous algorithm
- Defined domain of applicability
- Appropriate measures of goodness-of-fit
- Robustness and predictivity
- Mechanistic interpretation, if possible

There are many methods available for validating developed QSAR model.

6.9.1. Standard Deviation

Standard deviation is the easiest way to validate developed QSAR model. It measures distance from the mean thereby reflects the extent of deviation between data and model (equation 52). If deviation is large than model is not good on the contrary if standard deviation comes out to be small corresponding model is assumed to be goo model. Value of standard deviation lies between 0 and 1. It is calculated using following formula as shown below:

$$SD = \sqrt{\frac{\Sigma\left(Y_{observed} - Y_{calculated}\right)^2}{n - m - 1}} \tag{52}$$

Where n represents number of compounds, m represents number of descriptors.

If data is large and large number of descriptors is used to develop the QSAR model, there will be a less standard deviation, therefore predictability will be more.

Problem with Standard deviation: It is qualitative measurement, if the standard deviation is less it is considered equally well but how much good or bad is not well-defined.

6.9.2. Correlation Index (r^2)

It is the most frequently used indices for measuring the performance of a QSAR model i.e., squared correlation r^2. It measures the degree of correlation between the predicted activity values and experimentally determined activity values i.e., it tries to grab the trend between experimental and calculated values. Trend changes by adding more and more data. Correlation index lies between zero (0) and one (1). If $\mathbf{r^2}$ value is zero or close to zero, this means there is no correlation between experimental and predicted activity values of compounds, thereby model is defective. If $\mathbf{r^2}$ value is one or close to one this indicate perfect correlation between experimental and predicted activity values of compounds and the model is good. Mathematically r^2 is calculated by dividing the fraction of variance explained by the model (the "explained sum of squares", ESS) by the original variance (the "total sum of variance", TSS). ESS is the fraction of variance explained by model and is equal to the total variance (TSS) minus that portion of the variance which was not explained by model (Residual, RSS).

- Original variance (Total Sum of Squares):

$$TSS = \sum\left(y_i - \bar{y}\right)^2 \tag{53}$$

- Explained variance (Explained Sum of Squares):

$$ESS = \sum\left(y_{i,calculated} - \bar{y}\right)^2 \tag{54}$$

- Variance around regression line (Residual Sum of Squares):

$$RSS = \sum\left(y_i - y_{calculated,i}\right)^2 \tag{55}$$

Where i varies from 1 to N, N represents number of compounds, y_i is experimental activity values, $y_{i,calculated}$ is the value obtained from QSAR model and $\bar{y}$ is average value.

$$r^2 = \frac{ESS}{TSS} = \frac{(TSS - RSS)}{TSS} \quad (56)$$

$$r^2 = 1 - \frac{RSS}{TSS} \quad (57)$$

The problem with r^2 is that for different number of data correlation will be different. Also if number of data is increased for same equation, it will give different r^2 values.

6.9.3. T-Test for Single Descriptors and Significance of r^2

Correlation index (r^2) alone is not sufficient to determine whether the relationship has occurred by chance or not. Significance of r^2 is calculated using t-statistic for single descriptor as follows:

- Keep repeating the process of deriving QSAR equation and calculate resulting r^2 values, each one using a set of different descriptors.
- If number of molecules are large (>30), the sampling distribution of resulting r^2 values will have a normal shape (Gaussian curve).
- If number of molecules is low, it will have shape known as t-distribution.

For a set of two molecules we get r^2 value equal to 1 irrespective of descriptors used. Asnumber of molecules increases, the probability of obtaining large r^2 values with irrelevant descriptors decreases. This problem corresponds to the area under t-distribution curve away from the center. Therefore the shape of the t-distribution depends on the number of molecules used in the analysis.

Student t-test employs t-distribution to test whether the correlation coefficient obtained from QSAR is significantly different from zero (0). Large t-value corresponds to large probability that correlation significantly differs from zero i.e., large probability that descriptor used for analysis is relevant to the activity.

Procedure of performing T-test:

i) Estimate the value of t according to formula:

$$t = r\sqrt{\frac{(N-2)}{1-r^2}} \quad (58)$$

where r^2 is correlation coefficient, N is number of molecules.

ii) Next step is to select a significance level. For each t-value we have confidence level. It is a percentage that a relationship found in data is just due to unlucky sample. If the confidence level is X then 100 – (X / 100) is the total number of cases predicted by chance. For example, if X is 25 then 75 cases are correctly predicted while 25 cases are predicted by chance.

iii) Look up the t-distribution derived for correct number of data points (N) at significance level.
iv) If the value of calculated t-distribution is larger than listed t-value then regression equation is significant at this significance level.

6.9.4. F-test

F-test is an extension of t-test, only change is that the quantity depicting number of descriptors is added to formula. It tests the assumption that the model did not explain any of the original variance in the data set (ESS= 0). It uses F-distribution which, similar to t-distribution, depends on number of compounds and descriptors. F-distribution is applied to examine whether the correlation coefficient obtained from MLR analysis significantly differs from zero or not. If the calculated F-value is greater than the value derived from distribution table than larger is the probability that r^2 significantly differs from zero i. e. greater is the probability that descriptors used for analysis is relevant to the activity. However if the calculated F-value is small than the theoretical value than descriptors are not related to biological activity. Technical steps involved are shown in Figure 24.

Procedure of F-test:

(i) Estimate the value of F using formula mentioned in figure 24.
(ii) Select significance level (p).
(iii) Look for F value in the F-distribution table for values of N, k, p.
(iv) If $F_{calculated}$ is more than F_{table} then the correlation is significant.

6.9.5. Cross Validation Method

Cross validation is preferred when size of data is too small. Data is randomly divided into N equal parts. N-1 parts are used to build model which is then used for the remaining N^{th} part to predicted activities of corresponding molecules. The process is repeated until the activities of all compounds have been predicted independently (table 6).

Problem with cross validation:

QSAR model that is ultimately used to predict the activities of new compounds is derived from all N data points and is therefore different from N partial QSAR models. Therefore cross validation does not provide us with predictive power of specific QSAR equation. It gives an estimate of our ability to make predictions for compounds similar to those used in QSAR analysis.

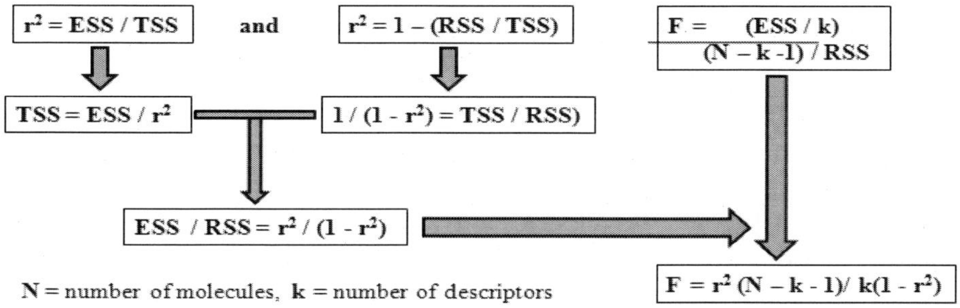

Figure 24. Schematic illustration of Derivation of F value.

Table 6. Cross-validation strategy for 50 compounds

	Stage 1	Stage 2	Stage 3	Stage 4	Stage 5
Compounds (1 - 10)	Training set	Training set	Training set	Training set	Test set
Compounds (11 - 20)	Training set	Training set	Training set	Test set	Training set
Compounds (21 - 30)	Training set	Training set	Test set	Training set	Training set
Compounds (31 - 40)	Training set	Test set	Training set	Training set	Training set
Compounds (41 - 50)	Test set	Training set	Training set	Training set	Training set

6.9.6. The Predictive Index Q^2

The predictive power of a model, termed Q^2 is computed by analogy with r^2. The difference is the use of PRESS (predicted sum of squares) rather than the RSS (residual sum of squares) in the numerator. PRESS is calculated as the difference between the measured activity and the predicted activity for the test set compounds.

$$r^2 = 1 - \left(\frac{RSS}{\sum (y_i - \bar{y})^2} \right) \Leftrightarrow Q^2 = 1 - \left(\frac{PRESS}{\sum (y_i - \bar{y})^2} \right) \quad (58)$$

where $RSS = \sum \left(y_{i,calculated} - \bar{y}_i \right)^2$ and $PRESS = \sum \left(y_{i,predicted} - \bar{y}_i \right)^2$

While discussing mathematical tools available for assessing the ability of a QSAR model, it was that:

1) The standard deviation is an isolated "absolute" index of local significance.
2) With r^2 it is possible to compare different models, but this indicator is entirely mathematical- not statistical.
3) t and F values have a statistical content that can be used for single and multiple linear regression respectively; however they only measure the ability of the QSAR model to reproduce the data from which it was constructed.
4) Q2 gives the predictability power of QSAR equation.

The ideal QSAR should:

1) Consider sufficiently large number of molecules for accurate statistical representation.
2) Have a wide range of quantified endpoint potency for regression models.
3) Be applicable to new compounds.
4) Allow to have mechanistic information on the modeled endpoint.

7. Three Dimensional (3D) Qsar

Traditional QSAR generates a model which attempts to relate physical and chemical properties of molecules to their biological activities using easily calculable descriptors e.g., Mol. wt, LogP, rotatable bonds and Multiple Linear Regression (MLR) to build a model. This model is then used to identify the activity of training set compounds and to predict the activities of test set compounds or any new compound whose activity is not known. Classical QSAR accurately predicted the potency of additional compounds and has lead to the development of several commercial drugs and pesticides.

Descriptors that are used in classical QSAR are simple to calculate and allow for relatively fast analysis, but they often fail to take into account the 3D structures of chemical structure.

Structural chemistry has explained why changing a substituent on a molecule might change its biological activity. Quantum chemistry changes the focus from traditional structure i.e., nucleus of atoms to electrons of molecules. Semi-empirical quantum methods allow one to calculate molecular structure and electronic properties of almost any organic molecules using less number of parameters. Physical organic chemistry provided methods for quantization of electronic, steric and hydrophobic effects of substituents on reactions. It has demonstrated that multivariate statistical analysis can suggest the physical basis of biological structure activity relationship. Molecular modeling in the form of molecular mechanics allowed incorporation of electrostatic and steric effects, generation and comparison of many conformers of the same molecules and comparison of three dimensional structures of different molecules. Development in the field of computer graphics enables the visual insight into 3D structure and allows comparing different molecules by superimposing their chemical structures. Since 3D QSAR uses insights from so many scientific disciplines, different implementations differ in concepts and strategies employed.

3D QSAR is a method based on the analysis and comparison of the three dimensional field (electrostatic / steric) that are produced in the surrounding of different compounds for the establishment of a correlation between the biological activities and the fields.

Principle of 3D QSAR: Biological receptor does not see a ligand as a set of atoms and bonds; rather it perceives it as a shape that carries complex forces. In 3D QSAR framework these forces are believed to be determined predominantly by electrostatic and steric interactions. 3D-QSAR involves mapping and comparison of electrostatic and steric fields around a set of ligands to establish a 3D QSAR.

7.1. Electrostatic Field

Electrostatic field is obtained by calculating electrostatic interaction energy between two molecules A and B using Coulomb's law, i.e.

$$F = k_e \frac{q_1 q_2}{r^2} \tag{59}$$

where k_e equals to $\frac{1}{4\Pi\varepsilon_0}$, q_1, q_2 are the charges, r is the distance between two charges.

The electrostatic forces can be attractive or repulsive. As they are expressed as inverse of distance, they are far from negligible even when the groups involved are far apart i.e., at long distances, electrostatic interactions drive the approach of ligand to an active site/receptor.

7.2. Steric Field

Steric field describes the non-electrostatic interaction between non-bonded atoms. They are short range forces and are obtained by calculating Van der Waals interaction energy between two atoms. Steric field plays an important role when the molecule/ligand is very close to the active site and controls final binding. Steric field is calculated by the formula given in equation 60.

$$E_s = \sum_{i=1}^{n} \frac{A}{r^{12}} - \frac{B}{r^6} \tag{60}$$

There are various other forces that are generated between ligand and biological receptor like interaction energies with functional groups, molecular lipophilicity field, H-bond donor, H-bond acceptor, hydrophobic effect *etc.* but electrostatic and steric fields are extensively studied. 3D QSAR uses *probe-based sampling* within a molecular lattice to determine 3D properties of molecules (electrostatic and steric values) and then correlate these 3D descriptors with biological activity.

It was not straight forward as that of Hansch analysis. It took nearly a decade to first formulate a lattice model to compare molecule by aligning them in 3D-space and by mapping their molecular fields to a three dimensional grid. 3D QSAR is generally applicable in situations when the structure of receptor is not known.

7.3. 3D-Qsar Model Generation

There are two original 3D-QSAR methods namely **GRID** and **CoMFA.**

7.3.1. Grid Approach

Grid approach, given by Peter Goodford in 1985, is first program based on the calculation of molecular interaction fields (MIF's) using a probe atom placed in 3D lattice which consists of regularly distributed grid points in space. Probes used should be of same type of field to be measured. Ex: *Van der Waal* probes are used for calculating steric field and charged probes are used to calculate electrostatic field.

It is a structure based method to analyze the active site of proteins by systematically exploring and calculating interactions between protein and probes at each point (equation 61). A typical GRID interaction energy function between protein and probe is:

$$E = \sum E_{ij} + \sum E_{es} + \sum E_{hb} + S \tag{61}$$

Where E_{ij} represents Leonard-Jones potential, E_{es} represents electrostatic potential, E_{hb} represents hydrogen bond potential and S stands for entropy term.

7.3.1.1. Principle of GRID

The molecular interaction fields are calculated using different probes. They contain relevant information about the nature of active sites of protein and forces involved in binding of ligand. Large number of probes is used and as a result one get huge data consisting of many tables listing numerical values of interactions energies at each grid point which can be analyzed by novel statistical methods and progress in computer graphics.

7.3.2. Outline of Grid Approach

GRID is molecular field analysis based method developed for the analysis of the macromolecule active site, to reveal "hot spots" in their binding regions. It paved way for the ideas that led to the development of 3D QSAR approaches, which retained molecular interaction field (MIF) concept and fully exploited it for the study of small molecule ligand, in projects where the 3D structure of the target protein is not known.

Deployment of GRID requires:

1) Three dimensional coordinates of atoms of protein
   Coordinates may be obtained from X-ray crystallography or NMR studies, Protein Data Bank or for newly synthesized sequences we carry out homology modeling.
2) Binding site to be exploited
   Space surrounding the surface of protein is huge and it is not necessary to explore entire space. Normally the exact location of the binding site is known thus calculation of interaction fields can be confined to a box containing active site to be explored.
3) Selection of Probes
   There are dozens of probes in GRID. Selection of probes depends on the nature of groups that are present in binding site of the protein. One can address particular types of favorable energy interaction such as hydrophobic, aromatic, salt-bridge interaction, polar etc.
4) Run of GRID leading to anticipation of favorable positions for each probe
   If probe used is a single atom probe, then the probe is placed at each position of lattice and molecular interaction fields are calculated. If probe used is multi-atom probe, then the probe is rotated at each grid point in order to find lowest-energy orientation (ex: essential for H-binding interaction), an optimization that is very demanding in terms of computing time.
5) Analysis of results with computer graphics
   The output of GRID consists of two types of files; printer and binary file. Both need to be used in conjunction with other software's. Binary file serves as input for programs such as CoMFA, GOLPE for statistical analysis of GRID maps.

Total GRID calculations are equal to product of number of compounds, the number of grid points and number of probes. This must also be multiplied by number of rotations, if several orientations at each grid point have been taken into consideration for multi-atom probes. Connecting a maximum of fragments in correct orientations into synthetically assessable molecule is not simple. GRID provides useful hints for creative structural design.

7.4. CoMFA: Comparative Molecular Field Analysis

CoMFA is introduced by Cramer in 1908 for comparison of molecular field analysis of different molecules. Since its introduction, it has quickly become one of the most popular methods of QSAR. Over the years, this approach has been applied to a wide variety of receptor and enzyme ligands. CoMFA methodology is based on the assumption that the changes in the biological activities or binding affinities of sample compounds correlate with the changes in steric and electrostatic fields of these molecules. The three dimensional distribution of molecular interaction fields of a compound and their comparison contains relevant information for understanding the biological activities of compounds and can also facilitate their optimization.

It also makes a linear equation, correlating the biological activities with the values of fields in each point. Each value calculated for a field on a given point is termed as a descriptor.

7.4.1. Outline of Comfa Calculation

1) A selection of set of related analogs/reference compounds.
   CoMFA starts by selecting a set of active/inactive molecules with their associated biological properties. It assumes that the set of molecules posses following properties:
   - Share same mechanism of action,
   - Active for same reason,
   - Bind in same manner,
   - Biological action is enthalpically driven,
   - Entropic terms and de-solvation energies are similar for all compounds.

   The data set is then separated into a training set for which a CoMFA model is derived and a test set that will prove the external predictivity of the resulting model.
2) Defining a rule for superimposing training set compounds.
   All molecules in the training set are then aligned to one another prior to molecular interaction field calculations. Typically used methods for alignment are based on superimposing their common chemical scaffolds or common pharmacophore. This is one of the critical and difficult steps in the CoMFA study as it is highly dependent on way molecules are aligned. There are several other methods for alignment like template or atom alignment, field fitting, electrostatic field based alignment, moment alignments, receptor based alignments, alignments from X-ray data. Whatever method is used for superimposing the molecules, they must be aligned in their bioactive confirmations.
3) Constructing a lattice of grid points and calculating molecular interaction fields at each grid point

A box is placed around the superimposed molecules in such a manner that the box is in all directions several Å larger than the combined volume of all molecules. A regular lattice is laid over the molecules to calculate different molecular fields at each grid point; the default distance between the grid points is 2Å. For each molecule, the molecular interaction fields are calculated using probe and at each grid point. In CoMFA two probes are used: Probe atoms or groups, such as a neutral carbon atom (for steric interactions) or charged atom (probe for electrostatic interactions) are used. Mathematical functions used for calculation of steric and electrostatic interactions are given in equations 59 and 60.

Both Lennard-Jones potential and Coulomb potential create relatively “hard fields”. They modify their values from close to zero to very large numbers within a few tenths of Angstroms. Thus cut off values have to be defined to avoid values that approach infinity at the atom positions.

4) Deriving a correlation function

The results of the field evaluation in every grid point for every molecule in the training set are placed in CoMFA QSAR table, which therefore contains thousands of columns.

Figure 25. Summary of 3D-QSAR.

$$Activity = f(3DMoleuclarfields) \tag{61}$$

The values obtained are then processed by sophisticated mathematical statistical methods, with the aim of revealing a linear relationship between field’s parameters and biological activities. The analysis of the CoMFA QSAR table by the means of standard multiple regression is practically impossible, as the number of descriptors accumulated are much larger as compared to traditional QSAR, moreover descriptors are highly correlated because many values of neighboring grid points are similar. Nevertheless, the application of special multivariate statistical analysis such as PLS analysis ensures the statistical significance of the final CoMFA equation (Figure 25).

5) Assessing the predictability of model

Once a model is formed it can be used to predict the biological activity of a molecule which is yet to be synthesized and tested. The same sequence is repeated; alignment, interaction fields and projection in PLS space to predict its activity. If a designed molecule is structurally new, care must be taken while aligning with the training set compounds.

7.4.2. Problems with CoMFA

Various studies revealed that CoMFA results can be extremely sensitive to a number of factors, such as alignment rules, overall orientation, lattice placement, step size and probe atom size. The problem of three dimensional alignments has been the most notorious among the others specially in case of structurally diverse compounds. There is no standard recipe as to how to align all molecules under consideration in a unique and unambiguous fashion.

Even after fixing the structural alignment, the resulting value of q^2 could also be sensitive to the orientation of rigidity of aligned molecules. The grid orientation in CoMFA is fixed in the coordinate system of a computer, thus every time when the orientation of the molecular aggregate is changed, the size of the grid may change but not its orientation. The orientation of the assembled molecules therefore affects the placement of probe atoms, which in turn, influences the field sampling process. This leads to the variability of the q^2 values.

In conventional CoMFA implementation, steric and electrostatic fields, which theoretically form a continuum, are sampled on a fairly coarse grid. As a result, they are not represented inadequately and the results are not strictly reproducible. It was demonstrated that decreasing the grid size from 2.0 to 1.0 Å increase the adequacy of sampling minimized the fluctuation observed in q^2 values. The reason for phenomena is that the decrease in grid spacing increases the number of probe atoms, which in turn should raise the probability of placing the probe atoms in a region where the steric and electrostatic field changes can be better correlated with the biological activity. However increase in number of probe atoms, also increases the noise in PLS analysis and leads to a less statistical significant q^2.

7.5. Partial Least Square Analyses

The resulting matrix contains several thousands of individual grid point values for each molecule. The entire data is huge and cannot be correlated by regression analyses.

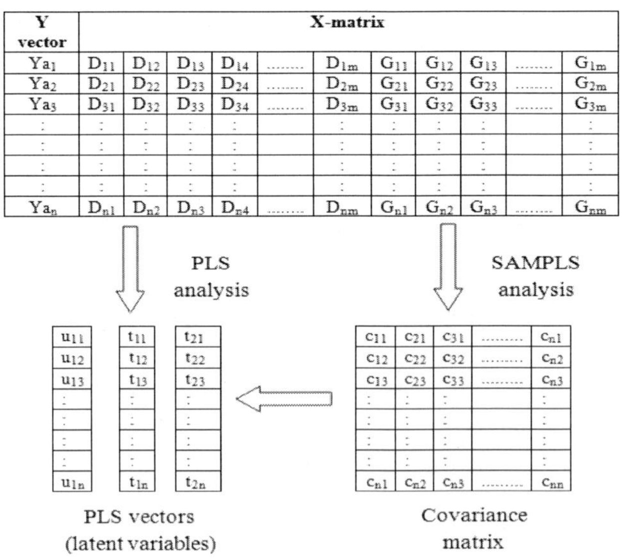

Figure 26. Partial least square (PLS)method generate latent variables (principal component like vectors) from biological activity data (Y vector) and calculated values of different molecular field at different grid positions (X matrix). SAMPLS analysis is a variant of PLS, which calculates a covariance matrix from X matrix followed by the derivation of latent variables. PLS and SAMPLS give absolutely identical results.

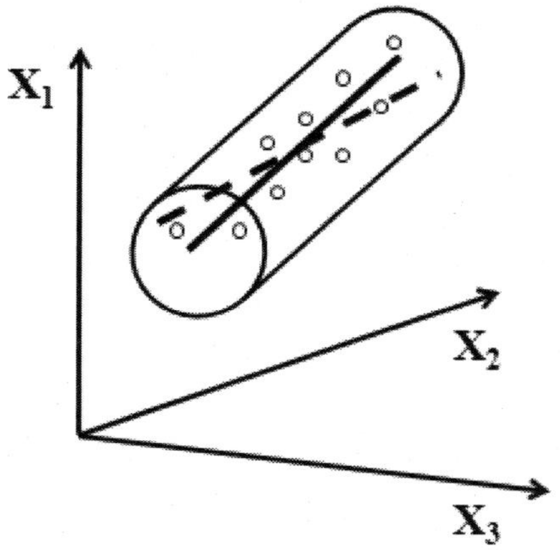

$$\mathbf{u} = \mathbf{kt} \quad \text{where } k = k_1, k_2, k_3\ldots\ldots\ldots, k_j$$

$$\Downarrow$$

$$Ya_1 = a_1S_{i1} + a_2S_{i12} + a_3S_{i3} + a_4S_{i4} + \ldots\ldots + a_mS_{im} + \\ + b_1E_{i1} + b_2E_{i2} + b_3E_{i3} + b_4E_{i4} + \ldots\ldots + b_nE_{im}$$

Figure 27. Relation between PLS vector and principal component.

Partial least analysis extracts a principal component-like vectors, the so-called latent variables from biological activity data (Y) and molecular field variables (matrix X) at different grids. The latent variables are then shifted within the confidence volumes of principal components, in such a manner that a maximum correlation between latent variables ('u' and't') is achieved (Figure 26). The optimum number of latent variables is determined by cross-validation technique [5, 57, 58]. The results of PLS analysis are a regression equation with thousands of coefficients which can further be used to predict new compounds outside training set. PLS results are presented as contour plots having favorable and unfavorable regions for certain properties, which are represented by different colors. The main advantage of PLS analysis is that the PLS vectors (dotted line) are shifted against the principal components (bold line), to achieve maximum correlation between Y vector and X matrix (Figure 27).

8. Difference between Traditional QSAR and 3DQSAR

There are many differences between traditional and 3D-QSAR. Few are listed below:

- 3D-QSAR saves time as compared to traditional QSAR.
- In 3D-QSAR no experimentation required, physical properties are studied by computer 3D-QSAR consider property of whole molecules not individual substituents as in case of traditional QSAR. These properties are known as fields – steric, electrostatic. Hydrophobic does not contribute significantly.
- Traditional QSAR is applicable to similar type of compounds (skeleton should be same) in 3D QSAR emphasis is on common pharmacophore.

- The key difference between traditional and 3D QSAR is the form of output. Although both provide the statistical evidence for the validity of proposed relationship, results of 3D QSAR are typically supplied as a graphic image superimposed on a molecule of the dataset.
- 3D QSAR is not typical analogues based as the structure of ligand and receptor is known to us but in case of traditional QSAR there is no idea about receptor structure.
- Another difference lies in the source of the descriptors of molecules. In traditional QSAR, molecular descriptors (electronic, steric, hydrophobic) are described by parameters that are not x, y, z dependent e.g., logP, MR, Es, σ, π whereas in 3D QSAR the molecular descriptors are represented by a set of values and are x, y, z dependent, measured at many different locations in space around molecule.
- The number of descriptors are very large in 3D QSAR as compared to traditional QSAR. To deal with such a large number of descriptors dimension reduction methodologies (partial least square (PLS) are used in 3D QSAR. Calculations are then executed on the transformed function of descriptors.
- Final limitation of traditional is that equations discovered by the traditional QSAR do not directly suggest a new compound to synthesize. One must be experienced with values of substituent constants in order to imagine which molecules will have desired properties.

References

[1] Free, S. M., Wilson, J. W. (1964). A mathematical contribution to Structure-Activity studies. *J. Med. Chem.,* 7, 395-399.

[2] Hansch, C., Fujita, T. (1964). Port Analysis. A method for the correlation of biological activity and chemical structure. *J. Am. Chem. Soc*., 86, 1616-1626.

[3] Kubinyi, H. (1997) QSAR and 3D QSAR in drug design. Part 1. Methodology, *Drug Discovery Today,* 2 (11), 457-467.

[4] Ramsden, C. A., ed. (1990). Quantitative Dntg Deszgn (Comprehenszve Medicinal Cbemistr 39, Vol. 4, Pergamon Press, United Kingdom.

[5] Kubinyi, H. (1993). QSAR: Hansch Analysis and Related Approaches. VCH, Weinheim.

[6] Hansch, C., Leo, A. (1995) Exploring QSAR. Fund~onentals and Applications in Chemist O' and 3ioloRv, American Chemical Society.

[7] Hansch, C., Leo. A., Hoekm:M., D. (1995). Exploring QSAR. Hydropbobic, Electronic, and Steric Constant, American Chemical Society, Washington, DC, USA.

[8] van de Waterbeemd, H, ed. (1995) Chemometrt'c Methods in Molecular Design, VCH, Weinheim.

[9] van de Waterbeemd, H., ed. (1995) Advanced Computer assisted Techniques in Drug Discovary, VCH, Weinheim.

[10] Hecker, E., Kubinyi, H., Bresch Eine neue Gruppe von , H (1995). Burger´s Medicinal Chemstry and Drug Discovery, 5th Edition, Vol. I, Principles and Practice, pp. 497-571, Wolff, M. E., Ed., John Wiley & Sons, New York.

[11] Sanz, F., Giraldo, J. and Manaut, F., Eds (1995). QSAR and Molecular Modelling Concepts. Computational Tools and Biological Applications (Proceedings of the 10th European Symposium on Quantitative Structure Activity Relationship, Prous Science Barcelona.

[12] Pliska, V., Testa, B. and van de Waterbeemd, H. Eds (1996). Lipophilicity in Drug Action and Toxicology, VCH, Weinheim.

[13] van de Waterbeemd. H., ed (1996). Structure Property Corelations in Drug Research, Academic Press, London.

[14] van de Waterbeemd, H. (1996). In The Practice of Medicinal Chemistry (Wermuth, C.G., ed.), pp. 367-389, Academic Press, London.

[15] Bohm, H. J., Klebe, G., Kubinyi, H. (1996). Wirkstoffdesign, pp. 363-380 and 399-436, Protein-Ligand Wechselwirkungen Spektrum Akademischer Verlag, Heidelberg.

[16] van de Waterbeemd, H., Testa, B., Folkers, G., Eds (1997). Computer assisted Lead Finding and Optimization (Proceedings of the 114th European Symposium on Quantitative Structure-Activity Relationships: Lausanne,), Verlag Helvetica Chimica Acta and VCH.

[17] Kier, L. B., Hall, L. H. (1976). Molecular connectivity in Chemistry and Drug Research. Academic Press, New York.

[18] Charton, M. (1971). The quantitative treatment of the ortho effect. *Prog. Phys. Org. Chem.*, 8, 235.

[19] Fujita, T., Nishioka, T. (1976). The Analysis of the Ortho Effect. *Prog. Phys. Org. Chem.*, 12, 49.

[20] Bolton, P. D., Fleming, K. A., Hall, F. M. (1972). Linear free energy enthalpy entropy relation for the ionization of benzoic acids. *J. Am. Chem. Soc.*, 94, 1033.

[21] Bergon, M., Calmon, J. P. (1981). A nonlinear hammett relationship as evidence for a change-over in mechanism in the alkaline hydrolysis of methyl carbanilates. *Tetrahedron Lett.*, 22, 937-940.

[22] Schreck, J. (1971). Nonlinear Hammett relationships. *J. Chem. Ed.*, 48, 103.

[23] Brown, H. C., Okamoto, Y. (1958). Rates of Solvolysis of Phenyldimethylcarbinyl Chlorides Containing Substituents (-NMe3+,-CO2-) Bearing a Charge. *J. Am. Chem. Soc.*, 80, 4979.

[24] Albert, A. (1985). Selective Toxicity: The Physicochemical Bases of Therapy, Ed. 7th , p. 379, Chapman and Hall, London.

[25] Meyer, H. (1899). Theory of alcohol narcosis. *Arch. Exp. Pathol. Pharmakol.*, 42, 109-110.

[26] Overton, E. (1901). Studien Uber die Narkose, Fischer, Jena, Germany.

[27] Hansch, C., Maloney, P. P., Fujita, T., Muir, R. M. (1962). Correlation of biological activity of phenoxyacetic acids with Hammett substituent constants and partition coefficients. *Nature*, 194, 178.

[28] Leo, A., Hansch, C., Elkins, D. (1971). Partition Coefficients and Their Uses. *Chem. Rev.*, 71, 525-616.

[29] Rekker, R. F. (1977). The Hydrophobic Fragmented Constant. Its Derivation and Application: A Means of Characterizing Membrane Systems, p. 131, Elsevier, Amsterdam.

[30] Kamlet, M. J., Carr, P. W., Taft, Linear solvation energy relationships. 13. Relationship between the Hildebrand solubility parameter, delta.H, and the solvatochromic parameter, .pi.*R. W., Abraham, M. H. (1981). *J. Am. Chem. Soc.*, 103, 6062-6066.
[31] Kamlet, M. J., Abboud, J. L., Abraham, M., Taft, R. (1983). Linear solvation energy relationships. 23. A comprehensive collection of the solvatochromic parameters, .pi.*, .alpha., and .beta., and some methods for simplifying the generalized solvatochromic equation *J. Org. Chem.*, 48, 2877-2887.
[32] Platts, J. A., Butina, D., Abraham M. H., Hersey, A. (1999). Estimation of molecular free energy relation descriptors using a group contribution approach. *J. Chem. Inf. Comput. Sci.*, 39, 835 -845.
[33] Ishihama, Y., Asakawa, N. (1999). Characterization of lipophilicity scales using vectors from solvation energy descriptors. *J. Pharm. Sci.*, 88, 1305-1312.
[34] Platts, J. A., Abraham, M. H., Butina, D., Hersey, A. (2000). Estimation of molecular linear free energy relation descriptors using a group contribution approach. *J. Chem. Inf. Comput. Sci.*, 40, 71-80.
[35] Taft in, R. W., Newman, M. S. Ed. (1956). Steric Effects in Organic Chemistry, p. 556, John Wiley & Sons, New York.
[36] Charton, M. in Charton, M., Motoc, I. Eds. (1956). Steric Effects in Drug Design, 57, Springer, Berlin.
[37] Tute, M. S. in Ramsden, C. A. Ed. (1990). Comprehensive Medicinal Chemistry.
[38] The Rational Design, Mechanistic Study and Therapeutic Application of Chemical Compounds, *Quantitative Drug Design*, 4, 18, Pergamon, Elmsford, New York.
[39] Verloop, A., Hoogenstraaten, W., Tipker, J. in Ariens, E. J., Ed. (1976). *Drug Design*, 7, 165, Academic Press, New York.
[40] Verloop, A. (1987). The STERIMOL Approach to Drug Design, Marcel Dekker, New York.
[41] Hall, L. H.; Kier, Lemont, B. (1976). Molecular connectivity in chemistry and drug research. Boston: Academic Press, London.
[42] González-Díaz, H., Vilar, S., Santana, L., Uriarte, E. (2007). Medicinal chemistry and bioinformatics--current trends in drugs discovery with networks topological indices. *Current Topics in Medicinal Chemistry,* 7 (10), 1015-29.
[43] King, R. B. (1983). Chemical applications of topology and graph theory: a collection of papers from a symposium held at the University of Georgia, Athens, Georgia, U. S. A., 18–22 April. Elsevier, Amsterdam.
[44] Hosoya, H. (1971), Topological index. A newly proposed quantity characterizing the topological nature of structural isomers of saturated hydrocarbons, *Bulletin of the Chemical Society of Japan,* 44 (9), 2332–2339.
[45] Rouvray, Dennis H. (2002). The rich legacy of half a century of the Wiener index", in Rouvray, Dennis H.; King, Robert Bruce, Topology in Chemistry: Discrete Mathematics of Molecules, pp. 16–37, Horwood Publishing, Chichester.
[46] Randic, M. (1975). On characterisation of molecular branching. *J. Am. Chem. Soc.*, 97, 6609-6615.
[47] Hall, L. H., Kier, L. B. (1977). Structure-activity studies using valence molecular connectivity. *J. Pharm. Sci.*, 66, 642.
[48] Kubinyi, H. (1997). QSAR and 3D QSAR in drug design Part1: methodology. *DDT,* 2 (11), 457-467.

[49] Renner, R. (2002). The Kow controversy, *Environ. Sci. TEchnol.*, 36, 410A-413A.
[50] Devillers, J. Balaban, A. T. (Eds) (1999). Topological Indices and Related Descriptors in QSAR and QSPR, Gordon Breach Sci. Pub. Amsterdam.
[51] Karelson, M. (2000). Molecular Descriptors in QSAR/ QSPR. Wiley-InterScience, New York.
[52] Tideschini, R. Consonni, V. (2000). Handbook of Molecular Descriptors, Wiley-VCH, Weinhein, Germany.
[53] Todschini, R., Consonni, V., Mauri, A., Pavan, M. (2006). DRAGON-Software for the calculation of molecular descriptors. Ver 5.4 for Windows, Talete srl, Milan, Italy.
[54] Katritzky, A. R., Lobanov, V. S. (1994). CODESSA: Version 5.3, University of Florid, Gainesville.
[55] MEkenyan, O., Bonchev, D. (1986). OASIS method for predicting biological activity of chemical compounds. *Acta. Pharm. Jugosl.*, 36, 225.
[56] Shalabi, L. A. (2006). Data Mining: A Preprocessing Engine. *Journal of Computer Science,* 2(9), 735.
[57] Paola Gramatics: A Short History of QSAR Evolution [URL: www.qsarworld.com].
[58] Van de Waterbeend, H. ed. (1995). Advanced computer-Assissted Techniques in Drug Discovery, VCH, Weinheim.
[59] Kubinyi, H. (1993). 3D QSAR in Drug Design. Theory, Methods and Applications, ESCOM Science Publishers, Netherlands.

In: Introduction to Drug Designing and Development
Editors: R. Kumar, A. Sharma and R. Kumar Tiwari
ISBN: 978-1-62948-556-0

Chapter 11

Pharmacophore Modeling

Rajnish Kumar*
Amity Institute of Biotechnology, AMITY University-Uttar Pradesh,
Lucknow, Uttar Pradesh, India

Summary

Pharmacophore modeling is a robust technique to rapidly identify novel potential therapeutic agents. There are numerous therapeutically relevant drug targets with undetermined active site geometries. Pharmacophore modeling provides an effective mechanism for designing the drugs. Pharmacophore modeling for drug designing is adopted when information about target is unknown. In this chapter we will try to understand various principles related to pharmacophore modeling and their applications in drug designing and development.

The essential geometric arrangement of atoms or functional groups necessary to produce a given biological effect is known as pharmacophore. According to the International Union of Pure and Applied Chemistry (IUPAC), 'A pharmacophore is the ensemble of steric and electronic features that is necessary to ensure the optimal supra-molecular interactions with a specific biological target structure and to trigger or block its biological response' [1].

Pharmacophores can also be described as a graph-theoretic or connectivity based structural fragment and geometric patterns. Drug activity prediction using three dimensional geometric molecular conformations (topographic patterns) is considered to be more realistic, even for the chemically dissimilar drug candidates with same biological activity. Atom type specifications and inter-atomic distances are used to define topographical patterns.

Conformational searching scheme is the first and foremost step towards pharmacophore designing. The second step is to define the common specific types of atom, general types of atom, associated functional groups and other properties that are common.

* Email address: 12.rajnish@gmail.com, rkumar2@lko.amity.edu.

The next step is the alignment and the superposition of molecules at specific positions. Least-squares fit calculation is made and superposition sites are joined by calculating distances. Minimum points of connection for pharmacophore are three (represented by a triangle) but it may contain more (may be presented by other geometries).

History of Pharmacophore

1903, Paul Ehrlich Devised method to develop chromospheres which can kill trypanosomes for treatment of African sleeping sickness.

1909, Term Pharmacophore was coined by Paul Ehrlich. "A molecular framework that carries (known as phoros) essential features responsible for the drug's (known as pharmacophore) biological activity"

1967, L. B. Kier. First to calculate pharmacophore. He used Roald Hoffmann's extended–Hückel–theory quantum mechanics package for the study of muscarinic agonists [2].

1977, Peter Gund, A set of structural features in a molecule that is recognized by the receptor site and is responsible for that molecule's biological activity (most widely accepted definition).

1998, Milne et al., Pharmacophore models constitute pharmacophore features, which are entities with specific chemical properties and characteristic 3D geometry giving its biological activity.

2000, S. M. Tasso et al. Pharmacophore searching for anticonvulsant drugs [3].

Pharmacophore Based Drug Designing

Pharmacophore based drug designing facilitates the generation of new lead molecules (mimic molecule) based on biologically active molecules which are already known (reference molecule). Operational strategy starts with mimicry of structural features of the reference compound to generate new lead molecule.

Pharmacophore based drug designing approach includes following three major steps:

1. **Collection of data**: Gathering all relevant information. Data can be collected from various sources such as patents, publications, conferences, biological activities, chemical formula, mechanism of action, X-ray data, kinetic studies etc. It is a very important step and development of new lead molecule is governed by information collected and it works on the principle of "Garbage in Garbage out".

2. **Analysis**: In-depth analysis of collected data. When the data is collected, additional data must be deduced from the existed data. Deeper analysis gives rise to knowledge and establishes a logical link between different components of information. The central goal of analysis is to develop a framework that connects knowledge extracted from structural elements that are required for biological activities to the stereo-chemical feature of the receptor.

3. **Design**: Design of new molecule using analysis of data. In this step we try to develop new molecules with desired structural requirements to interact with receptor site. Pharmacophore can be derived from known active molecules and can be incorporated into new lead molecule.

Golden Rule of Six

First rule: Consider two bioactive molecules. These two molecules have the same mechanism of action. When we superimpose these two molecules, common structural features can be identified and it can be assumed that these common features are essential for biological activity.

Second rule: When common structural features are identified, there is possibility that they all are essential or nonessential for biological activity. In that case number of working hypotheses can be considered.

Third rule: If we have two active and two inactive molecules, we can find out number of elements that needed to be present simultaneously to have any bioactivity. The number of molecular models we create more is the chance to get biologically active molecule.

Fourth rule: If we consider two chemical structure wise closely related molecules, in that case we cannot conclude a constructive bioactive molecule.

Fifth rule: If two bioactive molecules are structurally not similar, there is very difficult to find out common pharmacophore.

Sixth rule: Consider two structurally similar molecules in which one is active and another is inactive. The inactivity may be due to the extra volume of analogue present in the inactive molecule because it leads to a rejection of that molecule at the receptor active site. When such analogue is introduced to active molecule, it results in loss of bioactivity.

Hip-Hop Theory

Hip-Hop is feature-based alignment of a group of compounds without taking care of biological activity. Hip-Hop matches the chemical features of a molecule against drug candidate molecules. This results in the exploration of hypotheses that can be used in iterative chemical databases to find new lead candidates. Hip-Hop theory is conceptually similar to the constructive phase of HypoGen theory. Hip-Hop does an exhaustive search to find out common pharmacophore. It starts with two features pharmacophore and once all two feature are exhausted, three feature combination starts. This process continues until Hip-Hop cannot generate common pharmacophore anymore.

Hip-Hop Theory Procedure

1. Input a series of active compounds i.e., collection of conformational models of molecules and a selection of chemical descriptors, and production of a sequence of molecular alignments in a number of standard file formats.

2. Hip-Hopbegins by identifying configurations of features common to a set of molecules. It performs an exhaustive search starting with small sets of features and extends them until no larger common configurations are found.
3. Perform superpostioning of features via Root Mean Square (RMS) fit.
4. Score based on the mapping between the hypotheses and leads and the rarity of the pharmacophore.
5. The result of above four steps generates Pharmacophores.

HypoGen Theory

HypoGen theory is used to generate structure activity relationship model. It uses a set of molecules for which activity values are known for a given biological target. HypoGen is an algorithm which produces pharmacophore model and this model can be further used to predict the activities of new compounds. HypoGen optimizes the hypotheses that are available in highly active compounds but not present in least active/inactive compounds. It tries to find out simplest hypothesis to relate the structures and activities.

The prediction models are created by a HypoGen algorithm in three distinct phases:
(a) Constructive phase
(b) Subtractive phase
(c) Optimization phase

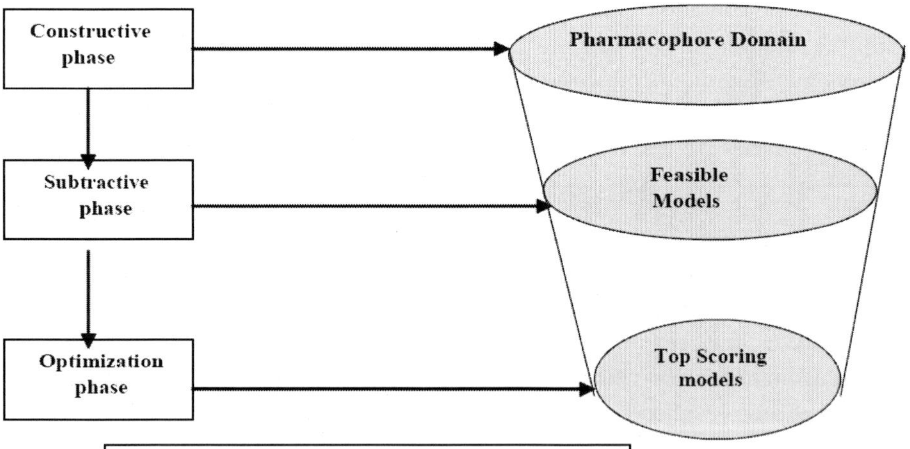

HypoGen Process Flow

Constructive phase: This phase finds out hypotheses that are common to a given set of compounds. The most active compound is derived by following equation:

$$MA*Unc_{MA} - A/Unc_A > 0.0$$

Where MA is an activity of the most active compound, Unc is uncertainty of the compound and A is activity of compound under investigation. If number of compounds is greater than eight then only top eight are used. This program finds out hypotheses using exhaustive search of all conformers just like Hip-Hop algorithm.

Subtractive phase: In this phase, hypotheses generated during the constructive phase are examined. If the hypotheses are common to the inactive compounds, they are removed from the data structure under consideration.

Optimization phase: This phase improves the score of hypotheses that were generated from the constructive and subtractive phase. For optimization of hypotheses HyoGen uses **simulated annealing algorithm.** Optimization phase considers the rotation of features, the addition of new features and removal of a feature etc. This phase accepts the hypotheses on the basis of probability function. 10 best scoring, unique and non-redundant hypotheses are selected.

Software/Tools for Pharmacophore modeling

First commercial software for pharmacophore modeling is **Catalyst.**

Catalyst creates three-dimensional (3D) models from collection of molecules having diversified structures and a range of activity. These three-dimensional models (also known as hypotheses) can be used as queries to search 3D databases to retrieve structures that fit the hypothesis. Hypotheses can also be used as models to predict the activities of new compounds.

Catalyst identifies possible binding features between a protein and a set of drug candidates that can explain variations in their activity. Catalyst specifies hypotheses in terms chemical features that are expected to be vital for binding to the active site of the protein.

Major highlights of catalyst:

- Constructs numerous hypotheses for a given hypothesis generation run, that explain the structure and activity data.
- Hypothesis features can be visualized and one can see the common features.
- Grouping of similar kind of data (cluster) and merging of hypotheses for developing more selective and refined models.
- Catalyst contains algorithms that can process large numbers of conformations and molecules.
- Hip-Hop's pharmacophore identification technology allows one to quickly and robustly handle flexible compounds that require investigation of a large number of conformational models3
- Thoroughly considers potential hydrogen bonding directionality, not just ideal lone pair positions [5].
- Identifies conformationally dependent features and checks surface accessibility. It ranks alignment hypothesis models by grouping to rank these configurations

according to a cost function that estimates the uniqueness and selectivity of each hypothesis [6].

DISCOtech automatically elucidates pharmacophore models using pre-calculated conformers. It uses clique detection methods to generate multiple pharmacophore hypotheses that can be compared and refined [7].

We get DISCOtech's models in a Molecular Spreadsheet that lists each model with its score, number of features, and distance tolerances. The scoring function reviews the quality of pharmacophore models by considering the number of molecules, the number of features, and inter-feature distances. Models are easily analysed using displays that show features in the form of colour coded spheres. Inter-feature distances are also mentioned. By superimposing the conformers on the models, distances are recorded in the spreadsheet for further analysis. An automated model refinement procedure selects conformers based on their similarity to a model. In next step it performs clique detection over the focused set of conformers [8].

Major highlights of DISCOtech:

- Generate and refine pharmacophore hypotheses for a set of ligands that bind to the same receptor.
- Build pharmacophore queries for use in 3D database searches.
- Predict the binding mode of a set of ligands.
- Identify functional group correspondences for molecules bound to the same receptor.
- Determine an alignment rule to enable 3D QSAR studies of a set of ligands.

Apex-3D methodology is automated identification of pharmacophores [1-3]. These pharmacophores can be used for building qualitative activity prediction rules and for creating search queries to identify new leads in a 3D-database. Identified pharmacophores can be used as starting points for constructing 3D-QSAR models when good quantitative data are available. The combination of a 3D pharmacophore with a quantitative regression equation is unique in the Apex-3D approach. Apex-3D generates pharmacophores queries for MDL Information Systems' databases [11] in order to find new compounds satisfying pharmacophores definition. The query generator converts internal pharmacophores representation to the query format using several built-in rules. Database hits can be loaded into Apex-3D and processed using the activity prediction module to eliminate any false positive hits resulting from the approximate nature of the pharmacophores query.

The automated identification of pharmacophore patterns according to the logico-structural approach involves the following steps:

- The compounds of the training set are separated into activity classes according to their activity type or level.
- Generation of a representative set of conformers for flexible compounds using a combination of such molecular modeling techniques as distance geometry, force field and quantum chemical geometry optimization, systematic conformational search, and molecular dynamics, all followed by conformer clustering.

- Generation of structural representations of compounds on the basis of property and distance matrices.
- The clique selection algorithm is implemented to identify common structural patterns in all pairs of compounds belonging to a given activity class. There are two available to find out pharmacophores from multiple conformers.

  Exhaustive search which matches all possible pairs of conformers of all compounds.

  Fast search which matches all conformers of each compound with only one conformer of all other compounds. This fast search algorithm produces the significantly lower number of pharmacophores without loss of the most frequently occurring biophoric patterns in most of the cases.
- Calculation of the number of occurrences of all identified structural patterns among compounds from each activity class of the analysed data sets.
- Biophores are selected as features having both probability and reliability higher than certain thresholds. These thresholds are established during training of the activity prediction system.
- Optimization of molecular superposition of compounds possessing a common pharmacophore. This procedure allows determination of superposition quality and can be used to filter pharmacophores producing bad alignment.
- Prediction of biological activity of novel compounds which have been synthesized, or suggested for synthesis, based on the identified pharmacophores [12].

Genetic Algorithm Similarity Program (GASP) performs pharmacophore elucidation. It does not require prior knowledge of pharmacophore elements or constraints. GASP automatically allows conformational flexibility and maps features among molecules using a genetic algorithm. In the absence of a three-dimensional protein structure, its active site model can be generated using ligands that bind to it. The most essential part in developing such a model are the finding out functional groups required for binding, their correspondence from one ligand to another, and the common spatial arrangement of these ligands when they are bound to the protein [13].

Major Highlights of GASP

- Allows full conformational flexibility of ligands, unlike methods that are limited to a pre-computed set of rigid conformers.
- Requires no advance knowledge of key functional groups or predefined correspondences between functional groups in different ligands.
- Automatically identifies rotatable bonds and key pharmacophore features. The only input required is a set of molecules.
- Intermolecular constraints can force correspondence between specific functional groups.

Phase is a high-performance program for ligand-based drug design tool by Schrödinger. Phase is a comprehensive package of pharmacophore modeling tools. It offers researchers and scientists great level of control at each step. It is comparatively fast, accurate, and highly configurable, Phase is a powerful tool for hit generation and lead hopping.

Major Highlights of Phase

The 'Phase' provides a standalone module for fast shape-based screening. One can screen number of molecules at a time. It stores pre-generated database for conformers. In addition user can generate conformers on the run. It has a graphical user interface that allows easy job submission along with extensive control of options.

Phase allows users to have precise control on job settings at each and every step such as pharmacophore scoring, Quantitative structure activity relationship (QSAR) building, database screening etc.

Phase can work for the projects where no receptor structure is available. It allows pharmacophores to be constructed with the aid of a crystal structure.

Phase finds out features using pattern matching which makes it easy to modify existing feature definitions and to create completely new custom features.

One can define regions of space that are assumed to be occupied by the receptor, and therefore it gives freedom for any ligand.

Schrödinger offers the Phase Commercially Available Compound Database (CACDB), against which a pharmacophore model can be screened for hit generation [14].

LigandScout is another completely integrated platform for accurate virtual screening based on 3D chemical feature pharmacophore models. It has seamless workflows, starting both from ligand and structure based pharmacophore modeling, and includes novel high performance alignment algorithms for excellent prediction quality with very good screening speed. In addition, they have included user friendly screening analysis tools, including the automated generation of Receiver operating characteristic (ROC) curves for performance assessments. All functions are accessible through a well elaborated graphic user. The algorithms are scientifically validated and based on pharmacophore research, while the application corresponds to state-of-the-art information technology.

Major Features of LigandScout

- Automatic interpretation of PDB ligands using geometry, dictionaries and rules.
- 2D view and hierarchical view directly linked to 3D interface.
- Fast alignment of molecules in their bio-active conformation of other molecules and 3D pharmacophores from several ligands and/or pharmacophores, shared feature pharmacophores can be derived to understand and model the relevant mode of action.
- Advanced handling of co-factors, ions, water molecules and covalently bound ligands.

- Pharmacophore export to Catalyst (tm), MOE (tm) and Phase (tm) for virtual screening.
- Extensive parameter control for more experienced users.
- Advanced PDB ligand perception and easy manual correction while modeling in the active site.
- Ability to treat co-factors and water molecules as part of the ligand or part of the macromolecule.
- Intuitive pharmacophore-based alignment of molecules.
- Support for most common file formats.
- Sophisticated file and repository management of edited and stored binding sites, molecules and pharmacophores.
- Smart enumeration of tautomers [15].

References

[1] Wermuth, C.G., Ganellin, C.R., Lindberg, P., Mitscher, L.A. (1998). Glossary of terms used in medicinal chemistry (IUPAC Recommendations 1998). *Pure and Applied Chemistry* 70 (5): 1129–1143.

[2] Kier L.B. (1967), Molecular orbital calculation of preferred conformations of acetylcholine, muscarine, and muscarone, *Mol. Pharmacol.***3**: 487–494.

[3] Tasso S.M., Bruno-Blanch L.E., Moon S.C., Estiu G.L. (2000), Pharmacophore searching and QSAR analysis in the design of anticonvulsant drugs, Journal of Molecular Structure (Theochem) 504: 229–240.

[4] Güner O.F. (2000), Pharmacophore Perception, Development, and Use in Drug Design, pp 177-178. USA: International University Line.

[5] Smellie A., Teig S., Towbin P. (1995), Promoting conformational variation, *J Comp. Chem.*16: 171-187.

[6] http://chipre.iqm.unicamp.br/~marcia/ACPHARM.pdf [accessed: 18-03-2013]

[7] Martin Y., Bures, M., Danaher E. et al. (1993) A Fast New Approach to Pharmacophore Mapping and Its Application to Dopaminergic and Benzodiazepine Agonist. *J. Comp. Aided Mol. Design* 7: 83-102.

[8] http://www.tripos.com/data/SYBYL/DISCOTech_072505.pdf [accessed on 18-03-2013]

[9] Golender V.E., Rozenblit A.B. (1983) Logical and Combinatorial Algorithms in Drug Design, Research Studies Press: Letchworth, U.K.

[10] Golender V.E., Vorpagel E.R. (1993) 3D QSAR in Drug Design: Theory, Methods and Applications, pp 137-149, ESCOM, Leiden.

[11] ISIS 3D Searching. (1994) New Features. Version 1.2. MDL Information Systems Inc. San Leandro.

[12] http://www.netsci.org/Science/Compchem/feature09.html [accessed on 18-03-2013]

[13] http://www.tripos.com/index.php?family=modules,SimplePage,,,&page=GASP [accessed on 18-03-2013]

[14] http://www.schrodinger.com/productpage/14/13 [accessed on 19-03-2013]

[15] http://www.inteligand.com/ligandscout [accessed on 21-03-2013]

In: Introduction to Drug Designing and Development
Editors: R. Kumar, A. Sharma and R. Kumar Tiwari
ISBN: 978-1-62948-556-0

Chapter 12

Drug Formulation and Dosage Forms

Prakash Deep [*] ***and Amrit Kumar Singh***
Amity Institute of Pharmacy
Amity University Uttar Pradesh, Lucknow Campus, India

Abstract

The present chapter gives an introduction and general overview on various dosage forms like solid, semi solid, liquid and gaseous dosage forms. The principal objective of dosage form design is to achieve a predictable therapeutic response to a drug included in a formulation which is capable of large scale manufacture with reproducible product quality. It gives brief idea about absorption, distribution, metabolism and excretion of drugs on which bioavailability of any drug depends. It is required to deliver the active drug molecule at an optimum rate and to an optimum extent. On the other hand, it should be easy to administer and have a required degree of acceptability for patients. The non medicinal components of a dosage form must have an acceptable extent of compatibility with the active drug molecule.

Introduction

The ultimate aim of a drug substance is; to show optimum therapeutic response in a desired manner. In the process of drug discovery when a number of Leads (drug candidates with desired pharmacological activities) are obtained out of several Hits (initial drug candidates), the next step is Lead optimization, which involves various modifications of active drug molecule to enhance its suitability to be developed as a drug candidate. During pre clinical phase of drug development, along with the establishment of an optimum level of safety and confirmation of efficacy of optimized lead molecule in animal models, there is also

[*] Corresponding author: Prakash Deep, E-mail: pdeep@lko.amity.edu.

a simultaneous development of suitable dosage form for further use in human volunteers in clinical trials.

It is a very rare event that a drug molecule is administered in its pure active form; instead, it is administered in a combined form along with some other non medicinal agents. There are various reasons for using these non medicinal agents. For example, because of highly potent nature, very minute amount of the drug molecules (in milligrams) are needed to produce the desired therapeutic effect and it may not be convenient enough to administer such low quantities to the patients. So an additional component in form of a diluent can easily overcome such problems. On the other hand, slight overdosing of such high potency drug molecules may cause serious side effects, in such cases also an additional agent may help in accurate and safe delivery of active drug molecule. Apart from these, such agents also help in protection of active drug molecules from surrounding factors like environmental, physical, chemical etc., these factors can influence the drug quality badly. These non medicinal agents ultimately help in getting optimum therapeutic response in a desired manner and are termed as pharmaceutical excipient/ ingredients/ additives. The pharmaceutical ingredients may act either as solubilizing agent, suspending agent, emulsifier, stabilizing agent, preservative, coloring agent, flavoring agent etc. or they may just be added as diluents or to enhance the patient compliance also. There is wide range of dosage forms according to various routes of administration e.g., tablets for oral administration, solutions for both oral and parenteral administration. [1, 13, 14]

A Suitable Dosage Form – Why?

Precipitation of a desired level of therapeutic response from a drug molecule requires optimization of a number of factors like physicochemical, pharmaceutical, pharmacological etc. Designing of a suitable dosage form is based on most of these factors. So, proper conversion of a drug molecule in a suitable dosage form enhances the possibility of getting desired therapeutic effect significantly. There are many important issues which indicate the need of a suitable dosage form; some of them are as follows: [4, 8, 12, 14]

1. To achieve a desired drug response e.g., parenterals are used for quick response.
2. To make the drug delivery more convenient.
3. To meet the specific requirements of various categories of patients e.g., syrups can be used more conveniently in children but solid dosage forms for geriatric use.
4. To enhance the reproducibility of the quality product on large scale production e.g., manufacturing on industrial scale.
5. To optimize risk/ benefit ratio in order to increase the developability of drug candidates e.g., sustained release, controlled release etc.
6. To provide a kind of protection to the active drug molecule from various physical, chemical, and even from pharmacological damages.
7. To enhance the patient compliance by making the non therapeutic aspects like visual appearance, palatability etc. of the drug molecule more pleasant.

8. To make the applicability of active drug molecule more patient oriented. For example, semisolid dosage forms are more preferable for topical application while solids are for oral administration.
9. To regulate the pharmacokinetic aspects of the drug molecule in order to enhance the therapeutic usefulness of the drug.

Above some points signify the need of a suitable dosage form. There are several other factors also, which can be used to acknowledge the need of suitable dosage forms for various drug molecules. [10]

Therapeutic Response and a Suitable Dosage Form

After discovery, the active drug molecule is required to be administered to the human body in a suitable combination so that it can produce the desired therapeutic response. When a drug molecule is administered to the human body, it undergoes mainly 4 different types of processes viz. absorbed to the systemic circulation (absorption), distributed to the actual site of action (distribution), metabolized through various enzymatic processes (metabolism) and ultimately gets eliminated through organs like kidney, lungs etc. (elimination). In these 4 processes, which are also known as ADME, a part of the drug molecule administered originally gets destroyed and only a fraction of administered dose actually reaches to the site of action.

In the process of absorption, the fraction of the administered dose that reaches to the systemic circulation in unchanged form, is called as Bioavailable dose. This Bioavailable dose depends upon the rate and extent of drug absorption i.e., Bioavailability. Maximum Bioavailable dose (100%) can be achieved through intravenous route of administration. With increase in the amount of Bioavailable dose, possibility of reaching a large fraction of administered dose to the site of action also increases.

In general, therapeutic response of a drug molecule increases if a large fraction of drug molecule reaches to the site of action and stay there for a long period of time. So, for getting a better therapeutic response, a large fraction of administered dose needs to reach the site of action which can be influenced by the bioavailability. Moreover, bioavailability of a drug molecule is related to the various characteristics of drug molecule (e.g., physicochemical properties, ADME etc.), dosage form designed to deliver the particular drug molecule and also to the route of drug administration. Study of these three parameters on bioavailability, is known as Biopharmaceutics. Also, these are the three major areas of biopharmaceutics which play crucial role in designing a suitable dosage form. The biopharmaceutical considerations are liable to change with change in any of these three areas. All these biopharmaceutical parameters are interlinked and must be optimized for obtaining an optimal therapeutic response. With these discussions, it can be said that the desired therapeutic response can not be achieved unless there is a suitable dosage form for delivering active drug molecule inside the human body. [7]

Salient Features of a Suitable Dosage Form

The most desired feature of a dosage form is to produce optimum therapeutic response in a required manner by delivering the active drug molecule at an optimum rate and to an optimum extent. However, it is very difficult since physiological and pathological conditions, of the individual patients, are likely to interfere with the bioavailability of active drug molecule. A dosage form must be stable and have the capability to be reproduced at large scale with desired level of quality standards. It should be easy to administer and have a required degree of acceptability for patients. The non medicinal components of a dosage form must have an acceptable extent of compatibility with the active drug molecule. They must not cause any kind of physical, chemical or pharmacological abnormality which may affect the qualitative aspects of the formulation, especially stability, safety and efficacy. [4]

Challenges in Developing Suitable Dosage Form

The challenges are different for different categories of dosage forms. For instance, it is very difficult to prepare a suitable dosage form for a drug molecule having very less water and /or lipid solubility since a certain level of hydrophilic / lipophilic balance is required for considerable bioavailability

Classification of Dosage Forms

Basically, there are following 4 types of dosage forms:

1. Solid
2. Semisolid
3. Liquid
4. Gas

Solid Dosage Form

Oral route for drug administration is the most preferred route because of ease of administration and patient acceptability. A major proportion of the available dosage forms for this route comprise of solids (powder, tablet, capsules) and liquids (solutions, emulsions, suspensions). Solid dosage forms are used more frequently than any other form and are safer for the patient to self administer. Capsules and tablets are two most common types and are inexpensive to manufacture. Generally drugs and pharmaceutical excipients are available in solid state. This gives one more reason to prepare solid dosage form. Solid dosage forms are divided into unit and bulk dosage forms. Example of unit dosage forms are tablets and capsules and bulk dosage forms are powders.

Powders: A powder is a homogenous mixture of more or less finely divided particulate material in dry form. Powders are starting material in the manufacturing of many dosage forms. Powdered drugs may be blended with powdered fillers and other pharmaceutical ingredients to prepare solid dosage forms as tablets and capsules; they may be dissolved or suspended in solvents or liquid vehicles to make various liquid dosage forms; or they may be incorporated into semisolids bases in the preparation of medicated ointments and creams. [12]

Medicated powders- Some medicated powders are made to be used internally and externally.

Divided powders: these are unit dosage powders normally packed in properly folded papers and dispensed in envelops.

Bulk powders: when accuracy of dosage is not critical, powder can be dispensed in bulk like antacids, laxatives, douche and dentifrices. [6]

The advantages of powder, are as follows:

1. Powder form is the most versatile and convenient to prescribe, compound and administer.
2. Powder can be manufactured at less cost hence product cost is very less as compare to other dosage forms.
3. Powders are stable and do not enter into reaction in solid state.
4. Particle size can be reduced to the desired range and thus facilitate rapid absorption.
5. Less incompatibility as compared to liquid dosage form.
6. Being small particles; they offer a large surface area for solvent action and hence dissolve rapidly. Thus the chances of irritation in gastrointestinal (GI) tract will be reduced.
7. In case of children and infants where they are unable to swallow tablets and capsules, drugs may be administered in powder form, making them palatable by mixing with milk, fruit juice or honey.

The disadvantages of powder are as follows:

1. Patient may misunderstand the correct method of use.
2. Patient can refuse to take bitter or unpleasant tasting drugs.
3. It is difficult to protect powders containing hygroscopic, deliquescent (tending to melt or dissolve in humid environment), or aromatic materials from decomposition.
4. Manufacturing cost increases when packing of uniform, individually wrapped doses of powders (sachets) is required.
5. In case, doses are not packed separately than chance of inaccurate dosing increases.
6. Powder must be a homogeneous blend of all of the components and must be of the most advantageous particle size otherwise the required effect will be compromised.

Tablets: tablets are solid, flat or biconvex discs, prepared by compressing a drug or a mixture of drugs with or without diluents. Today, tablets are most popular dosages forms intended for oral use. Advantages of tablets includes accurate dosing, ease and convenience to take, rapid bioavailability and onset of action, easy handling, masking of unacceptable taste, stability, controlled release (whenever required) and economical production. [2, 5, 3, 12]

Capsules: Capsules are solid dosage forms which contain one dose of the medicament enclosed within a small, water soluble shell of gelatin. Capsules are as popular as tablets. One extra advantage of capsule over tablet is that the drug having unpleasant taste or odour is completely enclosed in a practically tasteless shell. Rapid solubility of gelatin at gastric p^H gives the rapid release of drug and disintegration is not required so early onset of action can be seen. Solid substances can be enclosed in hard gelatin capsules and liquid or semisolid can be enclosed in soft gelatin capsules. [12]

The disadvantages of capsules are as follows:

Capsules are not suitable for highly soluble salts like Potassium chloride, Potassium bromide, Ammonium chloride as they can cause gastric irritation on rapid release.

Liquid Dosage Form

Two types of liquid dosage forms are available i.e., monophasic and biphasic liquid dosage forms. In monophasic system only one homogenous phase is present like solutions, waters, tinctures. In biphasic liquid dosage forms two distinct phases are present like emulsion and suspension.

Monophasic Liquid Dosage Forms

Solutions: solutions are liquid dosage forms containing one or more chemical substances usually dissolved in waters. Solutions can be used internally or externally for specific therapeutic effect of solute. [3, 11]

Aromatic waters: these are clear, saturated aqueous solutions of volatile oils or aromatic substances. Their odour and taste are similar to those of the drugs or volatile substances from which they are derived.

Syrups: Syrups are sweet, viscous, concentrated aqueous solutions of sucrose or other sugars. It contains pharmacologically active substances, flavoring agents. Syrups are more often used in the preparation of pediatric medicines. [6]

Spirits: Spirits are alcoholic or hydro-alcoholic solution of volatile substances. Generally it contains high percentage of alcohol. Spirits can hold the more amounts of aromatic or volatile substances in comparison to the aromatic water. It can be used internally and externally both. Flavoring agent, inhalations, external application are its important uses.

Eye Drops: eye drops are sterile, aqueous or oily solutions or suspensions meant for instillation into the eyes.

Lotions: Lotions are dilute aqueous solutions or suspensions which are used for external application. They are available for skin, hair or eyes. They are applied without friction. If cooling effect is required than solvent like alcohol should be added. Generally they are perfumed.

Inhalations: inhalations are solutions or suspensions of volatile, antiseptic substances which can be administered by nasal or oral respiratory route in the form of vapor produced on surface of hot water.

Biphasic Liquid Dosage Forms

Emulsion: Emulsion is biphasic liquid dosage forms in which one phase (internal phase, discontinuous phase) is dispersed in the other phase (external phase, continuous phase, dispersion medium) in the form of tiny droplets ranging the size from 0.1 micro meter to 100 micro meter in diameter. Emulsions are thermodynamically unstable system so it requires presence of emulsifying agent (emulsifier, emulgents) to be stabilized. [6]

Suspension: In this dosage form finely divided insoluble solid materials are suspended in a liquid medium. In most of the pharmaceutical suspensions average size of suspended particles ranges from 0.5 μm to 5 μm. [6]

The advantages of suspension are as follows:

1. It helps in the administration of insoluble substances.
2. In this form we can administer the substances which are not pleasant in taste.
3. This dosage form is also suitable for the application of dermatological materials to the skin as well as mucous membrane.
4. Parenteral preparations of insoluble drugs can be prepared.

Semi Solid Dosage Form

Generally semi solid dosage forms are meant for topical applications; they may be applied to the skin, surface of eye, nose, vagina and rectum. They may be of medicated or non medicated. Medicated preparations are used for the pharmacological effects (local and systemic) of the agents which they contain. Non medicated are used for their physical effects as protectants or lubricants. If this dosage form is designed to deliver the medicament into the skin, to treat dermal disorders, then it is called dermatological product. If it is designed to deliver the medicament through the skin to the general circulation for systemic effects, then it is called transdermal products and this type of absorption is known as percutaneous absorption.

Ointments: These are semisolid preparations meant for external application to the skin or mucous membranes. It may, or may not be medicated. Non medicated ointments are used for the physical effects as protectants, emollients or lubricants. Generally four types of ointments are used named topical, ophthalmic, rectal and vaginal. Ointment bases may be used for their physical effects or as vehicles. Ointment bases are generally classified as (a) oleaginous bases (b) absorption bases (c) water removable bases (d) water soluble bases.

It is also applied for percutaneous absorption i.e., passage of medicinal substances through the skin which reaches to blood stream. Some factors influence the percutaneous absorption like skin structure, diffusion, drug solubility characteristics, medicament concentration, skin hydration, vehicle, skin condition, penetration enhancers. [6, 9, 12]

Creams: Pharmaceutical creams are semisolid W/O or O/W emulsions which contain suspension or solution of one or more than one medicaments. Creams show pseudoplastic flow properties. They show very little yield value when applied but not flow under the influence of gravity. After application of the cream, the water evaporates, leaving behind a thin residue film of the oleaginous component. Primarily creams are used for topical application. [9, 12]

Gels: These are semisolid preparation consisting of dispersion of small or large molecules in an aqueous liquid vehicle rendered jellylike by addition of gelling agent like carbomer 934, carboxymethyl cellulose, hydroxyl propyl methylcellulose, tragacanth etc. [9, 12]

Pastes: Pastes are semisolid preparations intended for external application and contain larger proportion of finely divided powdered medicaments (about 25%) and hence these are stiffer than ointments. Because of stiffness they remain in place after application, require more force to apply and are effectively employed to absorb serous secretions. As they absorb serum secretions, pastes are used for acute lesions having a tendency to ooze. These are not suitable for application to hairy parts, like scalp because they form a sticky mass. [12]

Plasters: Plasters are solid or semisolid adhesive masses for external application. They bring medicament into close and prolonged contact with the surface of the skin. The adhesive material is a rubber base or a synthetic resin. Non medicated plasters are used for protection or mechanical support and to provide macerating action. Medicated plasters provide effect of incorporated medicament at the site of application. [12]

Glycerogelatins: These are plastic masses which contains gelatin (15%), glycerine (40%), water (35%) and an added medicament (10%). Gelatin is moistened with water for about 10 minutes then dissolved by heating on steam bath.

In next step medicament mixed with glycerine is added and mixture is allowed to cool with stirring until it gets congealed. Glycerogelatins are applied to the skin for long time. They are melted before application and then cooled to slightly above the body temperature and applied to affected area.

After some time it hardens, usually it is covered with bandage. [12]

Suppositories: Suppositories are solid or semi solid dosage forms meant for insertion into body cavities like rectum, vagina or urethral tract where they melt soften or dissolve and exert local or systemic effects. They have various shapes and weights. Vaginal suppositories are called pessaries and urethral suppositories are called bougies. Vaginal suppositories are used as contraceptives, antiseptics, to combat pathogens. Local actions of rectal suppositories are to relieve constipation or the pain, irritation, itching and inflammation associated with hemorrhoids or other anorectal conditions. They may contain number of components like local anesthetics, astringents, analgesic, vasoconstrictor, emollient and protective agents. Urethral suppositories may contain antibacterial substances or local anesthetics. On the other hand, in systemic effects the mucous membranes of the rectum and vagina permits the absorption of many soluble drugs. [6, 7] The advantages over the oral therapy are as follows:

a. Alternative route of administration for the patients suffering from nausea, vomiting and gastro intestinal disturbances.
b. Drugs are not exposed to the destructive environments of stomach like acidic p^H, Enzymes.
c. Drugs causing irritation to the stomach can be given by this way.
d. First pass metabolism can bypass.
e. Drugs can be given to patients who are unable to take it through oral route.
f. Faster onset of actions as compared to oral administration because drugs are absorbed from rectal mucosa directly into the venous circulation.

Gaseous Dosage Form

Aerosol: These are pressurized dosage forms which give a fine dispersion of liquid, semi solid, solid, fine mist, wet spray, quick breaking foam, stable foam in a gaseous medium. This dosage form is dependent upon the container, valve assembly and propellant. Two components are essentially required for any aerosol formulation i.e., propellant and active ingredient. Single or mixture of propellant can be used to give the desired vapor pressure, solubility and particle size. Concentrate component consists active medicament, solvent, surfactant, anti oxidants. [7]

The advantages of aerosol are as follows:

a. Required amount of medicament can be taken out without contaminating the rest amount thus the sterility would be maintained.
b. Being of completely closed dispensing system, drug can not be affected by atmospheric oxygen, light and moisture.
c. Medicament can be applied uniformly over the affected area without painful or irritating touching the area.
d. Delivery of amount of medicament can be controlled by using the metered valve.

References

[1] Swarbrick, J. (2007). *Encyclopedia of Pharmaceutical Technology.* edition 3, Informa Healthcare US, Inc.
[2] Parikh, D. M. (2005). *Handbook of Pharmaceutical Granulation Technology*, Taylor and Francis Group.
[3] Niazi, S. K. (2004). *Handbook of Pharmaceutical Manufacturing Formulations*, CRC Press LLC. Volume 1: Compressed Solid Products, Volume 2: Uncompressed Solid Products, Volume 3: Liquid Products, Volume 4: Semisolid Products, Volume 5: Over-the-Counter Products, Volume 6: Sterile Products.
[4] Banker, G. S., Rhodes, C. T. (2002). *Modern Pharmaceutics edition 4*, Marcel Dekker, Inc., New York.
[5] Liberman, H. A., et al., (1989). *Pharmaceutical Dosage Forms-Tablets.* Marcel Dekker, Inc., New York.
[6] Gennaro, A. R. Remington (2000) *The Science and Practice of Pharmacy.* Lippincott. William and Wilkins.
[7] Lachman, L., Lieberman, H. A., Kanig, J. L. (2000). *The Theory and Practice of Industrial Pharmacy.* Varghese Publishing Home.
[8] Aulton, M. E. (2005). *Pharmaceutics-The Science of Dosage form Design.* Churnchill Livingstone, London.
[9] Osborne, D. W., Amann, A. H. (2000). *Topical Drug Delivery Formulation*, Marcel Dekker Inc., New York.
[10] Bontempo, J. A. (1997). *Development of Bio-Pharmaceutical Parenteral Dosage Forms*, Marcel Dekker Inc., New York.

[11] Liberman, H. A., et al. (1984). *Pharmaceutical Dosage Forms-Parenterals*, Marcel Dekker Inc., New York.

[12] Allen, L. V., Popovich, N. G., Ansel, H. C. (2010). *Ansel's Pharmaceutical Dosage Forms and Drug Delivery Systems edition 9*, Lippincott Williams and Wilkins, Baltimore.

[13] Jones, D. (2008). *Pharmaceutics –Dosage Form and Design*, Pharmaceutical Press London.

[14] Ghosh, T. K., Jasti, B. R. (2005). *Theory and Practice of Contemporary Pharmaceutics*. CRC Press LLC, Florida.

In: Introduction to Drug Designing and Development
Editors: R. Kumar, A. Sharma and R. Kumar Tiwari
ISBN: 978-1-62948-556-0

Chapter 13

Drug Regulatory Affairs

Abhishek Kumar*
Amity Institute of Biotechnology, AMITY University Uttar Pradesh, Lucknow Campus, Uttar Pradesh, India

Abstract

Innovations are the result of tremendous effort and they are created with an interest to benefit the mankind whereas to make that endeavor a success sometimes rules and regulations are needed to make the process ethical. These regulations provide a competitive edge to the industry as well as the product, as they are extensively monitored at different levels e.g., efficacy, registration and marketing in pharmaceutical/ biotechnology industry. With the involvement of various steps, from scientific assessment to the management, the subject is day-by-day becoming more relevant for the industry. A close eye is kept on the product movement to make it spotless at every step, ensuring that the companies abide all the set norms pertaining to their business, track the changing business environment and reform accordingly.

The chapter details the importance of regulatory affairs in the pharma industry, various regulatory bodies, the drug regulatory process, and an introduction to ICH guidelines. A comprehensive note on the working physiology of the pharmaceutical industry will be delivered.

Introduction

Commercial engines i.e., industries are engaged day and night in the societal benefits and economical growth of countries. Every industry is producing varied goods and services in various categories. Amongst them all, pharma is recognized to be the most dynamic and regulated of all the industries. Regulations are put in order to develop the most efficient and

* Corresponding author: Abhishek Kumar, E-mail address: kumarabhishek1302@gmail.com, akumar2@lko.amity.edu.

safe pharmaceutical products. An input of around USD $800 million and a period of 8 – 15 years is invested to come out with a novel drug. To protect the advantages of this endeavor and innovation strategic guidelines are required to establish ethical practices in research.

Regulations are formed to provide an edge of ethics to the general practices whether common or business. Stringent norms and laws in biological and pharma industries are opted to safeguard the humankind from unethical practices and publicities specially RandD, marketing of drugs including their pricing issues. The new entity thus generated costs millions and years to progress and for protection of such endeavors strategic and technical practices right from the beginning of the development of a product are needed which would definitely make an important contribution in business. Regulations or the directives in pharma/ biotech are needed for extensive assessment of the product to ensure full protection of health, publicity, registration, marketing authorization and supplies.

1. Importance of Regulatory Issues

Regulatory affairs specially in drugs offers an insight where through different agencies wisdom collected in form of supervision, prior knowledge, market preference, etc. analyses the health of that particular product (drug) and its future prospects thus helps in reducing series of development failures. The pharmaceutical, biotech and medical devices industries are well known to be running with high regulations. The subject caters to all the regulatory requirements needed to get the new product(s) approved. Considering pharma/biotech, new products thus generated may be classified as New Active Substances (NAS), Biotech Products, Biological Products, Animal Products and medical/ diagnostics products.

New Active Substances (NAS)

This category includes chemical, biological, and even the radiopharmaceutical substances not previously available for therapeutic use in humans to be used for the cure, alleviation, treatment, prevention, or in vivo diagnosis of diseases in humans.

An isomer, blend of isomers, a complex/ derivative/ salt of a chemical substance previously available as a medicinal product but differing in properties regarding safety and efficacy from that substance previously available.

A biological substance previously available as a medicinal product but differing in molecular structure, nature of source material, or manufacturing process

A radiopharmaceutical substance that is a radionuclide or a ligand not previously available as a medicinal product; alternatively, the coupling mechanism linking the molecule and the radionuclide has not been previously available.

Biotech Products

Biotech products may include naturally occurring/ modified polypeptide, protein, DNA, or RNA product (*produced by recombinant DNA or hybridoma technology and expressed in cell lines, transgenic animals, or transgenic plants*) for therapeutic, prophylactic, or in vivo diagnostic use in humans; the only types of vaccines included in the biotech category are recombinant vaccines

Biological

A substance isolated from animal tissues (e.g., vaccines, hormones, and antigens) or plant alkaloids.

Medical Devices

Instruments or products used for treating or diagnosing disease (such as thermometers, artificial hearts implants, and pregnancy kits)

2. Global Regulatory Bodies

Regulatory is a vital organ of the industry, responsible to endorse whether a required drug can move for the clinical – trials and launch. The authority assesses the scientific and clinical data to ensure the consistency, potency, high purity, claimed clinical effects and along with the unaccepted side effects.

The regulatory authorities also check for quality control, manufacturing, licensing/ labeling, marketing factor, directions of use, we can say the DRUG IN TOTO. To comply with the norms, the worldwide nations have established regulatory bodies to look after the drug regulatory affairs. The various regulatory bodies are mentioned in Table No.1

3. Process of Drug Regulation

Globalization has strengthened the global business process through its cross fertilization of technologies thus creating a cutting edge competition in biopharmaceutical industries as well. Stringent rules and guidelines assist in complying with the quality norms and hence also build the brand in market.

The strategic process of drug regulation starts from the process of drug regulation starts with inception of the product from development for human use, receipt of scientific data to the complete review of data through registration, market viability and life cycle optimization.

Regulatory persons are exhaustively engaged right from the conceivement of product, initial developments, clinical trials submission, successful studies and results, exploring opportunities for the development such as orphan drug *(Global regulatory affairs—role in the biopharmaceutical industry, Role in the biopharmaceutical industry, Chapter 2)*[1] and fast track designations, discussions with regulatory agencies on drug development proposals,

[1] URL: (Global regulatory affairs—role in the biopharmaceutical industry).

protocol assessments, filing the marketing applications and regulatory reviews for product approval. The life cycle optimization of the product is also carried out to deliver better value of the product and maintain the product life cycle by additions and transformation in product.

The industry calls for innovative, breakthrough regulatory strategies for product development and registration process. There is a strong requirement to understand the biopharmaceutical environment, regulatory activity and its utilization along with global thrust with a focus on strengthening the relationship with the regulatory authorities and providing timely expert input into a new product, its manufacturing and further scope for registration.

Table 1. Regulatory Authorities established worldwide

Country	Name of Regulatory Authority
US	Food and Drug Administration (FDA)
UK	Medicines and Healthcare Products Regulatory Agency (MHRA)
Australia	Therapeutic Goods Administration (TGA)
India	Central Drug Standard Control Organization (CDSCO)
Canada	Health Canada
Europe	European Medicines Agency (EMEA)
Denmark	Danish Medicines Agency
New Zealand	Medsafe - Medicines and Medical Devices Safety Authority
Sweden	Medical Products Agency (MPA)
Netherlands	Medicines Evaluation Board
Ireland	Irish Medicines Board
Italy	Italian Pharmaceutical Agency
Nigeria	National Agency for Food and Drug Administration and Control (NAFDAC)
Ukraine	Ministry of Health
Singapore	Centre for Pharmaceutical Administration Health Sciences Authority
Hong Kong	Department of Health: Pharmaceutical Services
Paraguay	Ministry of Health
Sweden	Medical Products Agency (MPA)
Thailand	Ministry of Public Health
China	State Food and Drug Administration
Germany	Federal Institute for Drugs and Medical Devices
Malaysia	National Pharmaceutical Control Bureau, Ministry of Health
Pakistan	Drugs Control Organization, Ministry of Health
South Africa	Medicines Control Council
Sri Lanka	SPC, Ministry of Health
Switzerland	Swissmedic, Swiss Agency for Therapeutic Products
Uganda	Uganda National Council for Science and Technology (UNCST)
Brazil	Agencia Nacional de Vigiloncia Sanitaria (ANVISA)
Japan	Ministry of Health, Labour and Welfare (MHLW)

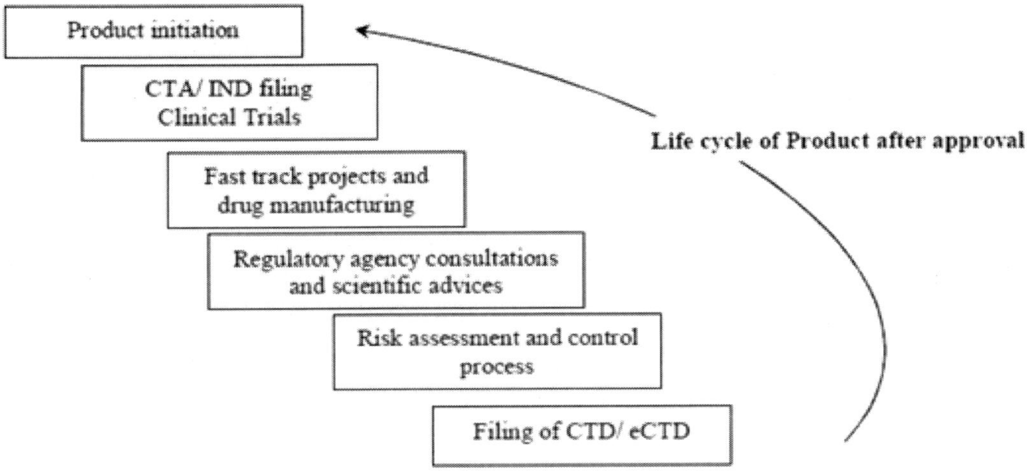

Figure 1. Regulatory Approval Mechanisms.

Regulatory affairs are a strategic process comprised of four major segments in the approval process:

- Receipt of data
- Scientific assessment
- Sponsor response authorization of product
- Marketing of labeled drug and communications/ laisionings

Global regulatory affairs include plays under mentioned important functions:

- Establishing strategic regulatory guidance and delivering regulatory strategy(s) globally for product development, manufacturing and registration
- The establishment and maintenance of a credible relationship with the regulatory authorities in communication.
- Making an efficient repository/ archives for objections/ complaints with regulatory standards for audits
- Maintaining high – quality, complete user friendly documents electronically
- Product details and labeling processing
- Process of regulatory intelligence, monitoring changes in regulatory policy with regulatory agencies
- Compliance with published information and promotions to meet regulatory requirement
- Functional units complying with regulatory requirements and good regulatory practices (GLP and cGMP norms).

To understand the functions of regulatory process we must also get into the key functional units of the industry:

a. Product Development Group

It comprises of subject technical experts that help in idea conceptualization, product development, manufacturing, registration and market acceptance. They also assist in making global regulatory strategies.

It reviews the regulatory documents for submission and is a nodal point for communication with the regulatory authorities.

This group is includes regulatory strategists, liaisons, scientists or other lexicons which extend their hands for technical contribution.

b. Chemistry, Manufacturing and Controls (CMC)/ Conformance/ Compliance Group

This is focused to the product/ process development, registration and manufacturing facility and site audits.

It ensures compliance to the current good manufacturing practices; good laboratory and clinical practices; and necessary audits and compliance seen at regulatory inspections.

c. Policy and Regulatory Intelligence

This team is vital organ of the industry responsible for product development, manufacturing and registration processes as they monitor the global regulatory environment for emerging trends, contributing in policy making, compliance to regulatory agency guidelines and analyzes and assesses precedents and standards to provide intelligence and preventive inputs to enable robust, proactive regulatory strategies.

d. The Marketing and Promotion

Works in association with the product developers and marketing personnel

Checks and ensures competitive healthy environment, promotional strategies.

Liaisons with regulatory agency on promotional and advertising resources.

e. The Regulatory Submissions

Caters to assembling, publishing and dispatching the regulatory documents to the global regulatory agencies.

Uses of electronic methods to ensure user friendly, complete submissions.

Application of e-technologies in dossier with careful coordination and considerations of global requirements for proper electronic submissions to the global regulatory agencies.

f. The Product Labeling Team

Stationed with the product development and regulatory teams and work in providing strategic directions in developing label content.

This panel furnishes label packages – (*inserts and literatures, container labels and packaging, and updating the product information*).

Ensures label contents, reviews for accuracy and ensures compliance to the specific regulatory norms, format and timelines for submission of the label information.

As a vital part of industry the regulatory team functions strategically in planned manner to ensure conformities, pre- and post-approvals, internal and external interfacing and communications.

4. Introduction to ICH Guidelines

The International Conference on Harmonization (ICH) is a significant technical requirement for registration of pharmaceutical products for Human Use. Its logo is designed in a manner which embodies the letters 'I', 'C' and 'H' in human abstract form.

ICH was established in 1990, to achieve greater harmonization in interpretation and application of technical guidelines and requirements for drug registration.

This regulation calls the drug regulatory authorities of Europe, Japan, and the United States, along with the pharmaceutical trade associations of these regions on a common platform to discuss on scientific and technical aspects of product registration.

ICH comprises of ICH Steering Committee, ICH Coordinators, ICH Secretariat, and ICH Working Groups. ICH Global Cooperation Group (GCG) and ICH MedDRA are components of Steering Committee. ICH Observers are actively associated with the ICH process to have a link with the non-ICH members/ regions.

ICH Expert Working Groups (EWGs) and Implementation Working Groups (IWGs)

Working groups elects *Official Representatives*, nominated from the 6 ICH (EU, EFPIA, MHLW, JPMA, PhRMA and FDA) and the ICH Observers (WHO, EFTA and Health Canada).

Table 2. Region wise government and industry based regulatory body

Region	Regulatory Body	Research Based Industry
Japan	MHLW: Ministry of Health, Labour and Welfare	JPMA: Japan Pharmaceutical Manufacturers Association
Europe	EU: European Union	EFPIA: European Federation of Pharmaceutical Industries Association
US	FDA: Food and Drug Administration	PhRMA: Pharmaceutical Research and Manufacturers of America

The official membership of EWG/ IWG comprises of *1-Topic Leader* and *1-Deputy Topic Leader* for the ICH Parties and *1-representative per ICH Observer* (EFTA, Health Canada, WHO). Experts are chosen by ICH regional Coordinators.

According to the topic under harmonization, experts may be called by ICH Steering Committee to nominate one representative to participate in ICH Working Groups.

On approval by Steering Committee, expert from ICH Regional Pharmacopeias, ICH Interested Parties (World Self-Medication Industry - WSMI, International Generic Pharmaceutical Alliance - IGPA, Biotechnology Industry, International Pharmaceutical Excipients Council – IPEC and Active Pharmaceutical Ingredient Industry - API) as well as Regional Harmonization Initiatives (RHIs), Individual Drug Regulatory Authorities (DRAs) and Department of Health (DoH) from non-ICH countries may be invited

ICH – Work Products

Common Technical Document (CTD)	Common structured format for application submission to the authorities eCTD (electronic mode of submission of documents)
Guidelines	Established 50 harmonized guidelines to reduce the duplication in development and registration
MedDRA	Medical Dictionary for Regulatory Activities (MedDRA) Terminology

ICH – Process

ICH harmonization process comprises of 4 significant steps with initiation of EWS working on draft guidelines to the confirmations and signing by Steering committee and finally ending with harmonized tripartite regulatory implementation.

Table 3. ICH Process of Harmonization

Step 1	Consensus building	EWG prepares a consensus draft of Guideline, based on Concept Paper. If endorsed by SC, EWG will also meet face-to-face at the biannual SC meetings. Interim progress reports provided to SC on a regular basis.
Step 2	Confirmation of 6 party consensus	Agreement is confirmed by at least one of the SC members for each of the six ICH parties signing their assent. The consensus text approved by the Steering Committee is signed off by the Steering Committee
Step 3	Regulatory consultation and Discussion	*Regional Regulatory Consultation*
		Discussion of Regional Consultation Comments
Step 4	Adoption of an ICH Harmonized Tripartite Guideline	Final Document is signed off by the SC signatories for the regulatory parties of ICH as an ICH Harmonized Tripartite Guideline
Step 5	Implementation	The harmonized tripartite Guideline moves immediately to the final step of the process that is the regulatory implementation. This step is carried out according to the same national/ regional procedures that apply to other regional regulatory guidelines and requirements, in the European Union, Japan and the US.

Source: ICH Guidelines, ICH Process of Harmonization, 2012.

What Is Good Manufacturing Practice (GMP)?

Products are consistently produced and controlled according to quality standards.

GMP covers all aspects of production; from the starting materials, premises and equipment to the training and personal hygiene of staff. Detailed, written procedures are essential for each process that could affect the quality of the finished product.

Risk assessment is done on: -

- unexpected contamination of products,
- causing damage to health or even death;
- incorrect labels on containers, which could mean that patients receive the wrong medicine;
- insufficient or too much active ingredient, resulting in ineffective treatment or adverse effects.

www.who.int/prequal/trainingresources/Training_gmp_info.htm

Conclusion

The industry is constantly dedicated to innovations with the intention to come up with something new for mankind. It exploits the scientific data generated during research and markets drugs effectively.

Regulatory Affairs (RA) is playing a vital role in the pharmaceutical industry with its involvement at every stage of drug development, including its inception, manufacturing, approval, registration, labeling or marketing. In this phase, the companies have to comply to an array of strict norms to ensure safety and efficacy of the drug in humans, sometimes animals. In such a highly regulated environment, regulatory affairs play a vital role, not only as an interface with health agencies but also as a link between various departments of the company. It also acts as the leading department that provides strategic advice on extremely difficult decisions through the life cycle of the product (drug).

In: Introduction to Drug Designing and Development
Editors: R. Kumar, A. Sharma and R. Kumar Tiwari
ISBN: 978-1-62948-556-0

Chapter 14

Recent Advances in Healthcare and Development of Biomedical Sensors

Prof. (Dr.) Ashok Kumar Mishra*
Department of Physics, Amity University Uttar Pradesh,
Lucknow Campus, India

Introduction: Biosensor Technology for Medical Applications

The biosensor technology is emerging as interesting area of research as various devices have already been reported for specific purposes e.g., detection of graft compatibility, detection of bitter taste of edibles etc. Recent development in Biosensor technology has provided the feasible means of health monitoring services and ubiquitous healthcare system. The one of the important aspects of the development of biosensor technology is human health monitoring. The technologies for ubiquitous solution comprise of "sensing", "monitoring", "analyzing" and "feedback". Population aging has become one of the most significant demographic processes of modern times. An inevitable consequence of the demographic transition and the shift to lower fertility and reduced mortality, the ageing of the world's population has many countries facing unprecedented numbers and proportions of older persons. In most of the world, populations are ageing at an extremely rapid pace. Providing a low cost and most convenient health facilities to the peoples have always been a great challenge for the Medical Physicist. Also fast changing lifestyle of the modern world and problem of an aging society puts an urgent need to renovate the healthcare facilities. There is an urgent need of devising a cheaper and smarter way to provide health care for sufferers of age related disease. Also emphasis has to be paid for providing health monitoring in out-of-

* E-mail: akmishra@lko.amity.edu.

hospital conditions for older people and patients who require regular supervision, particularly in remote areas.

In addition to the basic requirements of being wireless, future health care system based on wireless sensor network must have support for ad-hoc routing topologies, mobility and high degree of reliability. Also these systems need to be miniature in size and should be easily wearable so as to cause least inconvenience to the person. The health care system can be viewed as consisting of four major components namely sensing, monitoring, analyzing and feedback. Precisely designed and calibrated sensors and actuators perform the sensing of physiological data from the patient's body. The measured data can be monitored and recorded for later use. Monitoring component provides the graphical of the numerical representation of the data. Analyzing the components perform the specific analysis for particular diseases and studies their pattern for accurate diagnosis. Based on the results of analysis the feedback is sent to the other components to take the necessary course of action. The feedback can be behavior modification of system, emergency alert, or prescriptions to the patients.

Fabrication of Biosensors: Micromachining in Micro Electro Mechanical System (MEMS)

The Physics of the transistor has opened various interdisciplinary fields and many useful technological developments have taken place exploiting this effect in various ways. The term "micromachining" usually refers to the fabrication of micromechanical structures with the aid of etching techniques to remove part of the substrate or a thin film. Silicon has excellent mechanical properties, making it an ideal material for machining. One of the first pressure sensor based on silicon was isotropically micro machined by Honeywell in 1962. In 1966 Honeywell developed a technique to fabricate thin membranes using mechanical milling. Isotropic etching was used to produce membranes in 1970. Etchants dependent on crystal orientation led to a more precise definition of structures and increased interest. Anisotropic etching was introduced in 1976.

An early anisotropically etched silicon pressure sensor was made by Greenwood in 1984. In the 1960s the first surface micromachined structures using metal mechanical layers were presented. Surface micromachining involves the formation of mechanical structures in thin film formed on the surface of the wafer. The early 1980s saw the growth of silicon-based surface micromachining using poly silicon as the mechanical layer. In recent years a number of new technologies have been developed using both silicon and materials new to the semiconductor industry.

The formation of moveable structures needs extension of the 2-D fabrication process for the creation of patterned shape in the third dimension, perpendicular to the substrate. This is exemplified in silicon by four fundamental techniques namely Surface micromachining, Bulk micromachining, Deep reactive Ion etching (DRIE) and Single Crystal Silicon Reactive etch and Metal (SCREM), which are having their own advantages and disadvantages. In surface micromachining, 3-D mechanical structures are constructed in a layered fashion.

Two types of layers, based on their material composition/etching properties, are employed, namely sacrificial and structural layers. The former is ultimately dissolved via a process step named *release* and the latter remain, becoming part of the freestanding movable structure proper. In bulk micromachining, the substrate itself is sculpted to form a 3-D mechanical structure. The aspect ratio of the cavity or pit is determined by the etching properties of the atomic planes which, in turn, is a function of crystallographic properties and orientation of the wafer, in particular, the greater the number of atoms in a given plane, the slower its etching rate.

The dependence of aspect ratio on the crystallographic plane makes up the wall, motivated the development of techniques to increase it. In DRIE, the high aspect ratio trenches are achieved by a sequence of plasma etching and polymerization steps. Though DRIE is better than conventional micro machining yet it is an expensive one. The next process which is not so expensive as DRIE and better than conventional micro machining is SCREM. This process employs standard tools, is self-aligned, employs a temperature below 300 ^{0}C.

Nanotechnology Fabrication Elements: Nano Electro Mechanical System (NEMS)

The element of nanotechnology fabrication ranges from techniques to produce two-dimensional patterns with deep-submicron/nanometer-scale widths, to the techniques to produce atomic-thick layers/multi-layers of various material compositions, to the techniques to precisely manipulate atomic-size particles. These techniques, together with those presented previously, constitute the arsenal at the core of Nano-MEMS. Some of the available techniques have been summarized below.

Electron Beam Lithography

Electron beam lithography utilizes electrons, instead of the projection of a mask image illuminated by photons, to create directly the desired pattern on the photo resist as depicted in Figure 1.

Soft Lithography

The conventional IC fabrication processes, and the approaches to MEMS fabrication derived from them, have as their core step the photolithography definition of patterns on a planar substrate/wafer. Thus, as indicated previously, their application to create nanoscale devices becomes prohibitively expensive, as the development of the concomitant light sources and tools to create devices at these length scales is very expensive. This is of chief import, not just for research purposes but, more importantly, for the large scale production germane to commercial applications. Soft lithography, the production of nanoscale devices by creating elastic (soft) polymer masters that can then be used to print, mold, and emboss nanoscale structures, is a technique which has been the subject of much recent research of the inexpensive creation of nanoscale devices.

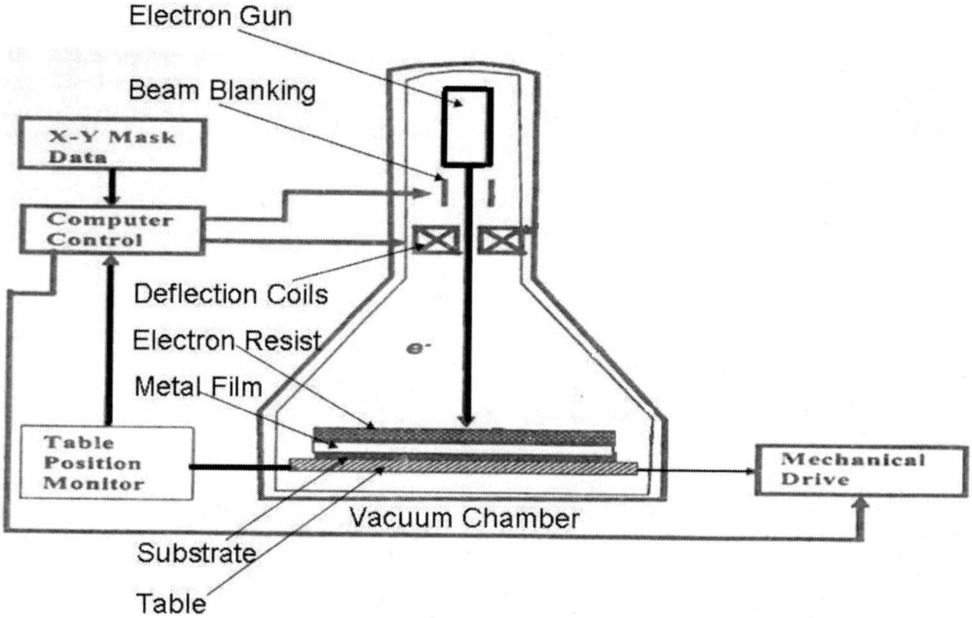

Figure 1. Sketch of electron beam lithography system.

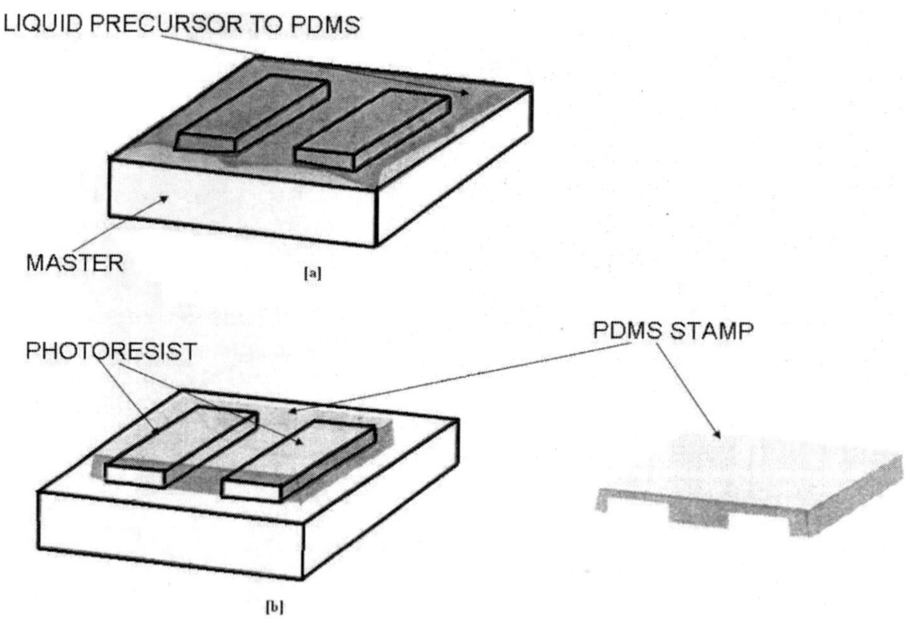

Figure 2. Soft lithography-Making an elastic stamp. (a) A liquid precursor to polydimethylsiloxane (PDMS) is poured over a bas-relief master produced by photolithography or electron-beam lithography. (b) The liquid is cured into a rubbery solid hat matches the original pattern. (c) The PDMS stamp is peeled off the master. The technique relies on first making an elastic stamp, shown in Figure 2, and appears to have been advanced by Whiteside, who applied it as an extension of his work on the creation of channels and chambers for micro fluidic systems.

Molecular Beam Epitaxy

The engineering of modem semiconductor device structures relies on the appropriate introduction and distribution of impurities via doping, together with band-gap engineering to effect electron confinement along the direction of transport. This latter gives rise to devices in which tunneling phenomena becomes manifest. The key to these types of structures is the technique for depositing down to mono-atomic-thick layers called molecular beam epitaxy (MBE). MBE underwent extensive progress during the 1990s and is now a well established production technology. The essentials of an MBE for growing a given structure are depicted in Figure 3.

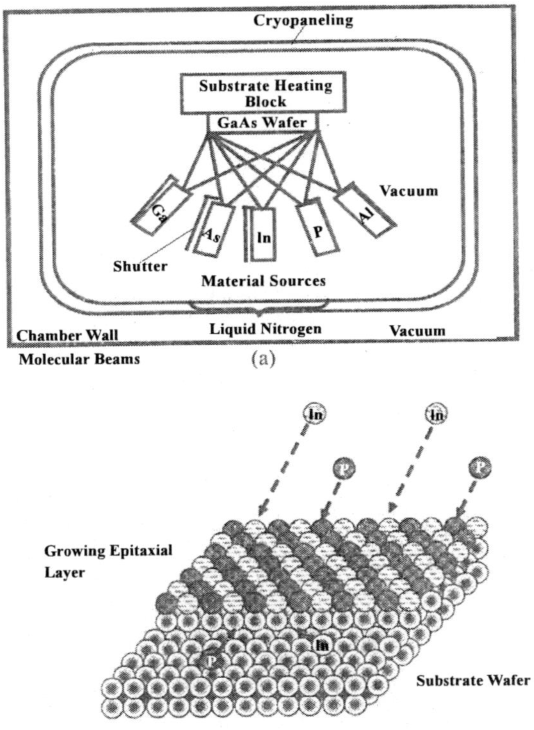

Figure 3. (a) Sketch of MBE system. The atomic sources may be either in the solid or the gaseous states, (b) Sketch of layered atomic deposition.

Scanning Probe Microscopy

Progress in Nanotechnology has been intimately related to the invention of a number of techniques for imaging and manipulating atoms/nano-particles at nano-scales. All of these techniques are based on a very fine tip (with atomic resolution), and the nature of what is imaged or manipulated is a function of the tip itself, i.e., whether it is conductive, insulating, magnetic, non-magnetic, etc. Excellent review articles summarizing advances in scanning probe microscopy have been published by Giessibl and Baski. In this section we focus on two of the main such techniques, namely: a) The scanning tunneling microscope (STM); b) The atomic force microscope (AFM).

a) Scanning Tunneling Microscope

In STM, a sharp metal tip is brought in very close proximity to a conductive sample, typically to a distance within a few Angstroms; see Figure 4.

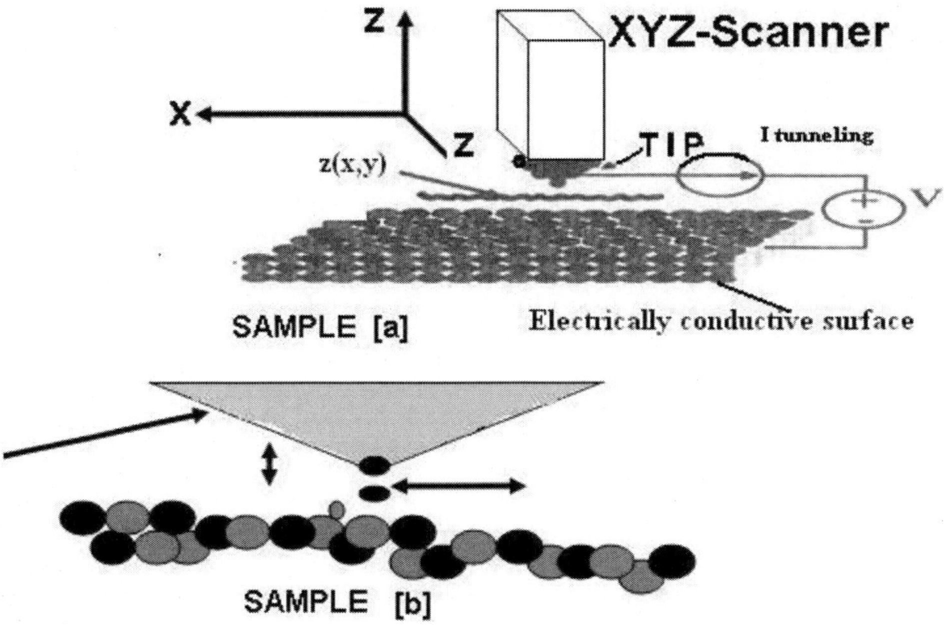

Figure 4. (a) Sketch of STM system. (b) Probe tip detail. The sample is held in ultra high vacuum.

b) Atomic Force Microscopy

In AFM, Figure 5, a sharp tip is also brought very close to the sample surface.

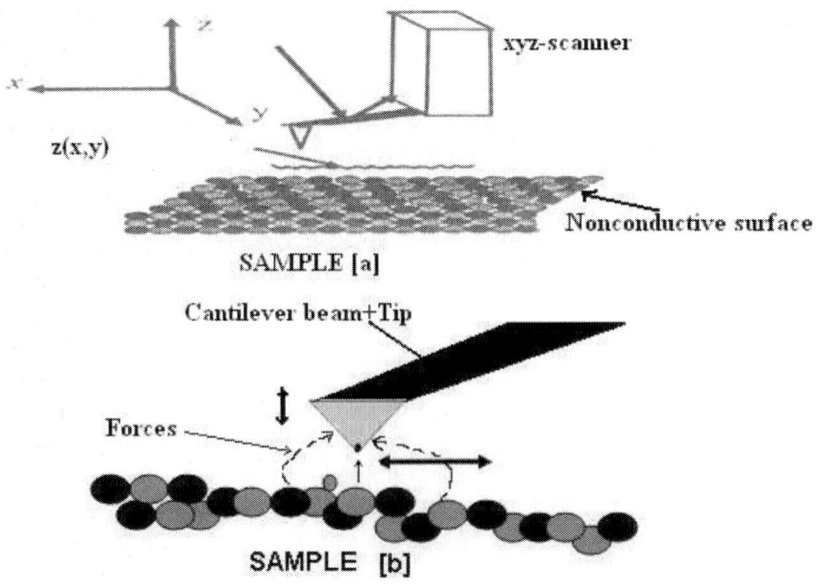

Figure 5. (a) Sketch of AFM system. (b) Probe detail. The sample may be held at ambient conditions.

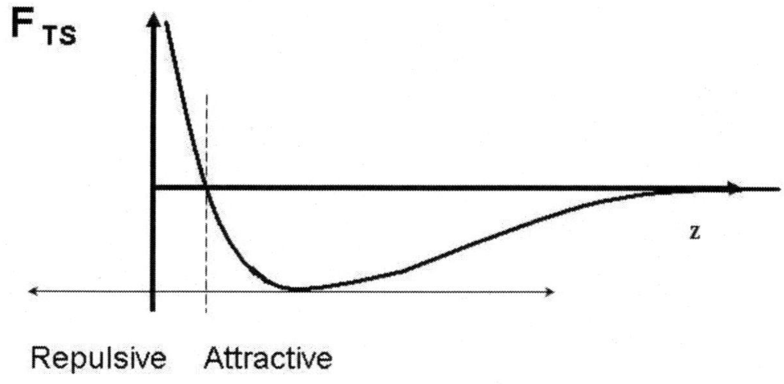

Figure 6. Sketch of AFM tip-sample force versus their separation z.

The image of the sample is then extracted by relating the cantilever beam deflection to the force required to produce it, F_{TS}. F_{TS} in turn, is related to the tip-sample (TS) potential V_{TS} via its negative gradient, $F_{TS} = -\partial V_{TS} / \partial z$ and is characterized by an effective spring constant $k_{TS} = -\partial F_{TS} / \partial z$. F_{TS} may be attractive or repulsive, as it embodies a variety of forces, each one varying differently with TS distance z, thus making it a nonlinear force, see Figure 6.

Nano-Engineering

The ultimate degree of control in nanofabrication is embodied in the ability to manipulate individual atoms/nano particles with precision. This is accomplished by two techniques, namely, exploiting AAFM to push particles, and DIP-Pen lithography.

AFM-Based Manipulation

In this technique, an oscillating AFM tip is brought close to a particle until, as a result of jump-to-contact, the oscillation amplitude goes to zero. The AFM approaches the nano particle via a fast X - Y scanning oscillation, in a plane perpendicular to the desired pushing direction, z, see Figure 7. Once contact of the AFM with the nano particle is established, motion proceeds in the z-direction at a slow scan rate.

DIP-Pen Lithography

This technique was developed by a Mirkin's group, see Fig. 8, and reminiscent of a goose-feather pen, a molecular "ink" is deposited over a gold surface according to a desired pattern. In one demonstration of the technique, an AFM tip was coated with a thin film of thiol molecules (the "ink") and moved two-dimensionally so as to inscribe the underlying gold surface.

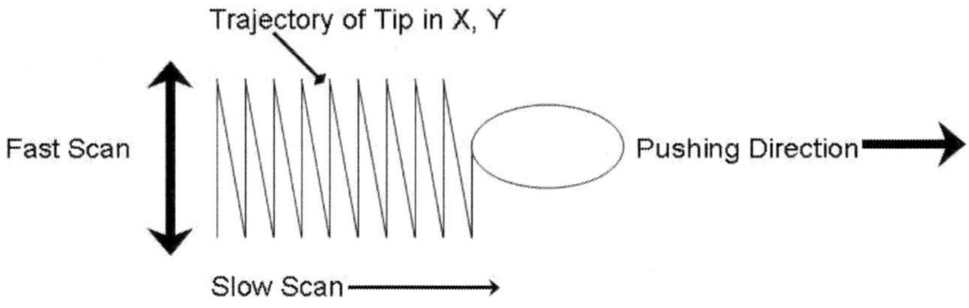

Figure 7. Pushing a nano-particle with AFM.

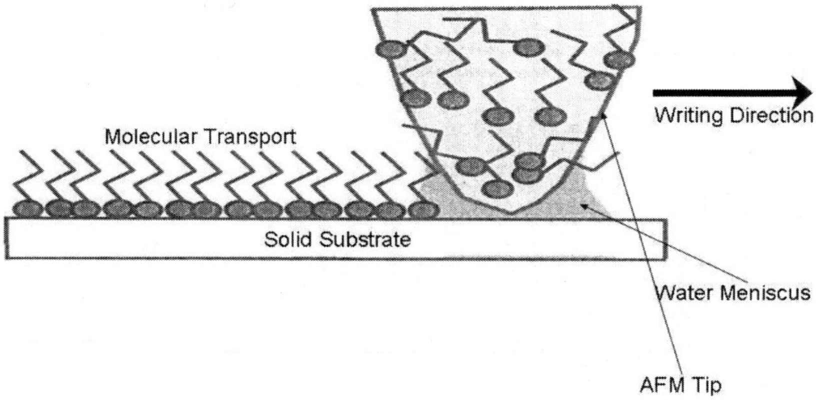

Figure 8. Close-up of inked AFM tip as molecules flow down the tip via water meniscus.

Since the thiol molecules can only attach to the gold surface in one particular orientation, a self-assembled monolayer of them, embodying the desired "writing," results. A variety of "inks" may be employed and, in of line width capability, lines few-nanometers wide have been demonstrated.

II. Description of Important Methods for Medical Applications

Healthcare field have been exposed of several technology innovations which varies from each other in some distinct features. On one hand there is a distinction in the manner the data are collected from the patient's body while some system differs in the technology used. Also some system differs from their application point of view.

Measuring Technique

The manner in which physiological data are collected from a patient's body varies from the direct access through sensor motes having actuators and transducers to the wearable type.

The former types are not wearable but can be carried in the pockets or attached to the patient's bed. Later types can be a small wrist wearable system which can measure ECG, Blood pressure or body temperature and can be used while performing daily activities. Convenient 'chest-belt' which is small and light can also measure some physiological parameters.

Sensing Methodology

Various physiological sensors can be embedded in our daily environments and systems which we use quite often. Without making the user aware of their presence these automatic sensors can measure the various types of health data when we interact with the environment or use these systems. Examples of such system include sensors embedded in toilet seats, sleeping beds or bath tubs. Such systems can be very useful in monitoring the daily health status of critical or elderly patients.

Tracking and Activity Test

One of the most important areas where the advantages of sensor networks can be exploited is for tracking mobile targets. Scenarios where such network may be deployed can be hospital (tracking the patient), home care (tracking the elderly person), tracking the activities of the suspicious person etc. This sensor based tracking is better that camera based as is requires less bandwidth for operation and does not need the patient to be in range of the camera every time. Also this technique is costly effective and can be deployed.

Fall Detection

Due to independent living of elderly persons, their activity & behavior monitoring has gained a significant importance in daily life. Body acceleration measurement can give the important information regarding person's daily activities i.e., walking, running and resting and particularly in the event of dangerous falling from stairs, bed or chair. As acceleration magnitude is different for different activities, it can be used for differentiating among the various activities.

Sensor Based Services for Continuous Health Monitoring

The two general classes of health monitoring applications are available for sensor networks. One class is patient monitoring in hospitals and includes tracking pulse and respiration rates via wearable sensors and sending the information to a personal computer for later analysis. This technology can be adapted to monitoring athletics performance on a running machine. The other class is home healthcare monitoring, for example, monitoring and elderly person's health or personal weight management. The patient's weight may be wirelessly sent to a personal computer for storage. Other examples are daily blood sugar monitoring and recording by a diabetic and remote monitoring of patients with chronic disorders.

Vital Signs Monitoring Using Sensor

A distributed healthcare monitoring system for clinical and trauma patients was developed using a wireless sensor network node. The proposed system aimed to measure various vital physiological health parameters like ECG and body temperature of patients and elderly persons and transfer his/her health status wirelessly in ad-hoc network, to remote base station which was connected to a doctor's PDA/PC or to a hospital's main to save the cost of health care facility for patients and the operating power of the system from the sensor to base station was shorter than in the general centralized system. The wireless data communication system will follow IEEE 802.15.4 frequency communication with ad-hoc routing thus enabling every motes attached to patients, to form a wireless data network to send data to base-station, providing mobility and convenience to the users in a home environment.

Sensor Based ECG Analysis of Signal

The sensor measure ECG-signals with a sampling frequency of 200 Hz. The signal is digitalized with 10 bits resolution, and continuous, transmitted it to a receiver module attached to PC/PDA, using a modulated RF radio link of radio chip. The sensors are sticky and attached to the patient's chest. It will continuously measure and wirelessly transmit sampled ECG-recording using of a built-in-RF-radio transmitter to the base station and then to PC/PDA through a RS-232 connector. After receiving the serial data received from the base station at the server, ECG data are analyzed, which includes searching the R-peak, ST-segment, P-wave and finding the beat rate, in real time. Server/Client software programs were developed in C# based on Net compiler for monitoring and ECG-recordings.

The doctor is able to change the scale-factor for the ECG-curves both in time scale and in amplification. Regular status-information is retrieved from the database and processed as a trend-analyze for 24 hours variations of R-R interval, T-wave, P-wave and ST-segment. The doctor can choose the desired time-interval, and the graphs can be printed out for documentation. In separate field the doctor can make his comments on the actual recorded curves and to the alarm-conditions detected by the system. Doctor can overview the latest alarm recordings and what time they occurred and can also save the ECG curve for further prediction or for previous record. For ECG analysis, the variant of the Pan-Tompkins algorithm is used for signal processing. These algorithms are improved according to our software analysis requirement and are developed in C# language based on net compiler. Pan-Tompkins algorithm proposes a real-time QRS detection based on analysis of slope, amplitude, and width of the QRS complexes. It includes a series of filters and methods that perform low pass, high pass, derivative, squaring and integration procedures. The algorithm adjusts the thresholds automatically and parameters periodically to adapt to changes in QRS morphology and heart rate.

Future Scope

The theory of Wave Behavior in periodic and aperiodic Media creates the new fields namely nanophotonics, quantum computing and advanced analytical methods, The ability to create patterns of very high precision, made available by nano-MEMS fabrication technology, will endow engineers with the ability to affect signal processing on a variety of wave phenomena, e.g., electronic, electromagnetic, acoustic, etc. Much of this functionality will exploit the phenomenon of band gaps; typically, domains of energies or frequencies in which wave propagation is forbidden. In what follows, the topics of electronic and photonic band-gaps, are of much interest and need to be addressed.

Exploiting the sensor technology we can design a movable sensing system embedded with suitable biosensor which can track the location information on RF signals and allow applications running on mobile and static nodes to detect the physical location. The tracking system based on senor technology may comprise RF and Ultrasonic hardware to enable a listener to determine their location in terms of space and position in three dimensions. The person to be tracked may be attached to the transmitter device. The position of the target can be calculated using the triangulation algorithm at the base station. The listener may be attached to a receiver device same in architecture of transmitter already attached to the target but distinguish each other in their programming domain. At the base station all the calculation can be set to be processed and the space and coordinate of the listener were determined. The location of the listener was displayed on the GUI and continuously updated as the target moves in the environment. Using this kind of architecture and technique of biosensors and associated devices can play a pivotal role in human tracking using distributed sensor network in the area of Medical Sciences.

Conclusion

The development of sensor technology has been substantiated as one of the important contributions of Science for the welfare of mankind through advancing many fields like Communication, Intelligence, Investigation and Medical Sciences etc. The extension of senor technology to detect the biological phenomenon leads to the development of biosensor which in turns could be exploited for sensing, monitoring, analyzing and feedback mechanism for health care services in the area of Medical Sciences. To establish the compatibility between biomaterials to be sensed and external electronic device is one of the design features of biosensor and needs to be addressed. Such compatible and smart sensor as well as actuator with additional features such as self-tests and self-calibration is developed with the help of micromechanical components integrated with electronic devices through micromachining termed as Micro Electro Mechanical System (MEMS). Since the discovery of the transistor effect in semiconductors, the possibility of making mechanical structures in silicon was studied and found that Silicon was an extremely good mechanical material for MEMS fabrication. The present chapter discusses the development of MEMS fabrication technique for biosensor development and its utility for the advancement of healthcare. services useful in the welfare of mankind.

References

[URL] http://www.veeco.com/learning/learning_molecularbeam.asp

Bardeen, J., Brattain, W. H. (1947). The Transistor, A Semiconductor Triode, *Phys. Rev.* 74(2), 230-231

Baski, A. A. (2002). Fabrication of Nanoscale Structures using STM and AFM, Advanced Semiconductor & Organic Nano-techniques, Part 3 (edited by Morkoc), Academic Press.

Bean, K. E. (1978). Anisotropic etching of silicon, *IEEE Trans. Electronic device*s, ED-25, 1185-1193.

Binning, G., Rohrer, H. (1982). Scanning tunneling microscopy, *Helvetica Physica Acta* 55, 726-735.

Chung, W. Y., Lee, Y. D. (2006). Wireless Sensor Network Technology for Ubiquitous Healthcare Applications, Proceedings of Second International Conference on Wireless Communication and Sensor Networks published in Macmillan Advanced Research Series of IEEE, Eds.(M.D. Tewari, U.S. Tewari, G.C. Nandi and M Radhakrishna) pp3-8.

Fan, L. S., Tai, Y. C., Muller, R. S. (1987). Pin Joints Gears, Springs, Granks and other novel micro mechanical structures. *Proc. Transducers* 87, 849-842.

Frazier, A. B., Warrington, R. O. et al., The Miniaturization Technologies: Past, Present and Future," *IEEE Trans. Ind. Electronics*, 42, 423.

Giessibl, F. J. (2003). Advances in atomic force microscopy, *Review of Modern Physics*, 75, 949.

Greenwood, J. C. (1984). Etched Silicon vibrating Sensor, *J. Phys. E. Sci. Instrum.* 17, 650-652.

Hamilton, P.S., Tompkins, W.J. (1986). Quantitative investigation of QRS detection rules using the MIT/BIH arrhythmia database, *IEEE Trans. Biomed Eng*, 33, 1157-65.

Hong, S., Zhu, J., Mirkin, C. A. (1999). Multiple Ink Nanolithography: Toward a Multiple-Pen Nano-plotter, *Science* 283, 661.

Howe, R. T., Muller, R. S. (1983). Polycrystalline and Amorphous Silicon micro mechanical beams: Annealing and Mechanical properties, *Sensors Actuators.* 4, 447-454.

Johansson, J., Volkar, M., Eliasson, J., Ostmark, A., Lindgren, P., Delsing, J. (2004). MULLE: A Minimal Sensor Network Device – Implementation and manufacturing challenges, Proc. IMAPS Nordic.

John, S. (1987). Strong Localization of Photons in Certain Disordered Dielectric Super Lattices, *Phys. Rev. Letts*, 58 (23), 2486-2489.

Jung, B.J. (2006), Report series of Ubiquitous society leader (in Korean), National Information Society Agency, Korea.

Katz, S., Ford, A.B., Moskowitz, R.W., Jackson, B.A., Jaffe, M.W. (1963). Studies of illness in theaged the index of adl: *A standardized measure of biological and psychosocial function journal of the merican Medical Association*, 185, 914-919.

Kittel, C. (1986). Introduction to Solid State Physics, John Wiley & Sons, Inc. New York.

Laermer, F., Schilip, A., Funk, K. Offenberg, M. (1999). Bosch Deep Silicon Etching: Improving Uniformity and Etch Rate for Advanced MEMS Applications, IEEE.

Laermer, F., Schlip, A. (1996). Method of Anisotropic ally Etching Silicon, Patent# 5501893, Issued: March26, Assignee: Robert Boch GmbH, Stuttgart, Federal Republic of Germany.

Lee, Y. D., Lee, D. S., Walia, G., Myllylae, R., Chung, W. Y. (2006). Query Based Duplex Vital Signal Monitoring System using Wireless Sensor Network for Ubiquitous Healthcare, pp. 388-391, World Congress on Medical Physics and Biomedical Engineering (WC 2006), Aug.27-Sep.I. 2006, COEX Seoul, Korea. In proceedings of Second International Conference on Wireless Communication and Sensor Networks, held in IIIT, Allahabad, India.

Malan, D., Fulford-Jones, T., Welsh, M., Moulton, S. (2004). Code Blue: An ad-hoc sensor network infrastructure for emergency medical care. In Proceeding of the International Workshop on Wearable and implantable Body Sensor Networks.

Mishra, A. K. et al. (2011). Model of an electronic biosensor applicable for bitter taste detection and food monitoring. *Proceedings of 16th National Seminar on Physics and Technology of Sensors*, Lucknow.

Mishra, A. K., Tiwari, S. N. (2012) Graft Compatibility and Plant growth through Electric Control: Developing an Electronic Biosensor for Graft Compatibility Detection. Published by Lap Lambert Academic Publishing GmbH and Co.KG, Germany.

Mishra, A. K., Tiwari, S. N. (2012). Biosensor based on signal transduction through electrical resistance of graft union in plants, *Proceedings of First International Symposium on Physics and Technology of Sensors held in University of Pune*, India.

Mishra, A. K., Tiwari, S. N., Dutta, R. (2006). Studies on the Development of an Electrical Biosensor to Detect the Graft Union Success Rate, Proceedings of Second International Conference on Wireless Communication and Sensor Networks published in Macmillan Advanced Research Series of IEEE, Eds. (M.D. Tewari, U.S. Tewari, G.C. Nandi and M Radhakrishna) pp3-8.

Mishra, A. K., Tiwari, S. N., Dutta, R., Tiwari, R. K. (2006). Electrical biosensor and measurement of graft union success rate in plant systems: A Review, *Journal of Applied Botany Abstracts*, 26, 355-365.

Nathanson, H. C., Wickstrom, R. A. (1965). A Resonant-Gate silicon Surface Transistor with High-Q band pass Properties, *Appl. Phys. Lett.* 7, 84.

Pan, J., Tompkins, W. (1985). A real time QRS detection Algorithm, *BME*-32, pp.230-236.

Petersen, K. E. (1982). Silicon as a mechanical material, *Proc. IEEE* 70, 420-457.

Purwar, A., Shin, K.S., Chung, W.Y. (2006). Wrist Type Sensor for Fall Detection and Bio-Signal measurement System for Elderly Person, *Proceeding of KIMICS*. pp. 477-480.

Requicha, A. (2003). Nano-robots, NEMS and Nano-assembly, *Proc. IEEE Vol.* 91, No. 11, November, pp. 1922-1933.

Santos, H. J. L. (2008). Principls and Applications of Nano-MEMS Physics, Springer, 16-17.

Singh, V. K., Lim, H., Myllylae, R., Chung, W. (2006). Passive and Cost effective People Location tracking System for Indoor Environments Using Distributed Wireless Sensor Net-work, *Proceedings of World Congless on Medical Physics and Biomedical Engineering*, pp.384-387, August 27-September 1, Coex Seoul.

Sze, S. M. (1983). VLSI Technology, Editor, New York: McGraw Hill.

Tufte, O. N. and Long, G. D. (1962). Silicon diffused element piezoresistive diaphram, *J. Appl. phys*. 33, 3322.

Whitesides G. M., Love, J. C. (2001). The art of building Small, Scientific American, September, pp 39-47.

Wood, A., Virone, G., Doan, T., Cao. Q. Selavo, I. Wu, Y., Fang, L., He, Z., Lin, S., Stankovic, J. (2006). ALARM-NET: Wireless Sensor Networks for assisted-living and

Residential Monitoring, "Technical report CS-2006-11, Department of Computer Science, University of Virginia.

Yablonovitch, E. (1987). Inhibited Spontaneous Emission in Solid State Physics & Electronics, *Phys. Rev. Letts*, 58 (20), 2059-2062.

Index

#

20th century, 6

A

Abraham, 175, 212
Absorption, 16, 23, 24, 27, 28, 112
abuse, 50
access, 28, 111, 146, 252
accessibility, 150, 219
accurate models, 19
Acetaminophen, 8, 25
acetic acid, 73, 165
acetone, 63, 74
Acetylation, 35
acetylcholine, 40, 47, 74, 96, 223
acid, 8, 10, 11, 12, 26, 27, 32, 33, 34, 40, 45, 46, 47, 48, 55, 59, 60, 63, 64, 73, 75, 76, 83, 88, 90, 94, 103, 124, 126, 144, 145, 151, 155, 156, 157, 165, 166, 167, 176
acidic, 26, 32, 36, 78, 232
acidity, 92
action potential, 46
activation energy, 167
active compound, 6, 50, 55, 73, 77, 142, 158, 217, 218, 219
active site, 113, 114, 123, 124, 125, 126, 127, 128, 129, 131, 133, 134, 135, 136, 137, 138, 204, 205, 215, 217, 219, 221, 223
active transport, 24, 25, 47, 103
activity level, 39
actual output, 120
actuators, 246, 252
acupuncture, 50, 52
acute asthma, 47
AD, 5, 53
adaptation, 56
additives, 226
adenosine, 46, 47, 59
adenosine triphosphate, 59
ADHD, 88, 94
adipose, 32
adipose tissue, 32
ADME, 1, 15, 16, 18, 31, 112, 227
ADMET, 112, 116
adrenaline, 82
adrenoceptors, 47
adults, 44
advancement(s), vii, 51, 55, 99, 255
adverse effects, 26, 39, 49, 243
advocacy, 97
Aerosol(s), 28, 233
aesthetic, 81
Affinity, 40, 114
AFM, 249, 250, 251, 252, 256
Africa, 79
age, 3, 29, 43, 44, 47, 245
agencies, 236, 243
aggregation, 89
aging society, 245
agonist, 7, 46, 47, 85, 7, 223
AIDS, 6
albumin, 26, 30, 32
alcoholism, 101
alcohols, 34, 152
aldehydes, 112
alertness, 75
algorithm, 107, 113, 114, 115, 116, 117, 119, 120, 122, 125, 126, 129, 131, 132, 138, 139, 198, 218, 219, 221, 254, 255
aliphatic compounds, 168
alkaline hydrolysis, 211
alkaloids, 5, 57, 72, 73, 74, 75, 78, 80, 85, 237
alkane, 179

alkylation, 103, 104
allergic reaction, 9, 13
almonds, 60
aloe, 58
alters, 126
alveoli, 28
AMBER, 133
amine(s), 57, 73, 109, 152
amino, 24, 33, 34, 35, 48, 55, 57, 73, 76, 80, 82, 83, 91, 92, 101, 103, 106, 124, 126, 127, 132, 144, 145, 146, 147, 152, 154, 155, 156, 159
amino acid(s), 33, 34, 35, 48, 55, 57, 73, 76, 82, 83, 91, 92, 101, 103, 106, 124, 126, 127, 132, 144, 145, 146, 147, 154, 155, 156, 157, 159
Aminomethyl resin, 152
amphibia, 96
amphiphilic compounds, 61
Ampicillin, 25
amplitude, 251, 254
analgesic, 69, 73, 93, 232
anatomy, 2, 3
anemia, 11, 58
Anesthetic, 10
anesthetics, 6, 36, 40, 45, 46, 74, 86, 232
angina, 11, 45
angiotensin II, 45, 85
angstroms, 127
anhydrase, 41
annealing, 115, 133, 138, 219
antacid(s), 10, 229
antagonism, 44
Antagonist, 7
Anthelmintics, 11
Anthraquinones, 57, 58, 67, 77
Antiallergic, 11
Antianemic, 11
Antianginal, 11
Antianxiety, 11
Antiarrhythmic, 11
antibiotic, 11, 67, 74, 106
antibiotic resistance, 74
antibody, 159
anti-cancer, 82, 91, 93, 94, 102
anticholinergic, 74
Anticholinergic, 11, 74
anticoagulant, 11, 58, 60, 89
anticonvulsant, 11, 216, 223
antidepressant, 11, 46, 67, 103
Antidiabetic, 11
Antidiarrheal, 11
Antidote, 11, 66
Antidysrhythmic, 11
Antiemetic, 11
Antiepileptic, 46
Antiflatulent, 11
Antifungal, 11, 106
antigen, 93, 159
Anti-glaucoma, 47
Antigout, 11
Antihistamine, 11
Antihyperlipidemic, 11
Antihypertensive, 11, 45, 103
Anti-impotence, 11
Anti-inflammatory, 11, 93, 103
anti-inflammatory agents, 47, 94
anti-inflammatory drugs, 46
antimalarials, 49
Antimanic, 11
Antimigraine, 11
Anti-migraine, 47
Antineoplastic, 11, 103
antioxidant, 62, 70, 71, 78, 79
Anti-Parkinson's, 47
Antiparkinsonian, 11
Antiprotozoal, 11
Antipsychotic, 11, 46
antipsychotic drugs, 6
Antipyretic, 11, 58
Antiretroviral, 11
Antispasmodic(s), 12, 58, 71, 74
Antituberculosis, 12
antitumor, 78, 105
Antitumor necrosis factor, 12
Antitussive, 12
Antiulcer, 12
Antiviral, 12
anxiety, 11
Apex-3D, 220
apoplexy, 85
apoptosis, 92
Apparent Volume of Distribution, 31
aqueous humor, 47
aqueous solutions, 230
Aristotle, 54
aromatic compounds, 62, 67, 168
aromatic hydrocarbons, 171
aromatic rings, 150, 170
arrhythmia, 45, 256
arteries, 5, 11, 13, 62
Artificial Neural Network (ANN), 117, 119, 127
Asia, 96
Aspirin, 8, 11, 12, 25, 26, 27, 35, 41, 44, 100
assessment, 110, 235, 236, 239, 243
assimilation, 25
asthma, 13, 82, 94, 102
astringent, 61, 69

atomic distances, 134, 215
atomic force, 249, 256
atomic force microscope, 249
Atomic Force Microscopy, 250
atoms, 124, 125, 129, 131, 133, 134, 136, 137, 138, 167, 175, 178, 179, 180, 181, 182, 183, 184, 189, 203, 204, 205, 207, 208, 215, 247, 249, 251
ATP, 59
Atropine, 5, 11, 27, 41, 42, 44, 75
attachment, 48, 145, 149, 152
audits, 239, 240
authority(s), 77, 237, 238, 239, 240, 241, 242
AUTODOCK, 133
automation, 111
Ayurveda, 2, 3, 50, 51, 81
Azathioprine, 13

B

Back-propagation, 120
Backward elimination, 192
bacteria, 48, 76
bacterial cells, 154
bacteriophage, 154
band gap, 255
bandwidth, 253
Barbiturates, 27, 34, 45
barriers, 24, 32, 33, 43, 171
base, 5, 26, 27, 86, 92, 103, 104, 114, 116, 128, 132, 151, 232, 254, 255
basic research, 159
Batrachotoxins, 85, 86, 89
BBB, 30, 31
beams, 256
beef, 82, 87
beer, 82
beetles, 89
behavior modification, 246
beneficial effect, 55
benefits, 49, 50, 235
Bengamide derivative, 91, 94
benzene, 74, 166, 175
Benzodiazepine(s), 40, 45, 46
Beta-Blockers, 45
bias, 119, 120, 138
bile, 26, 35, 36, 46, 82, 95
bile acids, 46
binding energy(s), 115, 135
bioassay, 108
bioavailability, 29, 30, 44, 62, 121, 163, 225, 227, 228, 229
Bioavailable dose, 227
Bioinformatics, vii, xi, 6, 120, 122, 138, 139, 212
biological activity(s), 6, 7, 49, 100, 108, 109, 142, 157, 161, 162, 165, 170, 172, 185, 186, 187, 188, 189, 191, 195, 196, 201, 203, 204, 206, 207, 208, 209, 210, 211, 213, 215, 216, 217, 221
biological systems, 170
biologically active compounds, 55, 163
biomaterials, 255
Biopharmaceutics, 227
Biosensor(s), 245, 255, 257
biosphere, 77
biosynthesis, 68
biosynthetic pathways, 56
biotechnology, 6, 235
Biotransformation, 16
bipolar disorder, 11
Blacks, 42
bleeding, 12, 64, 87
blood, 5, 11, 12, 13, 19, 22, 23, 24, 25, 26, 30, 31, 32, 33, 36, 37, 42, 45, 61, 64, 66, 72, 82, 86, 87, 231, 254
Blood brain barrier, 30
blood circulation, 33
blood clot, 11
blood flow, 19, 24, 25, 36
blood plasma, 86
blood pressure, 82
blood stream, 23, 231
blood supply, 22
blood vessels, 13, 64, 66
blood-brain barrier, 33
bloodstream, 32
Boc group, 153
body fluid, 37
body size, 43
body weight, 43
bonding, 114, 219
bonds, 77, 103, 114, 116, 128, 129, 131, 136, 178, 179, 180, 183, 203, 221
bone(s), 32, 86, 89, 93
Bone resorption inhibitor, 12
bowel, 13, 75
bradykinin, 85, 96
brain, 25, 30, 31, 32, 69, 163
branching, 149, 179, 212
Brand name, 7, 8
Brazil, 238
breast cancer, 48, 91
breast milk, 36
breastfeeding, 36
breathing, 36, 59
bromine, 175
Bronchodilator, 12
brothers, 13, 38, 48

Bryostatin I, 93, 94
building blocks, 134, 136, 137, 141, 142, 144, 146, 147, 148, 149, 152
business environment, 235
butyl ether, 153

C

cabbage, 66
caffeine, 1, 73, 75
calcium, 45, 46, 92, 101
calibration, 255
cancer, 6, 39, 48, 59, 65, 66, 85, 92, 93, 97, 102, 109, 159
cancer cells, 39
cancer therapy, 109
candidates, vii, 19, 81, 99, 111, 123, 215, 217, 219, 225, 226
capillary, 25, 28, 32, 60
capsule(s), 27, 228, 230
Captopril, 25
carbamazepine, 46
carbohydrates, 6, 57, 34, 106
carbon, 63, 64, 65, 74, 77, 174, 184, 207
carbon atoms, 74, 77
carboxyl, 144, 145, 157, 166
carboxylic acid(s), 34, 35, 70, 151, 152
carboxymethyl cellulose, 232
cardiac arrhythmia, 11
cardiac glycoside(s), 5, 12, 57, 58, 61, 68
cardiac output, 36, 45
cardiovascular disease(s), 62
cardiovascular risk, 85, 100
Caribbean, 88
catabolism, 76
catalyst, 219
Catalyst, 219, 223
catalytic hydrogenation, 153
catecholamines, 45
categorization, 58, 117
category a, 237
Catharanthus roseus, 55
cation, 45
cattle, 86, 87, 89
CAVEAT, 135, 136
cDNA, 154
CEE, 86
cell culture, vii
cell death, 68
cell differentiation, 102
cell division, 48
cell line(s), 91, 92, 237
Cell membrane(s), 6, 24, 30, 32, 106
cell surface, 102
cellulose, 156
Central Drug Standard Control Organization (CDSCO), 238
central nervous system (CNS), 12, 13, 31, 32, 33, 40, 71, 74, 75, 96
Centre for Pharmaceutical Administration Health Sciences Authority, 238
cerebral function, 31
challenges, 228, 256
Charak Samhita, 51, 81
chemical bonds, 13
chemical characteristics, 108
chemical interaction, 129, 132
chemical kinetics, 40
Chemical name, 7, 8
chemical properties, 40, 56, 165, 190, 203, 216
chemical reactivity, 192
chemical structures, 7, 57, 142, 186, 203
chemicals, 6, 83, 152, 188
Chemotherapy, 7
children, 226, 229
China, 50, 51, 238
Chinese medicine, 51, 53, 96, 97
Chloramphenicol, 34, 48, 106
cholesterol, 13, 24, 46, 61, 62, 72
choline, 48, 73
choroid, 32
chromatography, 142, 149, 158
chromosome, 133
Chronic tolerance, 44
circulation, 16, 24, 27, 28, 29, 30, 31, 33, 46, 227, 231, 232
City, 14
civil law, 54
civilization, 49
classes, 10, 45, 46, 74, 82, 117, 118, 220, 253
classification, vii, 1, 10, 40, 109, 117, 118, 120, 121
cleaning, 69
Clearance, 21, 36
cleavage, 34, 64, 83, 103, 105, 144, 145, 149, 151, 152
clinical trials, vii, 1, 92, 226, 237
CLIX, 129, 134, 135
cloning, 96, 109, 154
clozapine, 46
clustering, 115, 122, 130, 138, 220
clusters, 129
CMC, 240
CO_2, 211
coagulation process, 47
cocaine, 46, 50, 73, 109
Codeine, 5, 12, 27

CODESSA, 190, 213
coenzyme, 35, 46
colic, 75
colitis, 75
collagen, 66, 86, 87
colon cancer, 91
color, 56, 65, 67, 157
CombiChem, 141
Combinatorial libraries, 142, 144, 154, 157
combined effect, 44, 69
commercial, 203, 219, 247
Common Technical Document (CTD), 242
communication, 113, 121, 239, 240, 254
community, 95
comparative analysis, 106
compatibility, 129, 225, 228, 245, 255
competition, 30, 157, 237
compilation, 50
complement, 102, 107
complementarity, 137
complexity, 114, 134, 193
compliance, 226, 240, 241
complications, 9
composition, 29, 55, 79, 126, 247
computer, 130, 203, 205, 208, 209, 213, 253
computing, 93, 177, 205
conception, 12
conceptualization, 240
condensation, 57, 76
conductance, 46
conduction, 46, 74
conductivity, 157
configuration, 132, 133
confinement, 249
Congress, 257
conjugation, 34, 35, 169
connective tissue, 86
connectivity, 179, 182, 184, 211, 212, 215
consensus, 115, 121, 193, 242
conservation, 64, 96
constant rate, 16, 17, 20
constipation, 13, 232
constituents, 49, 69, 71
construction, 116, 132, 137
Constructive phase, 218
consumption, 94
containers, 243
contamination, 243
Contignasterol, 91, 94
contour, 209
Contraceptive(s), 12, 47, 232
controversial, 59
conviction, 192
COOH, 166
cooling, 133, 230
coordination, 240
correlation, 116, 133, 134, 161, 162, 167, 171, 176, 178, 185, 193, 199, 200, 201, 203, 207, 209, 210
correlation analysis, 161
correlation coefficient, 185, 200, 201
correlation function, 133, 207
cortex, 32
Corticosteroid, 12
cortisol, 82
cosmetics, 69
cost, 95, 111, 118, 220, 229, 245, 254
cotton, 87
cough, 12, 78
cough suppressant, 78
Coulomb potential, 207
Coumarinic heterosides, 60
coumarins, 57, 60
covalent bond, 151
COX-2 Inhibitor, 12
Creams, 231
crop, 78
crop production, 78
cross fertilization, 237
cross links, 150
Cross validation, 201
cross-validation, 187, 209
crystal structure, 222
crystalline, 58, 60, 68, 72, 78
crystallization, 142
CSD, 132
CSF, 33
CT, 78, 80
culture, 2
Cumarines, 64
cure(s), 1, 6, 11, 44, 48, 50, 54, 55, 81, 82, 89, 93, 96, 236
cyanide, 59, 85, 163
Cyanogenic heterosides, 59
Cyclic adenosine monophosphate (cAMP), 46
cycling, 36
Cyclodidemniserinol trisulfate, 91, 94
cyclooxygenase, 12, 46
cyclophosphamide, 48
cyclosporine, 47
cytochrome, 34, 59, 163
cytoplasm, 40, 41
cytotoxicity, 39

D

damages, 48, 226

dandruff, 69
Danish Medicines Agency, 238
data communication, 254
data set, 19, 117, 120, 180, 186, 187, 189, 190, 191, 201, 206, 221
data structure, 219
database, 50, 115, 131, 135, 136, 138, 164, 180, 220, 222, 254, 256
DDT, 212
decomposition, 229
Decongestant, 12
Decyclization, 34
Deep reactive Ion etching (DRIE), 246
Deer, 61, 82
defense mechanisms, 79
deficiencies, 39
deficiency(s), 39, 47
deficit, 88
delirium, 95
dementia, 88
demographic transition, 245
Dendrimer, 149
Denmark, 238
De-novo drug design, 123, 124
Department of Health
Pharmaceutical Services, 238
Dependence, 45, 48
deposition, 249
depression, 11, 39
depth, 132, 216
derivatives, 48, 61, 64, 68, 73, 74, 75, 80, 109
dermatitis, 36, 75
Descriptor, 116, 166, 175, 177, 189, 191, 192
Descriptor selection, 192
destruction, 12, 151
detection, 106, 220, 245, 254, 256, 257
developing countries, 81
deviation, 190, 198, 199
diabetes, 6, 11, 47, 62, 82, 83, 89, 102, 106
diarrhea, 11, 66, 77
diet, 3, 51
diffusion, 24, 25, 28, 32, 33, 178, 231
Digitoxin, 5
Digoxin, 5, 25, 31, 37
dilation, 42
diluent, 226
dimerization, 65
DIP-Pen Lithography, 251
direct measure, 106
directionality, 219
directives, 236
disability, 9
Discodermolide, 91, 94
DISCOtech, 220
discs, 229
disease progression, 12
Disease-modifying antirheumatic drugs (DMARDs), 12
diseases, 1, 2, 3, 6, 13, 43, 44, 51, 55, 79, 89, 93, 95, 100, 101, 108, 236, 246
disorder, 45, 88
dispersion, 16, 114, 177, 231, 232, 233
displacement, 30, 31, 139
dissociation, 7, 165, 166, 167, 169
distillation, 69, 142
distilled water, 59
distribution, vii, 15, 16, 19, 20, 21, 22, 26, 30, 31, 32, 33, 36, 37, 43, 56, 73, 112, 165, 166, 170, 178, 196, 200, 201, 206, 225, 227, 249
Diterpenes, 57, 68
Dithiocyanates, 91
diuretic, 12, 45, 58, 60, 69
diversity, 78, 81, 109, 132, 141, 154, 187, 188
diverticulitis, 75
DME, 227
DMF, 151, 152
DNA(s), 6, 47, 48, 62, 77, 101, 102, 103, 104, 105, 107, 128, 236
DOCK, 115, 127, 129, 131, 133
Docking, 113, 114, 115, 121, 122, 128, 129, 130, 131, 132, 133, 134, 138
Dolastatin 10, 94
donors, 30, 116, 189
dopamine, 46, 47, 73, 109
doping, 249
dosage, vii, 20, 27, 29, 43, 73, 121, 225, 226, 227, 228, 229, 230, 231, 232, 233
Dosage form, 233
Dose, 43
dosing, 229
double bonds, 77, 179
double helix, 103
draft, 242
DRAGON, 190, 213
drawing, 168
DRIE, 247
drug abuse, 9, 45
drug action, 5, 6, 7, 37, 39, 40, 42, 43, 44, 173
drug delivery, 27, 28, 29, 33, 226
drug design, vii, 1, 51, 55, 102, 107, 111, 116, 121, 123, 124, 127, 128, 210, 212, 215, 216, 221
drug discovery, 6, 15, 31, 38, 49, 81, 97, 99, 101, 102, 109, 110, 111, 120, 121, 159, 225
Drug effect, 7, 42
Drug Likeness, 114
drug metabolism, 34, 35

drug reactions, 8, 9, 14
Drug Receptor Theory, 40
drug targets, 42, 99, 100, 101, 102, 106, 109, 215
drug therapy, 8
drug withdrawal, 9
Drugs Control Organization, 238
drying, 50
duodenal ulcer, 12
dyes, 58, 64, 74

E

Ebers Papyrus, 3
ECG, 253, 254
eczema, 47, 82
ED_{50}, 7
education, 96
Efficacy, 7
Egypt, 3
electrical resistance, 257
electrolyte, 12
electrolyte depletion, 12
Electrolyte replacement, 12
electromagnetic, 255
electron(s), 31, 34, 104, 165, 166, 168, 169, 170, 182, 183, 186, 203, 247, 248, 249
electron beam lithography, 248
electron microscopy, 31
Electronic, 163, 165, 210, 256, 257
electronic structure, 170
Electrostatic field, 203
Eleuthrobin diterpene, 94
Elimination, 16, 19, 35
ELISA, 155
elucidation, 83, 221
emergency, 86, 246, 257
Emetic, 12
emulsion(s), 228, 231
encoding, 180
encouragement, ix
endangered, 82, 97
endangered species, 82, 97
endothelial cells, 30, 32
energy, 25, 34, 51, 81, 103, 113, 114, 115, 128, 131, 133, 134, 135, 137, 165, 167, 172, 179, 203, 204, 205, 212
engineering, 249
entropy, 115, 136, 169, 205, 211
environment(s), 51, 62, 229, 232, 238, 240, 243, 253, 254, 255
environmental factors, 3, 44
enzymatic activity, 115
enzyme(s), 6, 12, 29, 33, 34, 40, 41, 42, 47, 48, 62, 65, 85, 89, 101, 102, 107, 109, 113, 124, 127, 135, 137, 155, 163, 171, 206, 232
epilepsy, 85
epinephrine, 28, 185
epithelial cells, 32, 36
epithelium, 28, 33, 61, 72
epitopes, 155, 159
Eptifibatide, 85, 89
Equilenin Sulfate, 88
equilibrium, 7, 22, 30, 40, 51, 166, 167, 176, 196
Equilin Sulfate, 88
equipment, 158, 243
erosion, 51
Erythromycin, 25, 27, 106
ES-285(spisulosine), 94
Essential oils, 57, 68, 69, 80
ester, 68, 152, 167, 176
estrogen, 66, 87
Estrogen Sulfate, 88
etching, 246, 247, 256
ethanol, 150
ethics, 236
ethyl alcohol, 36
eucalyptus, 69
eukaryotic, 154
Europe, 5, 54, 238, 241
European Medicines Agency (EMEA), 238
European Union, 241, 242
evidence, 49, 210, 211
evolution, 79, 132
exclusion, 149, 158
excretion, vii, 12, 15, 16, 19, 31, 33, 35, 36, 43, 45, 112, 225
Exenatide, 83
exercise, 36
expectorant, 12, 61, 69, 78
experimental condition, 141
Expert Working Groups, 241
exposure, 44, 126, 157, 158
extinction, 77, 94
extraction, 55, 69, 73, 83
extracts, 49, 55, 64, 85, 107, 209
Eye Drops, 230

F

fabrication, 246, 247, 255
Fall Detection, 253, 257
false positive, 147, 220
families, 70, 71, 73, 99, 101, 137, 147
family members, ix
fat, 31

feces, 36
ferric ion, 163
fertility, 245
fetus, 30, 33, 82
fever, 11, 95, 163
FFT, 134
fibers, 92
fibrosarcoma, 85
Filamentous phage, 154
fillers, 229
films, 86
filters, 115, 254
filtration, 35, 36, 144, 145, 149
fingerprints, 165, 181
Finland, xi, 81
first generation, 6
First Pass Metabolism, 33
fish, 85
fitness, 132, 133
Flavonoids, 57, 58, 62, 65, 78, 79
flexibility, 29, 118, 128, 131, 135, 221
Flexible docking, 115, 128, 131, 139
flora, 49, 54
flora and fauna, 54
flowers, 65, 69, 75
fluctuations, 31, 43
fluid, 29, 32, 37
fluorescence, 64, 157
fluorine, 183
foams, 29
folate, 48
food, 24, 25, 26, 29, 44, 60, 69, 86, 257
Food and Drug Administration (FDA), 1, 83, 238, 241
food industry, 86
force, 12, 101, 102, 114, 115, 121, 133, 138, 144, 158, 177, 220, 221, 232, 251
Ford, 256
formation, 32, 34, 47, 48, 62, 63, 76, 83, 152, 153, 166, 167, 246
formula, 58, 116, 174, 180, 183, 190, 199, 200, 201, 204, 216
Fragment connection, 135
fragments, 114, 116, 124, 127, 131, 132, 134, 135, 136, 137, 173, 174, 180, 206
France, 5
free choice, 45
free energy, 167, 169, 171, 173, 175, 211, 212
free radicals, 47, 65, 78
Free Wilson analysis, 162, 186
freedom, 114, 129, 186, 222
friction, 230
frostbite, 78
fruits, 55, 65, 67
F-test, 187, 201
fungi, 11, 73, 76
fungus, 75
fusion, 124

G

GABA, 40, 46
Gastric acid-pump inhibitor, 12
gastric mucosa, 103
gastroesophageal reflux, 12
gastrointestinal tract, 28, 34
Gelatin, 86, 87, 89, 96, 232
Gels, 232
gene expression, 40
genes, 102, 110
Genetic algorithm, 114
genetics, 43, 107, 110, 138
genome, 84, 99, 107, 108
genomics, 6
Genomics, 108, 111
genus, 5, 89
geometry, 115, 134, 135, 165, 216, 220, 222
Georgia, 96, 212
Germany, 3, 38, 122, 211, 213, 238, 256, 257
germination, 76
gestation, 33
ginseng, 53, 62
gland, 33, 89
glaucoma, 6, 47, 101
Global indices, 179
Glomerular, 35
glucose, 12, 33, 34, 57, 61, 66, 103
Glucosinolates, 57, 62
Glucuronide conjugation, 34
glutamine, 153
glutathione, 35
Glutathione conjugation, 35
Glycerogelatins, 232
glycine, 34, 35
glycol, 150
glycoproteins, 41, 61, 72
glycoside(s), 12, 58, 59, 62
God, ix, 2, 3
GOLD, 115, 132
Golden rule, 197
GOLPE, 205
goods and services, 235
goose, 251
grafted copolymers, 150
granules, 32
graph, 129, 173, 179, 180, 182, 192, 212, 215

grass, 60, 61, 64
gravity, 231
Greeks, 54
GRID, 114, 127, 129, 135, 204, 205
grids, 127, 209
grouping, 219
growth, 11, 12, 55, 62, 78, 102, 235, 246, 257
growth factor, 102
guidance, ix, 121, 239
guidelines, 235, 236, 237, 240, 241, 242
Guinea, 91

H

habitat, 94
hair, 69, 230
hair loss, 69
half-life, 32, 36
Halichondrin B, 90, 91, 94
halogens, 175
Hansch model, 172, 173, 175
harmonization, 241, 242
Hartree-Fock, 170
healing, 5, 54, 82, 94
health, 1, 8, 14, 45, 50, 51, 55, 62, 163, 236, 243, 245, 246, 253, 254, 255
Health Canada, 238, 241, 242
health care, 8, 50, 52, 55, 245, 246, 254, 255
health care system, 50, 52, 246
health effects, 62
health status, 253, 254
heart disease, 65
heart failure, 44, 45
heart rate, 12, 45, 254
heavy metals, 66
hemorrhoids, 78, 232
Hemostatic, 12
hepatocytes, 32
herbal medicine, 50, 52, 55
herbal teas, 54
herpes, 12
Heterosides, 57, 58, 59, 60
high blood pressure, 11
HINT, 127
Hip-Hop Theory, 217
hippocampus, 95
Hippocrates, 3, 4, 13, 54
histamine, 11, 47
histidine, 153
history, 1, 2, 3, 51, 96, 102, 134, 143
Histrionicotoxin, 85, 86, 89
Hits, 225
HIV, 11, 91, 94, 101
Homeopathy, 50
homeostasis, 100, 102
Homogeneity, 188
Hong Kong, 238
HOOK, 114, 135, 136
hormone(s), 31, 39, 47, 68, 82, 86, 102, 237
Hormone replacement (HRT), 12
horses, 82, 89
host, 7, 40, 66, 154
hot spots, 205
human, 22, 49, 51, 56, 81, 83, 88, 91, 95, 99, 101, 102, 103, 106, 108, 109, 110, 226, 227, 237, 241, 245, 255
human body, 22, 51, 227
human genome, 99, 102, 103
human health, 88, 245
hunting, 82, 94
hybridization, 138, 175, 179
hybridoma, 236
hydrazine, 35
hydrocortisone, 47
hydrogen, 26, 29, 34, 45, 47, 66, 113, 114, 122, 128, 132, 133, 135, 137, 166, 170, 173, 174, 175, 177, 178, 182, 205, 219
hydrogen atoms, 182
hydrogen bonds, 29, 66, 122, 128, 132, 133, 135, 137, 179
hydrolysis, 34, 61, 167, 168, 176
hydrophobicity, 126, 165, 170, 171, 172, 173, 175
hydroxide, 47
hydroxyl, 57, 62, 63, 132, 153, 232
hydroxyl groups, 132, 153
hyperactivity, 88
hyperglycemia, 47
hypersensitivity, 9
hypertension, 74, 84, 101
hypnosis, 12
Hypnotic, 12
HypoGen Theory, 218
Hypoglycemic, 12
hypothesis, 31, 161, 185, 218, 219
Hypothyroidism, 82, 89, 96
hysterectomy, 87

I

iatrogenic, 8
ibuprofen, 37, 46
ICH, 235, 241, 242
ideal, 29, 31, 102, 127, 202, 219, 246
identification, vii, 7, 50, 99, 107, 108, 110, 124, 131, 192, 193, 219, 220
identity, 154, 184

idiosyncratic, 9
illumination, 157
image(s), 4, 21, 210, 247, 251
immune response, 12
immune system, 102
immunity, 13
Immunoglobulin, 102
Immunologic, 13
immunomodulator, 70
Immunosuppressant, 13
Immunosuppressive, 103
implants, 237
Implementation Working Groups, 241
impotence, 11
improvements, 74
impulses, 11, 86
impurities, 148, 249
in vitro, 65, 92, 109
in vivo, 121, 173, 236, 237
incompatibility, 229
independent living, 253
India, vii, xi, 1, 8, 15, 39, 42, 49, 50, 51, 52, 69, 78, 81, 96, 99, 111, 141, 161, 215, 225, 235, 238, 245, 257
Indians, 42
individuals, 34, 64, 132
induction, 107
industry(s), 19, 71, 78, 81, 86, 112, 235, 236, 237, 238, 239, 240, 241, 243, 246
infant colic, 75
infants, 229
infection, 65, 87, 91, 94, 95
inferences, 106
inflammation, 11, 12, 47, 68, 91, 232
information technology, 222
infrastructure, 257
ingredients, 55, 81, 226, 229
Inhalations, 230
inhibition, 47, 61, 85, 109, 162, 163
inhibitor(s), 12, 13, 47, 71, 89, 100, 102, 103
initial state, 132
initiation, 46, 65, 242
injections, 28, 33, 82
injury, 64
Innate tolerance, 44
insects, 68, 87
insertion, 232
inspections, 240
Insulin, 6, 11, 12, 39, 47, 82, 83, 84, 89, 96
integration, 18, 254
intelligence, 239, 240
Intercalation, 103, 104
interface, 154, 222, 243
intermolecular interactions, 121
intervention, 109
intestine, 27, 34, 46
intoxication, 66
intravenously, 27, 37
Intrinsic activity, 40
Inverse agonist, 7
inversion, 196
iodine, 29
ion channels, 40, 45, 46, 85, 101, 102, 103
ionization, 26, 33, 165, 169, 170, 211
ions, 26, 31, 68, 103, 222
Ipecac, 12
IPL-512602, 91
IPL-550260, 94
IPL-576092, 91
Ireland, 238
Iridoids, 70
Irish Medicines Board, 238
irradiation, 152
isobutane, 180
isolation, 7, 50, 55, 69, 77, 145
Isomerases, 103
isomers, 74, 179, 212, 236
isoprene, 67, 68
Isoquinolines, 74
issues, 121, 226, 236
Italian Pharmaceutical Agency, 238
Italy, 213, 238

J

Japan, 212, 238, 241, 242
joint pain, 61
joints, 12

K

K^+, 103, 109
Kahalilade F, 94
Kappa indices, 184
K_D, 7
Kernels, 118
ketones, 112
kidney(s), 22, 33, 35, 36, 45, 51, 60, 227
Kier and Hall, 182, 183
kill, 82, 216
kinetic studies, 216
kinetics, 6, 19, 21, 33, 36, 114, 196
Korea, 256, 257

L

labeling, 106, 237, 239, 243
lactation, 43
lactic acid, 73
Lactones, 70
Lamellarina 20 sulfate, 91, 94
L-arginine, 76
lasers, 64
Latin America, 82, 96
laws, 236
Laxative, 13, 67
laxatives, 41, 58, 67, 229
LDL, 62
lead, v, vii, 6, 8, 32, 34, 36, 37, 39, 41, 43, 49, 50, 55, 81, 82, 89, 93, 94, 100, 101, 104, 110, 111, 112, 124, 136, 143, 195, 203, 211, 216, 217, 222, 225
Lead compound, 6
Lead optimization, 225
leakage, 61, 68, 72
learning, 2, 96, 117, 119, 120, 121, 125, 256
learning process, 120
legs, 85, 87
leishmaniasis, 89
Lennard-Jones potential, 207
lesions, 232
leukemia, 6
Leukotriene receptor antagonist blocker, 13
life cycle, 237, 238, 243
life expectancy, 82, 93
ligand, 7, 99, 101, 112, 113, 114, 115, 116, 121, 123, 124, 125, 127, 128, 129, 130, 131, 132, 133, 134, 136, 137, 138, 154, 158, 177, 203, 204, 205, 210, 211, 221, 222, 223, 236
LigandScout, 222
Ligases, 103
LigBuilder, 138
light, 5, 6, 56, 73, 77, 102, 157, 177, 233, 247, 253
Lignanes, 65
lignans, 57, 66
lignin, 57
linear function, 40, 41
linear model, 193, 196
Linkers, 149, 151
Lipid carriers, 106
Lipid-lowering agent, 13
lipids, 11, 24, 55, 101
Lipophilicity, 170, 171, 211
lipoproteins, 41
liquid chromatography, 79
liquids, 228
lithium, 46
lithography, 247, 248, 251
liver, 22, 25, 26, 28, 29, 33, 34, 36, 46, 47, 51
livestock, 71
local anesthetic, 46, 64, 89, 232
localization, 73
location information, 255
lock-and-key, 128
loss of consciousness, 10
Lotions, 230
LSD, 45, 75
LTD, 14
lubricants, 231
LUDI, 129, 130, 134, 135
lung cancer, 93
Luvox, 13
lying, 117
lymphangiogenesis, 109
lysine, 76
lysosome, 92

M

machine learning, 117, 121, 127
macromolecules, 6, 62, 128, 165
magnesium, 47
magnitude, 169, 190, 253
majority, 35, 65, 73
Malaysia, 238
malignant cells, 102
malignant tumors, 62
mammalian cells, 158
mammals, 81, 86
man, 3, 51, 53
management, 9, 13, 82, 223, 235
manic, 11, 46
manic episode, 11
manic-depressive psychosis, 46
manipulation, 101, 106
Manoalide, 91
manufacturing, 58, 226, 229, 236, 237, 238, 239, 240, 243, 256
mapping, 101, 133, 134, 158, 203, 204, 218
marine species, 93
marketing, 235, 236, 237, 238, 240, 243
masking, 156, 229
mass, 40, 177, 232
materials, 49, 144, 229, 231, 243, 246
matrix, 24, 158, 185, 186, 195, 196, 208, 209
matter, 73, 136, 158
measurement(s), 107, 158, 169, 171, 199, 253, 257
meat, 95
mechanical properties, 246
MedDRA, 241, 242

medical, 3, 5, 13, 38, 48, 50, 51, 52, 54, 81, 83, 96, 236, 257
medical care, 257
Medical Products Agency (MPA), 238
medication, 1, 14
Medicinal plant, 49, 55, 79
medicine, 2, 3, 5, 14, 44, 50, 51, 54, 55, 60, 61, 69, 73, 82, 86, 95, 97, 243
Medicines and Healthcare Products Regulatory Agency (MHRA), 238
Medicines Control Council, 238
Medicines Evaluation Board, 238
Mediterranean, 91
Medsafe - Medicines and Medical Devices Safety Authority, 238
melanin, 64, 67
mellitus, 6, 62
melt, 229, 232
melting, 68
membership, 242
membranes, 24, 32, 33, 40, 43, 68, 77, 109, 170, 246
memory, 93, 97, 132
MEMS, 246, 247, 255, 256, 257
menopause, 12
menstruation, 43
mental illness, 50
Metabolic, 44, 80
metabolism, vii, 15, 16, 25, 28, 29, 31, 33, 34, 35, 36, 42, 43, 44, 55, 79, 80, 112, 196, 225, 227, 232
metabolites, 33, 34, 36, 39, 49, 55, 56, 57, 64, 68, 72, 76, 77, 78, 79, 80
metabolized, 6, 33, 34, 35, 42, 227
metabolizing, 29
meter, 231
methadone, 46
methanol, 63, 150
methodology, 114, 155, 161, 170, 206, 212, 220
methylation, 35
methylcellulose, 232
Mexico, 8
mice, 109
Micromachining, 246
microorganisms, 11, 65
microscopy, 249, 256
Middle East, 54
milligrams, 226
mimicry, 216
miniature, 246
Ministry of Health, 238, 241
Ministry of Public Health, 238
misuse, 45, 50
mitosis, 62
mixing, 146, 177, 229
models, vii, 19, 21, 49, 89, 101, 108, 130, 132, 161, 165, 176, 177, 193, 196, 201, 202, 216, 217, 219, 220, 222, 225
modernization, 82, 93
modifications, 107, 184, 195, 225
modules, 223
moisture, 233
Molar Refraction (MR), 177
molar volume, 177
mold, 247
molecular beam, 249
molecular beam epitaxy, 249
Molecular descriptors, 164
molecular dynamics, 137, 220
molecular structure, 65, 162, 164, 181, 182, 184, 203, 236
molecular weight, 25, 30, 66, 72, 173, 176, 177, 178, 189
monoamine oxidase inhibitors, 46
monolayer, 252
monomers, 66, 144
Monoterpenes, 57, 68
monoterpenoids, 70
Monte Carlo method, 134
Moon, 223
Morphine, 5, 35, 46, 49, 50, 55, 72
morphology, 69, 254
mortality, 245
MR, 165, 173, 176, 177, 192, 194, 210
mRNA, 6, 106
Mucolytic, 13
mucosa, 28, 33, 232
mucous membrane(s), 12, 61, 231, 232
mucus, 13
Multi-pin, 155
Multiple linear regression (MLR), 195
multiple regression, 207
muscarinic receptor, 47
muscle relaxant, 46
Muscle relaxant, 13, 71
muscles, 13, 31, 59
mustard oil, 62
mutagenesis, 124, 127
mutations, 102
mycobacteria, 12
myocardial infarction, 88, 94

N

Na^+, 61, 89, 109
Nano Electro Mechanical System (NEMS), 247, 257
Nano-Engineering, 251
nanofabrication, 251

nanometer(s), 247, 252
nanophotonics, 255
nanoscale structures, 248
Nanotechnology, 247, 249
narcotic, 50, 162, 171
NAS, 236
National Agency for Food and Drug Administration and Control (NAFDAC), 238
National Pharmaceutical Control Bureau, Ministry of Health, 238
natural laws, 51
nausea, 11, 232
necrosis, 12
nematode, 91
nephron, 35, 45
nerve, 11, 31, 46, 74, 86, 103
nervous system, 31, 73
Netherlands, 213, 238
neural network(s), 119
neuralgia, 61
neurodegenerative diseases, 62
Neuroleptic, 13, 46
Neuromuscular blocking agent, 46
neurons, 119, 120
neuropathy, 42
neurotransmitter(s), 40, 45, 46, 68, 74, 92, 103
neutral, 7, 73, 165, 170, 207
Neutral antagonist, 7
New Active Substances, 236
New England, 14
New Zealand, 14, 238
NEWLEAD, 135, 136
NH_2, 150, 183
nicotine, 73, 85
Nigeria, 79, 238
nitrogen, 57, 72, 73, 74, 76
NMR, 112, 205
Nobel Prize, 82, 143
nodes, 255
Non-linear model, 196
non-polar, 24, 127, 169
Non-protein amino acids, 57, 76
non-steroidal anti-inflammatory drugs, 26
Nonsteroidal anti-inflammatory drugs (NSAIDs), 46
norepinephrine, 13
Normalization, 190, 191
NP hard, 192
NSAIDs, 46
Nuclear receptors, 102, 109
nucleic acid, 48, 115, 127, 148
nucleic acid synthesis, 48
nucleotides, 149
nucleus, 41, 75, 166, 173, 203
nutrients, 31, 33

O

OASIS, 190, 213
obesity, 101
Occupation Theory, 40
oceans, 88
Octanol, 170
OH, 41, 62, 64, 150, 168
oil, 62, 64, 67, 69, 70, 78, 88, 95, 171
Ointments, 231
oligomers, 141, 149, 155
Omega -3 fatty acid, 88, 94
omega-3, 97
omeprazole, 103
open spaces, 137
operations, 148, 156
Ophthalmic anti-infective, 13
Opioid analgesics, 46
opportunities, 102, 237
optimization, 107, 114, 128, 132, 133, 139, 205, 206, 219, 220, 225, 226, 237, 238
Optimization phase, 218, 219
organ(s), 5, 13, 19, 30, 32, 39, 51, 55, 56, 82, 102, 227, 237, 240
organelles, 41, 69
organic compounds, 101, 143, 147, 171
organic solvents, 74
organism, 1, 6, 126
Original variance, 199
ornithine, 76
oscillation, 251
osteoporosis, 12, 62
Otic preparations, 13
overlap, 125, 130, 131
oxidation, 34, 62, 73
oxidative stress, 62
oxygen, 34, 47, 70, 103, 163, 233

P

pain, 10, 46, 55, 62, 85, 92, 94, 95, 101, 163, 232
Pakistan, 238
palliative, 11
pancreas, 82
Paracetamol, 8, 44, 46, 163
Paraguay, 238
parallel, 107, 132, 142, 148, 154, 156, 159
parallel processing, 132
paralysis, 6, 85
parasites, 39

parasitic infection, 5
Parenteral route, 42
Partial agonist, 7
partition, 27, 28, 33, 162, 170, 171, 175, 211
Partition coefficient, 170
Passive diffusion, 24
Pastes, 232
patents, 216
pathogenesis, 100, 108
pathogens, 59, 62, 232
pathophysiology, 101
pathways, 76, 101, 169
pattern recognition, 102, 106, 107, 130
Penicillin, 6, 27, 31, 36, 48, 106
peptic ulcer, 75
peptide(s), 45, 48, 57, 83, 85, 89, 91, 92, 96, 106, 101, 141, 143, 144, 145, 147, 149, 151, 152, 154, 155, 156, 157, 159
peptide chain, 48, 106, 145, 151, 156
Perceptron, 119
peripheral nervous system, 74
peristalsis, 11
permeability, 30, 31, 33, 38, 40, 89, 112, 121, 161
permeation, 29
permit, 152
peroxide, 13
personal hygiene, 243
pH, 24, 26, 27, 29, 32, 38, 230, 232
phage, 154, 159
phagocytic cells, 66
pharmaceutical(s), 19, 81, 86, 89, 99, 143, 226, 228, 229, 231, 235, 236, 241, 243
Pharmacodynamics, v, 6, 38, 39, 48
pharmacokinetics, v, vii, 6, 15, 16, 17, 19, 23, 29, 38, 44, 121, 196
pharmacology, 5, 13, 14, 38, 39, 48, 55, 82, 162
Pharmacophore, v, vii, 6, 112, 116, 123, 215, 216, 217, 219, 223
Pharmacotherapeutics, 7
Pharmacy, xi, 7, 14, 37, 225, 233
Phase I reactions, 34
Phase II reactions, 34
phenol, 62, 168
phenolic compounds, 63
Phenolics, 63
phenotype(s), 107
phenylalanine, 63, 64
Phenylbutazone, 27
Phenylpropanoids, 57
phenytoin, 18, 27, 34
Philadelphia, 14, 48, 109
Philippines, 8
phosphate, 63, 103
phospholipids, 170
photolithography, 157, 247, 248
photons, 247
photosynthesis, 55, 56
Phylogenetic, 125, 126, 127
phylum, 92
physical environment, 56
physical interaction, 106
physical properties, 162, 209
physicians, 5, 14
physicochemical properties, 6, 163, 227
Physiological, 24
physiological factors, 29
physiology, 3, 69, 102, 235
Phytochemical, 79
pigs, 82, 86, 89
Pilocarpine, 27
pKa, 26, 27, 32, 170
placenta, 30, 33
placental barrier, 30, 33
plant growth, 171, 172
plants, 49, 51, 52, 53, 54, 55, 56, 57, 58, 59, 60, 62, 63, 64, 65, 66, 67, 68, 69, 72, 73, 74, 76, 77, 78, 79, 80, 237, 257
plasma levels, 17
plasma proteins, 26, 30, 31, 32, 35
plasmid, 154
Plasters, 232
platelet aggregation, 85
Platelet inhibitor, 13
platelets, 13
platform, ix, 222, 241
playing, 243
pleasure, vii
plexus, 28, 32
PLS, 207, 208, 209, 210
poison, 85
polar, 34, 103, 169, 170, 171, 205
polar groups, 170, 171
polarity, 73
polarizability, 162, 177
policy, 239, 240
policy making, 240
polio, 6
Polyacetylenes, 57, 77
polydimethylsiloxane, 248
Polyethylene glycol (PEG), 150
Polyketides, 76, 77
polymer(s), 48, 63, 143, 144, 145, 150, 151, 155, 247
polymerase, 6
polymerase chain reaction, 6
polymerization, 247
polypeptide(s), 57, 83, 155, 236

polyphenols, 57, 62, 79
polypropylene, 155
Polysome, 154
polystyrene, 145, 150
population, 7, 50, 81, 94, 141, 245
portal vein, 25, 29
Pose Clustering, 130
positive feedback, 95
potassium, 46, 47, 82, 101
Potency, 7
precedent(s), 101, 240
predation, 76
predictability, 197, 198, 199, 202, 207
prediction models, 218
pregnancy, 33, 43, 237
preparation, 229, 230, 232
preservation, 96
preservative, 226
President, ix
prevention, 1, 6, 7, 42, 48, 50, 55, 62, 78, 79, 236
Primary metabolism, 55
principles, 2, 19, 32, 39, 50, 215
prior knowledge, 221, 236
probability, 115, 133, 134, 189, 200, 201, 208, 219, 221
probe, 125, 127, 159, 204, 205, 207, 208, 249, 250
Prodrug(s), 6, 33
product life cycle, 238
production technology, 249
professionals, 14
programming, 255
progress reports, 242
Proinsulin, 84
project, 139
proliferation, 47, 102
propagation, 120
propane, 65
prophylactic, 237
prophylaxis, 8, 45, 47
proportionality, 18, 169
propranolol, 45, 47
prostaglandins, 29, 46, 85
prostate cancer, 92
Protecting groups, 149, 152
protection, 144, 149, 152, 155, 157, 226, 232, 236
protein components, 32
Protein Data Bank, 205
protein family, 101
protein kinase C, 68, 93
protein structure, 127, 129, 131, 221
protein-coding sequences, 99
Protein-ligand docking, 128
proteins, 24, 26, 32, 41, 46, 65, 67, 73, 76, 77, 101, 102, 103, 106, 121, 123, 128, 141, 145, 149, 154, 170, 204
proteomics, 6, 111
prothrombin, 85
proton pump inhibitors, 110
protons, 165
prototype, 134
Prozac, 13
pruning, 132
Pseudopterosins, 94
psoriasis, 47, 64, 82, 91, 94
psychosomatic, 51
psychostimulants, 74
publishing, 240
punishment, 3
purification, 7, 55, 106, 142, 143, 149
purity, 237

Q

QRS complex, 254
Quantitative Structure Activity Relationship (QSAR), 7, 116, 161, 162, 163, 164, 165, 170, 171, 172, 173, 176, 177, 178, 185, 187, 188, 189, 190, 191, 192, 193, 194, 195, 197, 198, 199, 200, 201, 202, 203, 204, 205, 206, 207, 209, 210, 211, 212, 213, 220, 222, 223
QSAR equation, 161, 163, 170, 171, 173, 187, 192, 194, 195, 197, 198, 200, 201, 202
quality control, 7, 237
quality of life, 96
quality standards, 228, 243
quantization, 203
quantum computing, 255
quantum mechanics, 216
quaternary ammonium, 26
query, 130, 135, 220
Quinidine, 27
Quinine, 5, 27, 49, 75
Quinoline, 74, 75
quinones, 57, 67

R

race, 29, 43
radio, 7, 254
radius, 125, 126, 129
Ranunculosides, 58, 61
reactant, 18, 112
reaction mechanism, 165
reaction rate, 18, 165

reactions, 9, 18, 34, 35, 36, 146, 148, 150, 152, 167, 169, 170, 203
reactive groups, 149
reactivity, 67, 169
reagents, 40, 144, 145, 146, 149, 150, 155, 156, 169
real time, 254, 257
Receptor tyrosine kinases, 102
receptors, 6, 7, 14, 40, 41, 45, 46, 47, 62, 85, 96, 101, 102, 109, 125, 161, 170
recognition, 103, 134
recombinant DNA, 236
recombinant proteins, 101
recreational, 81
rectum, 231, 232
red blood cells, 61, 78
redistribution, 32
Reduction, 34
redundancy, 132
reform(s), 82, 235
refractive index, 177
refractive indices, 177
regression, 115, 117, 118, 137, 164, 169, 173, 175, 193, 195, 199, 201, 202, 208, 209, 220
regression analysis, 115, 117, 169, 175
regression equation, 137, 195, 201, 209, 220
regression line, 199
regression model, 202
regulations, 235, 236
regulatory affairs, vi, vii, 235, 237, 239, 243
regulatory agencies, 237, 239, 240
regulatory bodies, 235, 237
regulatory requirements, 236, 239
rejection, 13, 217
relaxation, 13, 47
reliability, 115, 221, 246
relief, 11, 78, 248
religion, 2, 3
renaissance, 50
repellent, 69
replication, 11, 48, 103
repressor, 159
Reproducibility, 197
reproduction, 55
requirements, 141, 149, 187, 217, 226, 240, 241, 242, 246
researchers, vii, 158, 175, 179, 222
reserves, 77
Residential, 258
residues, 83, 126, 127, 129
resins, 46, 68, 74, 144, 146, 150, 151, 154, 156
resistance, 47, 102, 103
resolution, 157, 159, 249, 254
resources, 51, 77, 86, 240
respiration, 5, 36, 59, 253
respiratory arrest, 59
response, 7, 8, 9, 20, 26, 40, 41, 42, 43, 44, 65, 103, 112, 170, 215, 225, 226, 227, 228, 239
rheumatoid arthritis, 12, 46, 47, 62, 82, 102
ribonucleic acid, 76
ribosome, 48, 106
rings, 29, 112, 116, 173, 180, 189
Rink amide resin, 152
risk(s), 8, 64, 65, 87, 132, 197, 198, 226
RNA(s), 48, 76, 101, 105, 106, 107, 236
RNAi, 107, 110
room temperature, 69, 72, 74, 78, 152
root(s), 54, 55, 62, 66, 69, 73, 75, 76, 82, 182, 198
rotations, 205
Route of administration, 42
routes, 27, 28, 42, 226
rubber, 232
rules, 135, 137, 197, 207, 220, 222, 235, 237, 256
rural population, 55

S

safety, 29, 108, 225, 228, 236, 243
salicylates, 18
saliva, 35, 36, 83
salts, 26, 66, 73, 230
sampling distribution, 200
SAMPLS, 208
saponin(s), 58, 61, 68, 72, 78
Saponosides, 61
saturated hydrocarbons, 212
savings, 19
Scaling, 190
scanning tunneling microscope, 249, 250
scattering, 197
scavengers, 66
scent, 78
schizophrenia, 6
school, 1
sciatica, 61
science, vii, 2, 7, 48, 50, 51, 92, 96, 97, 117, 143
scope, 238
SCREM, 247
search space, 132
secondary metabolism, 55
Secondary metabolites, 56, 57, 79, 80
secretion, 12, 26, 35, 36, 47, 85
sedative(s), 13, 44, 46, 60, 69
seed, 69, 76
Selective serotonin reuptake inhibitors (SSRIs), 13
selectivity, 6, 89, 220
semiconductor(s), 143, 246, 249, 255, 256

semi-empirical method(s), 170
senses, 51
sensing, 245, 246, 255
sensitivity, 9, 44, 106
sensor network, 246, 253, 254, 255, 257
sensors, 246, 253, 254
sequencing, 99
Serendipity, 101
serotonin, 13, 46, 103
Serotonin nonselective reuptake inhibitor (SNRI), 13
serum, 232
services, 245, 255
shape, 29, 122, 128, 133, 134, 165, 176, 177, 178, 183, 184, 197, 200, 203, 222, 246
sheep, 87, 89
showing, 19, 20, 21, 73, 87, 119
sialic acid, 24
side chain, 61, 64, 72, 124, 133
side effects, 9, 10, 28, 31, 49, 87, 226, 237
signal transduction, 257
signalling, 101, 102
signals, 92, 102, 254, 255
significance level, 200, 201
silicon, 246, 255, 256, 257
Simulated Annealing, 114, 133
simulation, 115, 133, 134
Singapore, 238
Single Compartment Model, 19
Single Crystal Silicon Reactive etch and Metal (SCREM), 246
skeletal muscle, 13
skeleton, 63, 93, 136, 187, 209
skin, 22, 36, 47, 58, 61, 69, 78, 86, 95, 230, 231, 232
sleeping sickness, 216
small intestine, 36, 87
smallpox, 5
smooth muscle, 47
snakes, 82, 84
society, ix, 14, 51, 256
sodium, 45, 46, 68, 85, 101
Soft Lithography, 247
software, 111, 121, 129, 132, 178, 190, 205, 219, 254
solid phase, 144, 145, 146, 147, 149, 150, 151, 154
Solid Phase Organic Synthesis (SPOS), 144
solid state, 145, 228, 229
Solid support, 145, 149, 150, 157
solubility, 26, 27, 29, 38, 112, 121, 161, 162, 165, 196, 212, 228, 230, 231, 233
solution(s), 26, 27, 87, 132, 144, 145, 148, 152, 155, 156, 158, 230, 231, 245
Solution Phase synthesis, 144
solvation, 114, 115, 151, 169, 206, 212
solvents, 73, 149, 150, 151, 156, 169, 173, 229
South Africa, 238
South America, 54
soybeans, 66
spastic, 75
spasticity, 46
SPC, 238
species, 5, 26, 34, 42, 43, 54, 56, 59, 74, 77, 81, 82, 88, 91, 94, 105, 165, 170
specifications, 119, 215
spinal cord, 92, 163
spindle, 62
Spirits, 230
spleen, 51
sponge, 88, 91, 97
SPOTS membrane, 155, 156
Squalamine, 88, 90, 94
Sri Lanka, 238
stability, 108, 127, 151, 228, 229
standard deviation, 185, 190, 198, 199, 202
standardization, 7
starch, 60
state(s), 1, 29, 31, 37, 44, 51, 55, 73, 82, 101, 106, 131, 132, 151, 162, 169, 179, 222, 249
State Food and Drug Administration, 238
Steric field, 204
sterile, 230
STERIMOL, 177, 212
steroids, 6, 26, 29, 47, 57, 61, 68, 72
stimulant, 71, 74, 75
stimulation, 39, 102
stimulus, 103
STM, 249, 250, 256
stochastic processes, 132
stomach, 12, 24, 25, 33, 44, 232
storage, 32, 50, 76, 164, 254
strategy use, 141
stress, 69, 79, 82
structural characteristics, 50
structural knowledge, 123
styrene, 150
substance use, 1
substitutions, 168, 186
substrate(s), 34, 42, 63, 103, 124, 127, 149, 150, 151, 152, 154, 157, 246, 247
Subtractive phase, 218, 219
success rate, 197, 257
sucrose, 230
Sulfadiazine, 25
sulfate, 34, 35, 87, 91, 94
Sulfathiazole, 27
Sulfisoxazole, 25
sulfonamides, 6, 32, 35

sulfur, 85, 89
Sun, 82, 95
superimposition, 116
supervision, 236, 246
support staff, ix
Support Vector Machine (SVM), 117, 127
Suppositories, 28, 232
surface area, 28, 31, 43, 116, 189, 229
surfactant, 233
survival, 55
Suspension, 231
suspensions, 28, 29, 228, 230, 231
suture, 87, 97
sweat, 35, 36
Sweden, 238
swelling, 12
Swissmedic, Swiss Agency for Therapeutic Products, 238
Switzerland, 8, 238
symptoms, 6, 11, 12, 46, 65
synapse, 119
synaptic transmission, 46
syndrome, 14
synthesis, 7, 35, 45, 46, 47, 48, 56, 76, 78, 84, 95, 109, 112, 141, 142, 143, 144, 145, 146, 147, 148, 149, 150, 151, 152, 154, 155, 156, 157, 158, 159, 221
Syrups, 230

T

T cell, 102
T cell receptor, 102
Tablets, 229, 233
Taiwan, 85
tannins, 57, 62, 63, 66, 78
tantra, 2
target, vii, 32, 99, 100, 101, 102, 105, 106, 107, 108, 111, 112, 113, 114, 115, 120, 121, 123, 124, 128, 158, 171, 205, 215, 218, 255
target identification, 99, 106, 107
Target validation, 110
tau, 138
TAU descriptors, 179
Taxol, 49
t-distribution, 200, 201
Tea bag, 155, 156
teams, 241
techniques, 42, 50, 83, 107, 111, 112, 115, 116, 117, 124, 141, 142, 154, 164, 187, 190, 220, 246, 247, 249, 251, 256
technological developments, 246
technology(s), vii, 77, 83, 102, 111, 112, 117, 121, 155, 159, 219, 236, 237, 240, 245, 246, 252, 253, 255
temperature, 8, 56, 69, 133, 232, 247, 253, 254
tendons, 86, 87
tension, 11, 61, 72
Tentagel, 150
Teprotide, 84, 89
terminals, 103
terpenes, 67, 68
Terpenoids, 57, 67
test data, 197
testing, 5, 77, 107, 157, 187
Tetracycline, 27
textbooks, 5
TGA, 238
Thailand, 91, 238
theoretical approaches, 190
therapeutic agents, 50, 101, 215
therapeutic benefits, 50
Therapeutic Goods Administration (TGA), 238
therapeutic use, 227, 236
therapy, 6, 8, 19, 81, 86, 232
thermodynamics, 114
third dimension, 246
three-dimensional model, 219
thrombin, 85
Thrombolytic, 13
thromboxanes, 46
thrombus, 13
thyroid, 82
thyroid gland, 82
time frame, 131
time series, 118
tin, 61
Tirofiban, 85, 89
tissue, 7, 30, 31, 32, 91
TNF, 12
Tolbutamide, 27, 34
Tolerance, 44
tonic, 58, 60, 64
Topic Leader, 242
topology, 120, 212
torsion, 133
total cholesterol, 46
toxic effect, 73
toxicity, 1, 6, 7, 61, 62, 71, 107, 108, 112, 121, 163, 211
toxicology, 162
toxin, 96
Tracking, 253
trade, 82, 83, 241
traditions, 51

training, 117, 118, 120, 175, 178, 187, 190, 191, 193, 195, 197, 198, 203, 206, 207, 209, 220, 221, 243
traits, 170
transcription, 47, 102, 104
transcription factors, 102
transduction, 100
Transferase, 103
transformation, 130, 152, 238
transistor, 246, 255
translation, 5, 48, 76, 133
transport, 24, 25, 29, 30, 32, 36, 61, 76, 103, 196, 249
transportation, 176, 178
trauma, 254
treatment, 1, 2, 6, 7, 9, 11, 12, 13, 33, 42, 43, 44, 45, 47, 48, 50, 51, 54, 55, 59, 93, 94, 101, 106, 190, 211, 216, 236, 243
trial, 91, 102
triangulation, 255
tricyclic antidepressant(s), 46
trifluoroacetic acid, 152
triggers, 7
Triterpenes, 57, 68
Trityl chloride, 152
T-test, 187, 200
tuberculosis, 6, 12, 81
tumor(s), 11, 12, 59, 65, 66, 78, 89, 91, 92
tumor cells, 59
tumor necrosis factor, 12
tunneling, 249, 256
Two-compartment model, 22
type 1 diabetes, 47
type 2 diabetes, 47
tyrosine, 102, 109

U

Uganda National Council for Science and Technology (UNCST), 238
Ukraine, 238
ulcer, 47
ulcerative colitis, 82
Unani, 50, 54
United Kingdom (UK), 8, 79, 210, 238
United Nations, 48
United States (USA), 1, 8, 38, 159, 210, 223, 241
universe, 51
universities, 5
updating, 241
uric acid, 11
urine, 5, 12, 86
usual dose, 9
UV, 65, 152, 171
UV light, 152
UV radiation, 65

V

vaccine, 5
vacuole, 61
vacuum, 177, 250
vagina, 231, 232
valence, 182, 183, 212
validation, v, vii, 42, 99, 107, 108, 110, 122, 161, 187, 198, 201, 202
valve, 233
van der Waal, 121, 125, 176, 177
vapor, 171, 230, 233
variables, 118, 189, 208, 209
variations, 219, 254
varieties, 5
vascular diseases, 109
vasoconstriction, 11, 12
vasodilation, 45
Vasodilator, 13, 103
vasomotor, 12
Vasopressor, 13
vector, 118, 119, 130, 195, 196, 208, 209
vegetables, 66, 67
vehicles, 229, 231
velocity, 16, 177
Venezuela, 8
Verloop, 177, 178, 212
very low density lipoprotein, 46
vessels, 47
Viagra, 11
Virtual Screening, 111, 112, 113, 115, 122
viruses, 6
viscosity, 13, 165
vision, 130
vitamin B1, 73
Vitamin C, 58
vitamin K, 12, 47
vitamins, 33, 89, 96
volatility, 156
vomiting, 11, 12, 232
vote, 131

W

walking, 253
Wang resin, 152
Washington, 38, 210

water, 26, 32, 33, 34, 51, 54, 58, 63, 65, 66, 69, 72, 74, 86, 125, 127, 150, 162, 165, 170, 171, 222, 223, 228, 230, 231, 232, 252
wave propagation, 255
weakness, 60
web, 115
websites, 96
weight management, 254
Weiner index, 179, 180
welfare, 255
wells, 155, 156, 158
West Africa, 89
white matter, 32
withdrawal, 45, 169
wood, 51, 69, 71
workers, 73
World Drug Index (WDI), 112
World Health Organization (WHO), 1, 48, 49, 51, 241, 242
worldwide, 237, 238

X

X-ray, 112, 115, 205, 206, 216

Y

yeast, 87
yield, 142, 197, 231

Z

Ziconotide, 93, 94
Zoloft, 13